TRENDS IN BASIC AND THERAPEUTIC OPTIONS IN HIV INFECTION - TOWARDS A FUNCTIONAL CURE

Edited by **Bartholomew Ibeh**

Trends in Basic and Therapeutic Options in HIV Infection - Towards a Functional Cure

http://dx.doi.org/10.5772/58666
Edited by Bartholomew Ibeh

Contributors

José Miguel Azevedo-Pereira, Pedro Canhão, Pedro Barroca, Quirina Santos-Costa, Marta Calado, Enrique Valdes, Wan Suriana Wan Ab Rahman, Wan Majdiah Wan Mohamad, Carmen Rodríguez, Teresa Blasco, Celso Spada, Joel Da Cunha, Luciana Morganti Ferreira Maselli, Sérgio Bydlowski, Bartholomew Ibeh, Naoki Yamamoto, Jeremiah Stanley, Josiah Habu

Published by InTech

Janeza Trdine 9, 51000 Rijeka, Croatia

Publishing Process Manager Iva Lipovic

Technical Editor InTech DTP team

Cover InTech Design team

First published August, 2015

Printed in Croatia

Additional hard copies can be obtained from orders@intechopen.com

Trends in Basic and Therapeutic Options in HIV Infection - Towards a Functional Cure, Edited by Bartholomew Ibeh

p. cm.

ISBN 978-953-51-2157-2

For EU product safety concerns:
IN TECH d.o.o., Prolaz Marije Krucifikse Kozulić 3, 51000 Rijeka, Croatia,
info@intechopen.com or visit our website at intechopen.com.

Meet the editor

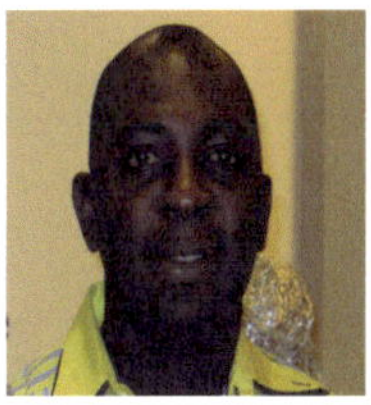

Ibeh Bartholomew MSc, Ph.D is currently Assistant Director of Medical Biotechnology Department, National Biotechnology Development Agency, Abuja. He has obtained several grants and awards. Dr. Ibeh has served as an external examiner and supervised over 30 university students on various HIV research topics. Though his work on HIV serodiscordant infection in blacks is widely acknowledged, his current research interest is on development of efficient immunodeficient mouse models using current genetic engineering tools. He is a member of the International Union of Biochemistry and Molecular Biology and the Nigerian Society of Biochemistry and Molecular Biology.

Contents

Preface IX

Section 1 HIV Transmission, Distribution, Prevention and Study Appraoch 1

Chapter 1 **Spatiotemporal Dynamics of HIV Distribution Pattern and Application of Indigenous Bioresources and Microbicides in Expanding Preventive Options 3**
Habu Josiah Bitrus and Ibeh Bartholomew Okechukwu

Chapter 2 **HIV Infection — A Sociological Approach to the Prevention of the HIV Pandemic 27**
Carmen Rodríguez Reinado and Teresa Blasco Hernández

Chapter 3 **Vertical Transmission of HIV — Medical Diagnosis, Therapeutic Options and Prevention Strategy 51**
Enrique Valdés Rubio and Rodolfo Guiñez Gahona

Section 2 Replication, Resistance, Treatment Options and Therapy Responses 73

Chapter 4 **Inhibition of HIV Replication by Host Cellular Factors 75**
J.M. Azevedo-Pereira, Pedro Canhão, Marta Calado, Quirina Santos-Costa and Pedro Barroca

Chapter 5 **Immunological and Haematological Changes in HIV Infection 105**
Wan Majdiah Wan Mohamad, Wan Suriana Wan Ab Rahman, Suhair Abbas Ahmed Al-Salih and Che Maraina Che Hussin

Chapter 6 **The Impact of Modern Antiretroviral Therapy on Lipid Metabolism of HIV-1 Infected Patients 129**
Joel da Cunha, Luciana Morganti Ferreira Maselli, Sérgio Paulo Bydlowski and Celso Spada

Chapter 7 **Oxidative Stress, Redox Regulation and Elite Controllers of HIV Infection: Towards a Functional Cure 183**
Ibeh Bartholomew Okechukwu

Chapter 8 **Novel Prospective Treatment Options 209**
Jeremiah Stanley and Naoki Yamamoto

Preface

This book is a collection of expert assays on various aspects of HIV prevention and treatment strategies for which there is evident need for scientific focus and review of current trend. The organization of the book is unique and organic because it brings to the fore the implications of HIV basic science, clinical, social and implementation aspects as well as pathogenesis and treatment options as an integral component defining modern therapeutic interventions. A visible objective of the book is to provide a wider readership of scientist, clinicians, social workers/HIV caregivers, trainers and vaccine developers a multidisciplinary approach to HIV treatment and intervention strategy by presenting current trends in the development of therapeutic options and its attendant challenges. It is of note that the antiviral drugs currently in use for the management of the infection have shown various haematologic, viremic and immunologic discordance in response from patients undergoing treatment. Also, this decade has witnessed naturally resistant individuals in different races of the world and an emerging host cellular antiviral proteins as well as the use of specifically designed preventive microbicides. Therefore, the chapters are organized from the simple sociological perspective and transmission to the more complex host antiviral proteins, redox activity, global circulating forms and functional cure.

Several factors have limited the success of a vaccine for HIV, including high mutation rates which result in various evasive circulating forms and lack of global immune response elicitation to the viral antigens. It is then obvious that in spite of the progress and huge financial resources from various governments and international agencies dedicated to HIV infection, there are still major challenges facing successful vaccine development, preventive and control mechanism of the infection. This book covers major aspects of HIV infection x-raying useful research and intervention approaches, challenges and future dimension of research in the field while bringing to limelight a comprehensive narrative of HIV treatment options.

Sincere appreciation to contributors who have extended full cooperation with the publisher INTECH to present their expert opinion as contained in the book.

Ibeh Bartholomew, Ph.D
National Biotechnology Development Agency,
Abuja, Nigeria

Section 1

HIV Transmission, Distribution, Prevention and Study Appraoch

Chapter 1

Spatiotemporal Dynamics of HIV Distribution Pattern and Application of Indigenous Bioresources and Microbicides in Expanding Preventive Options

Habu Josiah Bitrus and
Ibeh Bartholomew Okechukwu

Additional information is available at the end of the chapter

http://dx.doi.org/10.5772/61000

1. Introduction

HIV infection has maintained a high number of infections in human population. Currently, there are growing population changes and corresponding challenges including new recombinant circulating forms. The infection is endemic in sub-Saharan Africa with peculiarities in the distribution pattern.

Similarly, distinct transmission models have emanated over the years thus forming a special focal point in the management and prevention of HIV/AIDS. In resource poor settings, management of the disease remains a task as financial, infrastructure, and committed human resources are remarkably low. The current treatment options though widely accepted is still marred with issues of accessibility, resistance, toxicity, and financial burden on the recipient patients. This chapter discusses and brings to concept the current HIV distribution pattern and microbial bioresources deployed as a preventive and treatment option.

2. Global HIV population distribution pattern with emphasis on Africa

The global population of the virus infection has maintained an alarming rate, with record values of more than 34 million people currently living with HIV [1,2] compared to less than 30 million observed in 2002 [3]. The geographical spread of the disease has been astronomical in sub-Saharan Africa, with Nigeria having an estimated amount of 8% of the total global burden of the infection [4].

The distribution and spread of the infection globally is entirely non-uniform and non-homogenous, with more concentrated cases (over 70%) of occurrence observed in Africa alone [5] (Figure 1A/1B and Figure 2). This estimate is extremely significant, given the fact that Africa accommodates approximately 15.3% of the world population [6]. As previously observed in the global spread of the disease, correlation between disease prevalence and social behaviours such as sexual practices and use of intravenous drugs are existential. The spread of infection in Africa is more pronounced and is relative to cultural practices. For example, HIV population is seen to be least prevalent in the northern African countries and the Middle East (Figure 2), which are typically known to practice less of cultural deeds that predispose individuals to HIV infection. Conversely, the spread is dramatically highest in the southern region of the continent [3] where HIV infection appears to have been densely concentrated amongst injection drug users, gays, sex workers, partners of sex workers, etc. [7]. Not only is the prevalence of the disease highest in Africa per global scale, but the rate of rise of occurrence has also been astronomical on the continent, with estimated seven-fold increase in the number of occurrences between 2005 and 2012 [4].

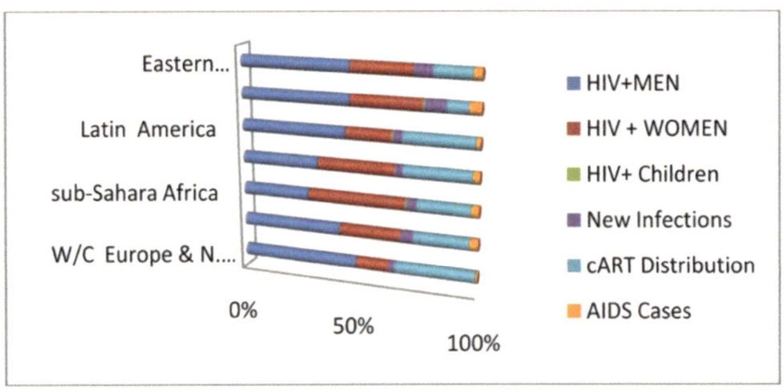

(A)

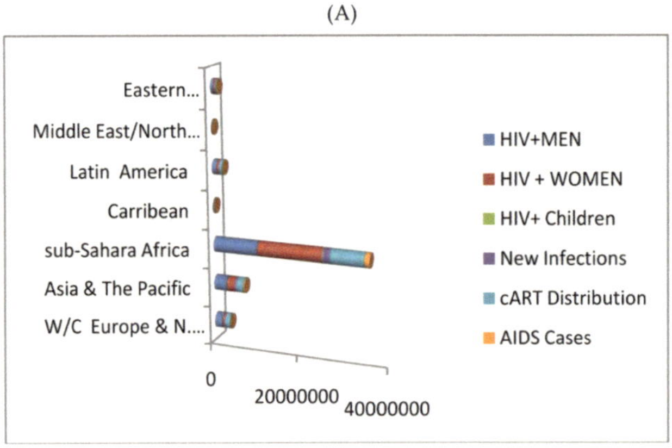

(B)

Data presented in Figures 1A and 1B are based on 2014 ECDC report [8], 2014 UN women report [9], and 2014 UN-AIDS Gap report [10]

Figure 1. (A) Regional HIV Population distribution pattern expressed as relative percentage based on 2013 data. (B): Regional HIV Population distribution based on 2013 data.

3. Transmission dynamics models

3.1. Routes of transmission, geographical and racial distribution

In sub-Saharan Africa, the major route of transmission is through heterosexual contact rather than homosexual interaction. In an endemic country like Cameroon, for example, whereas at 2012, the HIV prevalent rate amongst adults was 4.3% (4.0%–4.6%), the infection is concentrated within the 15–49 age bracket in which over 50% of the infected population are women [11]. The major mode of transmission identified by UNAIDS is largely heterosexual, with high occurrence amongst groups such as commercial sex workers, long distance truck drivers, injection drug users, and gay partners [12] with more than half of new HIV infection occurring through heterosexual activity [13]. The transmission of HIV infection is geographic as well as racial (as exemplified by cultural and social values) dependent (Figure 2). Differing factors has been adduced for infection rates in Africans, Asians, Americans, and Europeans which includes social values [14], economic stability/poverty [15, 16], level of awareness [17], and host genetic factors [18].

The three main established routes of transmission of the infection are sexual contact [19], blood transmission [20], needle sharing [21], and vertical (mother-to-child) [22] transmission. Heterosexual transmission seems to be the most common means of infection in Africa with over 60% of the global HIV infections [23] in contrast to other regions of the world, such as in USA which has homosexual transmission and needle sharing as the dominant means [19] (Figure 3). Sharing needles and injection instruments is thought to be three times more likely to transmit HIV than sexual intercourse.

The increased burden of HIV prevalence amongst women in endemic regions have been opined to be due to certain reproductive tract/biological susceptibility [24], social, physical, economical, and even psychological factors which women especially in sub-Saharan Africa are subjected to [25,26].

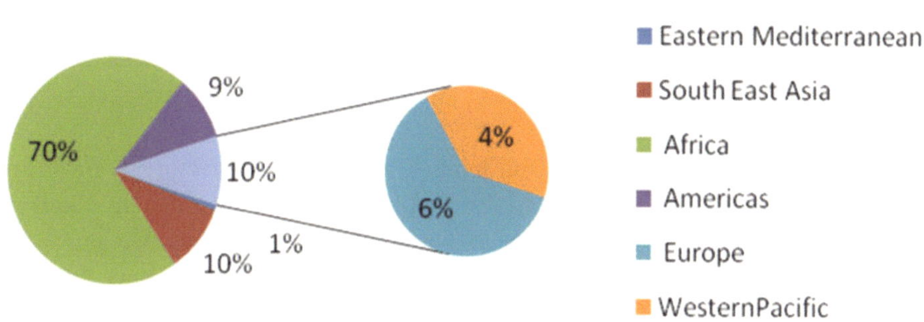

Figure 2. Estimated number of people (all ages) living with HIV based on 2013 WHO data

Available data shows that men who have sex with men (MSM) remain the group with the highest prevalence of HIV infection in the USA, accounting for up to 78% of total infection, as observed amongst men [27] (Figure 3). The prevalent rates amongst MSM are also recorded to increase in the order, Hispanic MSM (6,700), black MSM (10,600), and white MSC being the highest (11,200) [27]. Up to 16% of total HIV reported cases are due to intravenous drug users (IDUs) in which they represent 8% of new cases [28]. Similarly, Europe has a high number of HIV occurrences from MSM [29]. It could be observed that in high income countries HIV epidemics is highly associated with MEM sexual networks [30, 31,32] while heterosexual contacts prevail in low income regions [33,34,35] (Figure 3).

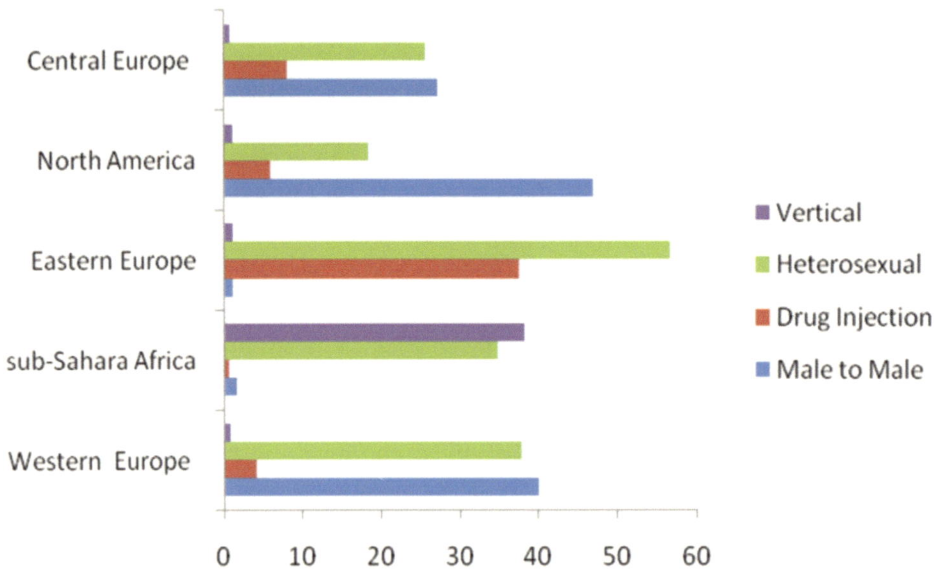

The data shows the prevalence based on 2013 United Nations Office on Drugs and Crime data from the annual report questionnaire and national Government reports, 2013 UNAIDS report and CDC publications. Note: IDUs stands for injecting drug users.

Figure 3. Regional distribution of HIV routes of transmission in HIV positive population

3.2. Exploring transmission models

Since both heterosexual and homosexual behaviour is a potent factor for increased HIV transmission rate, exploring the dynamics of this mode perhaps could be a sure way of providing and discovering a lasting HIV treatment option and drug design. A number of HIV epidemic models have emerged, particularly the modes of transmission (MOT) model recommended by the Joint United Nations Programme on HIV/AIDS (UNAIDS) [36,37]. The MOT model as developed in 2002 aims to identify persons at risk of HIV infection [38] with subsequent prevention policies and programmes [39]. This model was recommended for country-wide studies in the year 2008 as part of a synthesis process supported by UNAIDS and the World Bank Global HIV/AIDS Monitoring and Evaluation Team [40], with emphasis on local content and immediate environment prevailing circumstances. The MOT model utilizes accurate information on recent prevalence of HIV infections in a given population and the assumed patterns of risk behaviour within different risk groups (MSM, prostitutes, etc.) to calculate the expected distribution of new adult HIV infections the next year in terms of the mode of exposure. Certain considerations are necessary for a comprehensive and adequate utilization of this model either at country or community level studies. These considerations as noted by WHO are the proportion of the adult male and female population that belongs to each of several risk groups identified, such as commercial sex workers and their patronizers, injection drug users, men who sex men (MSM), persons of multiple heterosexual sex partners, the low risk group such as partners of persons with higher-risk behaviour and married or cohabiting couples with one monogamous heterosexual partner in the last year [41]. The model tends to resolve issues such as complexity in risk groups, for example, a prostitute who is a drug injection user. Secondly, the prevalent rate of HIV infection and of a generic sexually transmitted disease (STI) identified in each risk group [41]. Thirdly, the average numbers of sexual or injecting partners and exposures per partner with considerations of personal level protective behaviour (such as condom use or the use of new needles), for individuals in each risk group and lastly the probability of HIV transmission per exposure act in each risk group, taking into account the effect of STIs and the prevalence of male circumcision [41].

4. Recombinant circulating forms and distribution pattern

The capacity of HIV to exhibit a unique high genetic variability has posed a major challenge to its treatment [42]. The genetic diversity is also attributed to a high error rate of the HIV genome during transcriptase reaction and also high genetic recombination rate [43].

Recombination is defined as the process whereby various subtypes or strains of the HIV shuffle their genomic characteristics to form an entirely new strain. This recombination tactic, a system of alteration of the HIV genetic constitution, is mostly common with the HIV subtype-1 (HIV-1) and it is commonly called new circulating recombinant forms (CRFs) (Table 1). There also exists the HIV subtype-2 (HIV-2), which is relatively less pathogenic in comparison to HIV-1 [44]. The occurrence of CRF is closely linked to the dynamism of the HIV infection and epidemic and obviously to failure of most specific therapeutic target in eliminating the virus [45-47]. The study of the distribution pattern of the various subtypes is therefore highly crucial for effective HIV management especially in endemic regions of the world. Recombination occurs at a very rapid rate estimated to be in the order of 2.8 cross-over per genome per cycle [48]. Recombination events between subtypes lead not only to an ever increasing diversity of the HIV strains [49] but also presents astonishing scenarios of emerging strains with resistance to the common antiviral drugs [50,51]. The numbers of CRFs are increasing astronomically global, partly because of the emergence of recombinants of the various subtypes in various local epidemiological regions [46]. There has also been a correlation between the emergence of divergent subtypes in a population and the teeming occurrence of disease cases. For example, in Cameroon, the number of newly infected individuals increased from 8,596 to 10,625 between 2006 and 2007 as the number of recombinant subtypes increases in the studied population [47]. Criteria set to define a new subtype, sub-subtype, or CRF include having the representative strain identified in at least three individuals who have no direct epidemiological relationship. Three full-length genomic sequences are required but two complete genomes together with partial sequences of a third strain could also define a new subtype, sub-subtype, or CRF. CRFs are derived from recombination between viruses of different subtypes which are each given a number. CRF12_BF, for example, is a recombination between subtypes B and F.

HIV type	GROUP (%)	SUBTYPE(sub-subtype)	CRFs	GEOGRAPHICAL SPREAD
I	M: Major (90%)	A(A_1,$A_2$$A_3$)	CRF19_CPX,CRF01_AE,CFR14_BG,CRF03_AB, 31_BC,CFR06/18_CPX	West Africa ,Cuba[52,53,54]
		B	CRF07/8_BC,CRF15/48/51/52/53/54/55/58/59_01B	Europe, Japan, Thailand, Australia, the Americas [55]
		C	CRF10/41_CD, CRF11/45/49/37/36_CPX	S/E Africa, India, Nepal, China [55]
		D	CRF05_DF,CRF13_CPX, CRF16_A2D,CRF19_CPX	Eastern and Central Africa [55]
		E	CRF01_AE*	Africa [55]
		F (F_1 F_2)	CRF12_BF1,CRF22_01A1,CRF25_CPX,CRF26_AU	Central Africa, S. America, Eastern Europe [56]
		G	CRF02_AG,CRF09/56/65_CPX,CRF20/23/24_BG	Africa and Central Europe [56]
		H	CRF32_06A1,CRF33/34_01B,CRF35_AD,CRF38/39/40/42/44/46/47/70/71/72_BF,CRF43_02G	Central Africa [56]
		I	CRF04_CPX	Only in central America [57]
		J	CRF50_A1D,CRF60/61/62/64_BC,CRF17_BF1CRF49_01B,CRF63_02A1	North, Central and W. Africa Caribbean [56]
		K	CRF04/06/18/27_CPX,CRF21_A2D	Congo DR and Cameroon [56]
	N:Non- M,Non-O			
	O:Outlier			Cameroon [58]
II	P:Pending			West-Central Africa, Cameroon [59]
	A			None

HIV type	GROUP (%)	SUBTYPE(sub-subtype)	CRFs	GEOGRAPHICAL SPREAD
	B			W. Africa, Angola, Mozambique, India, Brazil[60]
	C-H			West Africa [61,62] Liberia, Sierra Leone, Ivory Coast [61,62]

* Recombine only with A, G, H, K, U, CPX=complex recombination of several subtypes (ADG)

Table 1. HIV Classification and global CRFs

5. HIV/AIDS prevention strategies, how well have they worked?

There are three major strategies of HIV prevention, namely, education or knowledge base, contraceptives, and antiretroviral treatment.

5.1. Peer education

Amongst the many ways of curbing the onslaught of the HIV, one of the most vital is educating the populace about the disease and its transmission dynamics. This significantly prevents re-infection and protects those who are not already infected [63, 64, 65]. Therefore, inadequate knowledge of the disease transmission equals resultant failure of all the measures originally put together to tackle the spread of the disease. In a research conducted in 2006 to access the effect of prior knowledge of HIV transmission relative to the number of occurrence of the infection in Boston, USA, it was found that a significant proportion of the infected people are those with significantly little or no knowledge of the disease or its mode of transmission [66]. Increase in HIV education, particularly amongst young people, remains the most effective way of tackling the HIV onslaught. Where this form of education is limited, the disease is known to prevail [67, 68] as also noted from various data in sub-Saharan Africa. Education on HIV/AIDS plays a major role in controlling the spread of the disease amongst young people, which consequently determines the global spread of infection. HIV infection has been captured as the second most prevalent killer amongst young people. As of 2012, one-third of the global new HIV infection was discovered to be amongst young people, with total infection of about 780,000 and concentrated within 15–24 age group [69]. This number has obviously dropped down from 2012 to present due to vigorous and continuous education campaigns but, even so, HIV/AIDS deaths amongst the young people worldwide are still at an alarming rate [70, 71]. Proper education enables young people and married adults to better protect themselves against the sexually transmitted route of HIV infection, vertical transmission, and also behaviours such as intravenous drug use [72]. So significant was the global implication of HIV/AIDS infection on young people that it was opined that HIV education should be dispensed even to healthy ones.

5.2. Antiretroviral prophylaxis

In poor-resource settings, it is not uncommon to use antiviral therapy as a means of controlling the spread of infection. Experiments however showed that the administration of antiviral therapy, although it has a considerable control rate on HIV infection, is limited in its cost. Many HIV populations do not have access to ART [73] and to others are very expensive [74]. In Nigeria for instance the price of generic ART reported in 2001 could be over 10 times more expensive in comparison with Asian countries and about 79% lower in some European countries [75]. When antiviral therapy is considered as a chosen measure for HIV treatment, an additional use of these therapeutic agents serves as a preventive measure rather than a treatment option. The application of ART at a specific stage of disease progression (measured by computerised simulation incorporating CD4 count and HIV RNA level) has proved to be cost effective [76]. HIV prophylaxis treatment refers to the institution of measures taken to protect a person from HIV infection to which the individual has been anticipated or is liable to be exposed to HIV. HIV prophylaxis could either be post or pre-treatment option based. According to the US CDC, pre-exposure prophylaxis (PrEP) is designed for individuals who do not have HIV but who are at substantial risk of getting it to prevent HIV infection by taking an antiretroviral drug every day [77]. Truvada which contains two HIV drugs (tenofovir and emtricitabine) is usually prescribed [78]. On exposure to HIV through sex or injection drug use, these drugs can work to keep the virus from establishing a permanent infection. PrEP has been shown to reduce the risk of HIV infection in people who are at high risk by up to 92% when adhered to for at least 3 months [77]. Similarly, WHO describes post-exposure prophylaxis (PEP) as contrasted by PrEP as a short-term antiretroviral treatment to reduce the likelihood of HIV infection after potential exposure, either occupationally or through sexual intercourse [79,80]. Post-exposure prophylaxis (PEP) involves taking a 28-day course of ARVs, for adults Tenofovir combined with either lamivudine (3TC) or emtricitabine (FTC) is prescribed. The recommended third drug by WHO is ritonavir-boosted lopinavir (LPV/r), which is also a preferred drug for HIV treatment. Zidovidune (AZT) and lamivudine (3TC) backbone drugs are used for children aged 10 or below, with ritonavir-boosted lopinavir (LPV/r) recommended as the third drug choice [81-84]. As effective as this preventive option may be, it faces challenges of adherences which has reduced its efficacy to less than 56%. Another challenge is the accessibility of the drug to individuals and accurate timing of exposure.

Limited studies on supply and distribution of antiviral drugs in poor-resource areas indicated that the mechanisms of supply and delivery of these drugs are not cost-effective [85-87]. The most significant concern is rural population having access to HIV antiviral drugs and the availability of laboratory facilities to monitor viral loads of patients on antiviral drug as response to therapy and for full HIV clinical management. One of the standard laboratory interventions used in the developed countries to monitor patients receiving antiviral drugs is the plasma viral load monitoring assay [88] which is not readily accessible to the wider population of HIV patients in resource-poor regions [89].

5.3. Contraceptives

Contraceptives may simply be understood as devices or pills used to prevent unwanted pregnancies and diseases mostly sexually transmitted. These can be in the form of drugs, hormones, or devices such as condoms and intrauterine devices (IUD). Evidently, hormonal contraceptives and pills do not protect against HIV or other sexually transmitted infections (STI). At present there are no contraceptives, with the exception of condoms (male and female), that protect against HIV infection [90]. Since the only forms of birth control that will protect against HIV are abstaining from vaginal (and anal) sex or using condoms while having sex, WHO therefore recommends dual protection technique for unwanted pregnancy and HIV prevention [91]. Birth control options that do not protect against HIV infection include oral contraceptives, birth control shot (injection of the hormone Depot Medroxyprogesterone Acetate (*DMPA*) in the arm to release progestin)/Depo-provera, morning after pill (Levonorgestrel or Ulipristal acetate) used after sexual activity, implants (implanon/norplant), IUDs which release progestin, female condoms such as diaphragm/vagina ring/sponge/cervical cap, withdrawal and spermicides. Currently, a new intravaginal ring that helps prevent pregnancy while simultaneously releasing low doses of an antiretroviral drug that reduces a woman's risk of contracting both HIV and genital herpes has been designed [92,93]. This device releases doses of the contraceptive Levonorgestrel and the antiretroviral HIV medication tenofovir after being inserted in the vagina for 90 days and has demonstrated a 39% protection against HIV infection in women [93]. It is obvious that many contraceptive pills may not be compatible with ARTs, the widely prescribed antiretroviral drug efavirenz substantially reduces levels of the hormonal contraceptive Levonorgestrel [94] and increases the risk of HIV infection [95,96].

6. Development of bioresources for HIV management

Bioresources relate to the total biological variation manifested in individual plants, animals, or their genes, which could be utilized by humans for beneficial use such as drugs, food, livestock feed, etc. It also refers to the development of improved crops and animals for higher yield and tolerance to biotic and abiotic stresses. However, despite the global investment in bioresources and machinery to curb the spread of HIV, weak health systems and inadequate human resources are continuing to be major barriers to the elimination of the disease [5]. There is therefore need for an upgrade of the existing methods of disease control and prevention to include local biological resources such as herbs and other plant materials. Several biological organisms mostly plant species have been employed in preventing and managing HIV infection in developing or resource poor countries. Recently, this has metamorphosed into an institutional traditional medicine sector with growing patronage and herbal formulations. Though active antiretroviral therapy (ART) is the principal method for preventing immune deterioration, about 80% estimated Africans still use herbal remedies [97]. In addition, prophylaxis for specific opportunistic infections is indicated in particular cases. There has been increased use of local resources in the treatment of HIV/AIDS known as alternative or complementary therapy [98] with growing scientific journals that publish its procedure and outcome. Some herbal remedies have been found to inhibit one or more steps of HIV replication (Table 2). Though most herbal preparations treat HIV opportunistic infection [99], many research groups are exploring the biodiversity of the plant kingdom to find new and better anti-HIV drugs with novel mechanisms of action. Since some plant substances are known to modulate several cellular factors, such as NF-kappa B and TNF-alpha, which are also involved in the replication of HIV. Their role as potential anti-HIV products should therefore be a desirable focus of attention. In conclusion, several plant-derived antiviral agents are good candidates for further studies, with a view to exploring their potentials and application in systemic therapy and/or prophylaxis of HIV infections and most probably in combination with other anti-HIV drugs. Plant resources in the form of herbal preparations provide cheaper and accessible antiretroviral therapy to the poor populations.

6.1. Selected plant resources with anti-HIV activity

Plant	Identified Compound	Mechanism
Daphne acutiloba (Rehder Thymelaeaceae)	Wikstroelide M	Inhibition of HIV1/2 reverse transcriptase activity and integrase nuclear translocation through disrupting the interaction between integrase and LEDGF/p75 [100]
Dracontium peruviuanum (jergón sacha)	D-tubocurarine and Phytochemicals	Possibly as a protease inhibitor [101]
Croton tiglium	Phorbol esters	Inhibitory effects on HIV-1 proliferation and its protease [102]
Mangosteen	Mangostin and gamma-mangostin	Inhibitory activity against HIV-1 protease [103]
Licorice	Glycyrrhizin	Inhibits HIV replication [104,105]
Andrographis paniculata	Diterpene lactones: (andrographolide)	Inhibit cell-to-cell transmission, viral replication and syncytia formation in HIV-infected cells [106]
Acer okamotoanum	Flavonoid gallate ester	Anti-HIV-1 integrase Activity [107]
Rhus succedanea L. Garcinia multiflora	Biflavonoids, robustaflavone, and Hinokiflavone	Inhibits HIV-1 reverse Transcriptase [108]
Ancistrocladaceae Ancistrocladus korupensis	Michellamines A and B	Inhibits reverse transcriptase, cellular fusion, and syncytium formation [109]
Annonaceae Polyalthia suberosa	Lanostane-type triterpene, suberosol	Anti-HIV replication activity [110]
Apiaceae Lomatium suksdorfii	Suksdorfin	Suppresses HIV-1 viral Replication [111]
Asteraceae Achyrocline satureioides (Lam.) DC (Marcela);	Dicaffeoylquinic acids: 3,5-dicaffeoylquinic acid, and 1-methoxyoxalyl-3,5-dicaffeoylquinic acid, Wedelolactone, a coumarin derivative;	Irreversible inhibition of HIV-1 integrase [112]
Arctium lappa (Burdock)	Orobol (an isoflavone derivative)	Inhibits HIV-1 replication;

Plant	Identified Compound	Mechanism
		blocks cell-to-cell transmission of HIV-1 [113]
Combreataceae Combretum molle R.Br. ex G.Don	Gallotannin	Inhibits HIV-1 reverse transcriptase [114]
Terminalia chebula, Euphorbia pekinensis	Gallic acid and galloyl glucose	Inhibits HIV reverse transcriptase and integrase [115]

Table 2. Selected plant resources with antiviral activity

6.2. Challenges of HIV Bioresources Development and Bioprospecting in Developing Nations

Several challenges face development of bioresources effective in enhancing antiretroviral development in low and mid-income countries. Such problems are mostly institutional highlighted as follows:

1. Lack of appropriate framework for deployment and exchange of bioresources materials within and amongst countries
2. Weak genetic banking infrastructure
3. Absence of advanced analytical and simulation laboratories
4. Weak linkage of existing bioresources centres to local industries
5. Absence of effective communication channel to supposed end users/beneficiaries of the eventual product
6. Weak standardization and evaluation procedure for products emanating from bioresources
7. Absence of a bioprospecting policy

7. Microbicides as preventive/treatment options

Microbicides are applications applied inside the vagina or rectum that protects against sexually transmitted infections (STIs) including HIV. These types of chemical applications could be formulated as gels, creams, films, or suppositories. Microbicides are potential HIV prevention options which can reduce the spread of HIV especially among women in developing countries. Without a preventive HIV vaccine, microbicides [116] offer an alternative to condoms as the most feasible method for primary prevention of HIV. Microbicides- intravaginal/intrarectal topical formulations of anti-HIV agents have also been proposed to prevent HIV transmission. Currently, antiretroviral-based microbicides have been achieved for the prevention of HIV new infections among women after many years of failed trial. More than 60 candidate agents have been identified to have *in vitro* activity against HIV, several of which have advanced to clinical testing stage.

At least 10 reverse transcriptase inhibitors and 16 entry inhibitors have been or are in the process of being investigated in clinical or preclinical trials. Ideally, these compounds are characterized by high potency, low absorption from the vagina to the blood to minimize development of resistance, and have a long half-life in order to remain active over a long period. Tenofovir has also been formulated as a topical vaginally applied gel and assessed for its protective effect against Simian immunodeficiency virus (SIV) in macaques. The results indicated that the macaques receiving the tenofovir gel were completely protected from infection [117] and in human trials [118]. The results of the human trial were released in July 2010 and showed that use of the gel reduced acquisition of HIV infection by 39% overall, and by 54% in women who were highly adherent to gel use [118].

Topical microbicides are grouped into five classes of agents, based on their mode and site of action [119] (Table 3)

Microbicides type	Mechanism	Formulation and year	Countries of clinical trial
Surfactants/membrane disruptors-based microbicides	Virucidal action through disrupting the viral envelope	1.Nonoxynol-9 (N9) 1985 [120] 2. C31G(cetylbetaine and myristamine oxide)1997 [121] 3. Sodium lauryl sulphate (Invisible Condom)2002 [122]	Kenya, Cameroon Ghana,
Vaginal milieu protector based microbicides	Enhance the natural protective mechanisms within the vaginal canal through altered pH range	BufferGel, PRO 2000 Gel [123]	Malawi; South Africa; Hlabisa, South Africa; Zambia; Zimbabwe; USA
Microbicide based on inhibition of HIV entry in the host cell	Negative charge, anionic polymers interact with HIV's viral envelope proteins and interfere with the attachment and fusion of HIV to target cell	CMPD167, Maraviroc (MVC), cyanovirin-N, Cellulose sulphate, SPL7013.2010 [124,125]	USA, Kenya Benin, India, Uganda, South Africa
Microbicides that act after entry of HIV in the host cells	Prevention of replication and release through inhibition of the virus-encoded reverse transcriptase (RT) or integrase (IN)	Tenofovir 2010 [126-128]	South Africa, Uganda, Zimbabwe
Microbicides based on inhibitors with unknown mechanism of action	Combination of extracts prepared from plants with anti-retroviral properties of unknown mechanism	Praneem 2005 [129] Basant	India

Table 3. Microbicides and their mechanism of action

For development of acceptable microbicide, researchers must develop not only the active ingredient but also a socially acceptable, affordable, and easy to apply microbicide providing protection for several days and/or weeks. Other major issues include how a microbicide might affect sperm and the possibility of causing adverse effects in women reproductive health. In Table 3 the listed microbicides failed to achieve the desired results except for tenofovir gel which showed 39% less likelihood for users to become infected with HIV than women who received a placebo gel. For women who adhered to tenofovir gel prescription correctly, HIV infection was 54% less likely than the placebo group.

8. Conclusion

HIV is widely distributed globally. Strong effort and interpersonal encouragement should be channeled on exploring and developing bioresources with antiretroviral potential to serve as a springboard for cheaper and locally available HIV drugs in addition to developing appropriate bioprospecting policies. Behavioural change and abstinence remain a sure means of HIV prevention, but need to be complemented with additional biomedical options especially in the populations most vulnerable to HIV infection.

Author details

Habu Josiah Bitrus[1*] and Ibeh Bartholomew Okechukwu[2*]

*Address all correspondence to: josiahabu@gmail.com; barthokeyibeh@yahoo.com

1 Bioresources Development Centre, Odi, Bayelsa State, Nigeria

2 Medical Biotechnology Department, National Biotechnology Development Agency, Abuja, Nigeria

References

[1] Joint United Nations Programme on HIV and AIDS, UNAIDS report 20 2012.

[2] UNAIDS. Global Fact Sheet, Joint United Nations Programme on HIV and AIDS, 2010.

[3] UNAIDS Report on the Global AIDS Epidemic 2010. http://www.unaids.org/globalreport/Global_report.htm

[4] UNAIDS 2012 report. http://www.unaids.org/sites/default/files/en/media/unaids/contentassets/documents/epidemiology/2013/gr2013/20130923_FactSheet_Global_en.pdf (accessed December 2014).

[5] United Nations, World populations. http://www.prb.org/Publications/Datasheets/2012/world-population-data-sheet.aspx. (accessed September 2014).

[6] Samuels F, Wagle S. Population mobility and HIV and AIDS: review of laws, policies and treaties between Bangladesh, Nepal and India. London: Overseas Development Institute, 2011.

[7] European Centre for Disease Prevention and Control/WHO Regional Office for Europe. HIV/AIDS surveillance in Europe 2013. Stockholm: European Centre for Disease Prevention and Control, 2014.

[8] UN Women Fact Sheet: Promoting the Legal Empowerment of Women in the Context of HIV/AIDS. 2014. http://www.unwomen.org/en/what-we-do/hiv-and-aids/facts-and-figures#notes (accessed 20 February 2015).

[9] UNAIDS. The Gap Report, 2014. http://www.unaids.org/sites/default/files/en/media/unaids/contentassets/documents/unaidspublication/2014/UNAIDS_Gap_report_en.pdf.9a(accessed 20 February 2015).

[10] Rapport National De Suivi De La Declaration Politique Sur Le Vih/Sida Cameroun. Global AIDS Response Progress (GARP), 2014. http://www.unaids.org/sites/default/files/country/documents/CMR_narrative_report_2014.pdf (accessed 22 February 2015).

[11] Gouws E, White PJ, Stover J, Brown T. Short term estimates of adult HIV incidence by mode of transmission: Kenya and Thailand as examples. Sex Transm Infect 2006; 82(iii): 51–55.

[12] CDC. Monitoring selected national HIV prevention and care objectives by using HIV surveillance data – United States and 6 U.S. dependent areas – 2012. HIV Surveillance Supplemental Report 2014; 19(No. 3).

[13] UNAIDS. FINAL SYMPOSIUM REPORT on Social norms and collective behaviour: How education needs to transform to better contribute to HIV prevention, treatment, care and support. ED/UNP/HIV/IATT/REPORT/2010/3.UNAIDS Inter-Agency Task Team on Education, May, 2010. http://unesdoc.unesco.org/images/0018/001888/188894E.pdf

[14] Dinkelman T, Lam D, Leibbrandt M. Linking poverty and income shocks to risky sexual behaviour: evidence from a panel study of young adults in cape town. The South African Journal of Economics 2008; 76(suppl): s52–s74.

[15] Durevall D, Lindsko A. Economic Inequality and HIV in Malawi. Department of Economics School of Business, Economics and Law at University of Gothenburg Vasaga-

tan 1, PO Box 640, SE 405 30 Göteborg, Sweden. https://gupea.ub.gu.se/bitstream/2077/21669/1/gupea_2077_21669_1.pdf

[16] Chirwa E, Malata A, Norr K. HIV prevention awareness and practices among married couples in Malawi. Malawi Medical Journal: The Journal of Medical Association of Malawi 2011; 23(2): 32–37.

[17] Chatterjee K. Host genetic factors in susceptibility to HIV-1 infection and progression to AIDS. Journal of Genetics 2010; 89(1): 109–116.

[18] Boily MC, Baggaley RF, Wang L, Masse B, White RG, Hayes RJ, et al. Heterosexual risk of HIV-1 infection per sexual act: systematic review and meta-analysis of observational studies. Lancet Infectious Disease 2009; 9(2): 118–129.

[19] Kleinman SH, Lelie N, Busch MP. Infectivity of human immunodeficiency virus-1, hepatitis C virus, and hepatitis B virus and risk of transmission by transfusion. Transfusion 2009; 492454.

[20] Kaplan EH, Heimer R. A model-based estimate of HIV infectivity via needle sharing. Journal of Acquired Immune Deficiency Syndrome 1992; 5(11): 1116–1118.

[21] Ioannidis JP, Abrams EJ, Ammann A, et al. Perinatal transmission of human immunodeficiency virus type 1 by pregnant women with RNA virus loads <1000 copies/ml. <1000 copies/ml. The Journal of Infectious Diseases. 2001; 184(4): 539–545.

[22] Joint United Nations Programme on HIV and AIDS, UNAIDS report 2011; 20–30.

[23] Rodriguez-Garcia M, Barr FD, Crist SG, Fahey JV, Wira CR. Phenotype and susceptibility to HIV infection of CD4 Th17 cells in the human female reproductive tract. Mucosal Immunology 2014; 7: 61375.

[24] Caldwell B, Pieris I, Ichuda B, Caldwell J. Sexually regimes and sexual networking: the risk of an HIV/AIDS epidemic in Bangladesh. Social Science and Medicine 1999;48: 1103–1116.

[25] Higgins JA, Hoffman S, Dworkin SL. Rethinking gender, heterosexual men, and women's vulnerability to HIV/AIDS: time to shift the paradigm. American Journal of Public Health 2010; 100(3): 435–445.

[26] CDC. Estimated HIV incidence among adults and adolescents in the United States, 2007–2010. HIV Surveillance Supplemental Report 2012; 17(No. 4).

[27] CDC. 1981. Kaposi's sarcoma and Pneumocystis pneumonia among homosexual men —New York City and California. MMWR Morbidity and Mortality Weekly Report 1981; 30: 305–308.

[28] Lucy P, Emma J, Vivian H, Alisher, Ford H, Lucy R, Tim R. HIV in the European region: vulnerability and response. World Bank, Washington, DC. © World Bank 2013. https://openknowledge.worldbank.org/handle/10986/16517 License: CC BY-NC-ND 3.0 IGO

[29] van Griensven F, van Wijngaarden JWDL, Baral S, Grulich A. The global epidemic of HIV infection among men who have sex with men. Current Opinion in HIV and AIDS 2009; 4(4): 300–307.

[30] Beyrer C. Global prevention of HIV infection for neglected populations: men who have sex with men. Clinical Infectious Diseases 2010; 50(supplement 3): S108–S113.

[31] Likatavicius G, van de Laar M. HIV and AIDS in the European Union, 2011, Eurosurveillance 2011; 17(48): Article ID 20329, 2012.

[32] Beyrer C, Baral SD, Walker D, Wirtz AL, Johns B, Sifakis F. The expanding epidemics of HIV type 1 among men who have sex with men in low-and middle-income countries: diversity and consistency. Epidemiologic Reviews 2010; 32(10): 137–151.

[33] McIntyre JA. The need for HIV prevention interventions for men who have sex with men in Africa. Sexually Transmitted Infections 2010; 869(20): 82–83.

[34] Baral S, Sifakis F, Cleghorn F, Beyrer C. Elevated risk for HIV infection among men who have sex with men in low- and middle-income countries 2000–2006: a systematic review. PLoS Medicine 2007; 4(12): article e339.

[35] Gouws E, White PJ, Stover J, Brown T. Short term estimates of adult HIV incidence by mode of transmission: Kenya and Thailand as examples. Sexually Transmitted Infectections 2006; 82(iii): 51–55. doi: 10.1136/sti.2006.020164

[36] Joint United Nations Programme on HIV/AIDS & The World Bank Global HIV/AIDS Program. Zambia HIV prevention response and modes of transmission analysis. Lusaka; 2009.

[37] Pisani E, Garnett GP, Grassly NC, Brown T, Stover J, Hankins C, et al. Back to basics in HIV prevention: focus on exposure. BMJ 2003; 326: 1384–1387.

[38] Brown T, Peerapatanapokin W. The Asian epidemic model: a process model for exploring HIV policy and programme alternatives in Asia. Sexually Transmitted Infections 2004; 80(i): 19–24.

[39] Colvin M, Gorgens-Albino M, Kasedde S. Analysis of HIV prevention response and modes of HIV transmission: the *UNAIDS-GAMET-supported synthesis process*. Johannesburg: UNAIDS Regional Support Team Eastern and Southern Africa; 2008. http://www.unaidsrstesa.org/sites/default/files/modesoftransmission/analysis_hiv_prevention_response_and_mot.pdf (accessed 27 November 2014).

[40] Case KK, Ghys PD, Gouws E, Eaton JW, Borquez A, Stover J, Cuchi PP, Abu-Raddad JL, Garnett GP, Hallett TB. The HIV modelling consortium: understanding the modes of transmission model of new HIV infection and its use in prevention planning. Bulletin of the World Health Organization 2012; 90: 831–838A.

[41] Robertson DL, Hahn BH, Sharp PM. Recombination in AIDS viruses. Journal of Molecular Evolution 1995; 40(3): 249–259.

[42] Martin DP, Williamson C, Posada D. Rdp2: recombination detection and analysis from sequence alignments. Bioinformatics 2005, 21(2): 260–262.

[43] Kannangai R, David S, Sridharan G. Human immunodeficiency virus type 2-A milder, kinder virus: an update. Indian Journal of Medical Microbiology 2012; 30(1): 6–15.

[44] Vijay NNV, Vasantika, Ajmani R, Perelson AS, Dixit NM. Recombination increases human immunodeficiency virus fitness, but not necessarily diversity. Journal of General Virology 2008; 89(6): 1467–1477.

[45] Kotaki1 T, Khairunisa SQ,Witaningrum AM,Yunifiar MQ, Sukartiningrum SD, Diansyah MN, Rahayu1 RP. Nasronudin13 and Masanori Kameoka HIV-1 transmitted drug resistance mutations among antiretroviral therapy – Naïve individuals in Surabaya, Indonesia. AIDS Research and Therapy 2015, 12: 5.

[46] Sampathkumar R, Shadabi E, Luo M. Interplay between HIV-1 and host genetic variation: a snapshot into its impact on AIDS and therapy response. Advances in Virology 2012; 2012: Article ID 508967, 16 pages. doi:10.1155/2012/508967.

[47] Zhuang J, Jetzt AE, Sun G, Yu H, Klarmann G, Ron Y, Preston BD, Dougherty JP. Human immunodeficiency virus type 1 recombination: rate, fidelity, and putative hot spots. Journal of Virology 2002; 76: 11273–11282.

[48] Konings FA, Haman GR, Xue Y, Urbanski MM, Hertzmark K, Nanfack A, Achkar JM, Burda ST, Nyambi PN. Genetic analysis of HIV-1 strains in rural eastern Cameroon indicates the evolution of second-generation recombinants to circulating recombinant forms. Journal of Acquired Immune Deficiency Syndrome 2006; 42: 331–341.

[49] Moutouh L, Corbeil J, Richman DD. Recombination leads to the rapid emergence of HIV-1 dually resistant mutants under selective drug pressure. Proceedings of the National Academy of Sciences USA 1996; 93: 6106–6111.

[50] Ragupathy V, Zhao1 J, Wood O, Tang S, Lee S, Nyambi P, Hewlett I. Identification of new, emerging HIV-1 unique recombinant forms and drug resistant viruses circulating in Cameroon. Virology Journal 2011; 8: 185.

[51] Zhang M, Foley B, Schultz A, Macke JP, Bulla I, Stanke M, Morgenstern B, Korber B, Leitner T. The role of recombination in the emergence of a complex and dynamic HIV epidemic. Retrovirology 2010, 7: 25.

[52] Mbanya D, Sama M, Tchounwou P. Current status of HIV/AIDS in Cameroon: how effective are control strategies? International Journal of Environmental Research and Public Health 2008; 5(5): 378–383.

[53] Bobkov AF, Kazennova EV, Selimova LM et al. Temporal trends in the HIV-1 epidemic in Russia: predominance of subtype A. Journal of Medical Virology 2004; 74(2): 191–196.

[54] Robertson DL, Hahn BH, Sharp PM, Hahn, Goudsmit S, Jaap. Viral sex; the nature of AIDS. Oxford University Press. New York, 1997, 51–58.

[55] Buonaguro L,Tonesello ML,bvuonaguro FM.Human immunodeficiency virus type 1subtype distribution in the worldwide epidermic:Patogenic and Therapeutic implications.Journal of virology 2007,81,19:10209-10219.

[56] Kouri V,Khouri R, Alemán, Y, Abrahantes Y, Vercauteren J, Pineda-Peña A, Theys K, Megens S, Moutschen M, Pfeifer N, Van eyenbergh J,. Pérez AB, Pérez J, Pérez L, Van Laethem K, Vandamme A., CRF19_cpx is an Evolutionary fit HIV-1 variant strongly associated with rapid progression to AIDS in Cuba. EBioMedicine 2015; 2(3): 188–189.

[57] Yamaguchi J, Coffey R, Vallari A, Ngansop C, Mbanya D, Ndembi N, Kaptué L, Lutz G. Gürtler, Bodelle P, Schochetman G, Devare SG, Brennan CA. Identification of HIV Type 1 Group N infections in a husband and wife in Cameroon: viral genome sequences provide evidence for horizontal transmission. AIDS Research and Human Retroviruses 2006; 22(1): 83–92.

[58] Peeters M, Gueye A, Mboup S, Bibollet-Ruche F, Ekaza E, Mulanga C, Ouedrago R, Gandji R, Mpele P, Dibanga G, Koumare B, Saidou M, Esu-Williams E, Lombart JP, Badombena W, Luo N, Vanden Haesevelde M, Delaporte E.Geographical distribution of HIV-1 group O viruses in Africa. AIDS 1997; 11(4): 493–498.

[59] Plantier JC, Leoz M, Dickerson JE, De Oliveira F, Cordonnier F, Lemée V, Damond F, Robertson DL, Simon F. A new human immunodeficiency virus derived from gorillas. Nature Medicine 2009; 15(8): 871–872.

[60] Santiago ML, Range F, Keele BF, Li Y, Bailes E, Bibollet-Ruche F, Fruteau C, Noë R, Peeters M, Brookfield JFY., Shaw GM, Sharp PM, Hahn BH. Simian Immunodeficiency virus infection in free-ranging sooty Mangabeys (Cercocebus atys atys) from the Taï Forest, Côte d'Ivoire: implications for the origin of epidemic human immunodeficiency virus Type 2. Journal of Virology 2005; 79(19): 12515–12527.

[61] Marx PA, Alcabes PG, Drucker E. Serial human passage of simian immunodeficiency virus by unsterile injections and the emergence of epidemic human immunodeficiency virus in Africa. Philosophical Transactions of the Royal Society B; Biological Sciences 2001; 356(1410): 911–920.

[62] Medley A, Kennedy C, O'Reilly K, Sweat M. Effectiveness of peer education interventions for HIV prevention in developing countries: a systematic review and meta-analysis. AIDS Education and Prevention 2009; 21(3): 181–206.

[63] UNAIDS. Peer education and HIV/AIDS: concepts, uses and challenges. http://www.unicef.org/infobycountry/files/PeerEducationUNAIDS.pdf. (accessed 2 December 2014).

[64] Tolli MV. Effectiveness of peer education interventions for HIV prevention, adolescent pregnancy prevention and sexual health promotion for young people: a systematic review of European studies. Health Education Research 2012; 27(5): 904–913.

[65] Smith Fawzi MC, Jagannathan P, Cabral J, Banares R, Salazar J, Farmer P, Behforouz H. Limitations in knowledge of HIV transmission among HIV-positive patients accessing case management services in a resource-poor setting. AIDS Care 2006; 18(7): 764–771.

[66] UNESCO report. Education for all by 2015, will we make it: regional overview of sub Saharan Africa. http://en.unesco.org/gem-report/sites/gem-report/files/157229E.pdf (accessed 25 February 2015).

[67] Baxen J, Breidlid A. Researching HIV/AIDS and education in Sub-Saharan Africa: examining the gaps and challenges. Journal of Education 2004; 34: 9–29.

[68] WHO. Health for the world's adolescents: a second chance in the second decade. 2014.

[69] Suzuki PTC, Gillespie A, Kasedde S, Idele P. Disparities and trends in AIDS mortality among adolescents living with HIV in low- and middle-income countries. 20th International AIDS Conference, Melbourne, abstract MOAC0101, July 2014.

[70] Idele P, Gillespie A, Porth T, Suzuki C, Mahy M, Kasedde S, Luo C. Epidemiology of HIV and AIDS among adolescents: current status, inequities, and data gaps. Journal of Acquired Immune Deficiency Syndrome 2014; 66: S144–S153.

[71] Paul-Ebhohimhen VA, et al. a systematic review of school-based sexual health interventions to prevent STI/HIV in sub-Saharan Africa. BMC Public Health 2008; 8: 4.

[72] WHO Library Cataloguing-in-Publication Data Access to antiretroviral drugs in low- and middle-income countries: technical report July 2014. http://apps.who.int/medicinedocs/documents/s21630en/s21630en.pdf (accessed 16 January 2015).

[73] Ford N, Ananworanich J, Ruxrungtham K, Simmons B, Hill A. Is the pricing of antiretrovirals equitable? Analysis of antiretroviral drug prices in 20 low- and middle-income countries. 7th IAS Conference on HIV Pathogenesis Treatment and Prevention, 30 June–3 July 2013, Kuala Lumpur, Malaysia. Oral abstract 2013.

[74] Coalition of Civil Society Groups on Access to Essential Medicines. A price comparison of selected HIV/AIDS drugs in Nigeria. Reports and Studies. Journalist against AIDS publication 2001. http://www.nigeria-aids.org/reports.cfm?read=75

[75] Goldie SJ, Yazdanpanah Y, Losina E, Weinstein MC, Anglaret X, Walensky RP, Hsu HE, Kimmel A, Holmes C, Kaplan JE, Freedberg KAN. Cost-effectiveness of HIV treatment in resource-poor settings – the case of Côte d'Ivoire. England Journal of Medicine 2006; 14; 355(11): 1141–1153.

[76] CDC. Pre-exposure prophylaxis (PrEP). http://www.cdc.gov/hiv/prevention/research/prep/ (accessed August 2014).

[77] CDC. Preexposure prophylaxis for the prevention of HIV infection in the United States – 2014 a clinical practice guideline. 1–67. http://www.cdc.gov/hiv/pdf/PrEPguidelines2014.pdf

[78] WHO. Supplementary section to the 2013 WHO consolidated guidelines on the use of antiretroviral drugs for treating and preventing HIV infection, Chapter 5 – Clinical guidelines across the continuum of care: HIV diagnosis and ARV drugs for HIV prevention.

[79] WHO. Guidelines on post-exposure prophylaxis for HIV and the use of co-trimoxazole prophylaxis for HIV-related infections among adults, adolescents and children. Recommendations for a public health approach – December 2014 supplement to the 2013 consolidated ARV guidelines.

[80] Agaba PA, Agaba EI, Ocheke AN, Daniyam CA, Akanbi MO, Okeke EN. Awareness and knowledge of human immunodeficiency virus post exposure prophylaxis among Nigerian Family Physicians. Nigerian Medical Journal: Journal of the Nigeria Medical Association 2012; 53(3): 155–160.

[81] Rutland E, Sundaram S, Mani R. The awareness of postexposure prophylaxis for HIV infection following sexual exposure in emergency departments in a regional HIV network. International journal of STD & AIDS 2010; 21(9): 636–637.

[82] Anon. Guidelines on Post Exposure Prophylaxis for HIV. Recommendations for a Public Health Approach. World Health Organization, Geneva, 2014.

[83] WHO. Post-exposure prophylaxis to prevent HIV infection Factsheet 2014. http://www.who.int/hiv/topics/prophylaxis/pep_factsheet_dec2014.pdf (accessed 29 December 2014).

[84] Schouten EJ, Jahn A, Ben-Smith A, et al. Antiretroviral drug supply challenges in the era of scaling up ART in Malawi. Journal of the International AIDS Society 2011; 14(Suppl 1): S4.

[85] Chandani Y, Felling B, Allers C, Alt D, Noguera M, Zuber A. Supply chain management of anitretroviral drugs: considerations for initiating and expanding national supply chains. DELIVER, for the U.S. Agency for International Development, Arlington, 2006.

[86] Waning B, Diedrichsen E, Moon S. A lifeline to treatment: the role of Indian generic manufacturers in supplying antiretroviral medicines to developing countries. Journal of the International AIDS Society. 2010; 13: 35.

[87] Hammer SM, Schechter M, Montaner JS, et al. International AIDS Society-USA panel. Treatment for adult HIV infection: 2006 recommendations of the International AIDS Society-USA panel. JAMA 2006; 296: 827–843.

[88] Badri M, Lawn SD, Wood R. Utility of CD4 cell counts for early prediction of virological failure during antiretroviral therapy in a resource-limited setting. BMC Infectious Diseases 2008; 8: 89.

[89] UNAIDS/WHO. HIV and hormonal contraception Frequently asked questions. 2012. http://www.unaids.org/sites/default/files/media_asset/JC2309_HIV_hormonal_contraception_en_0.pdf

[90] Philips GMSJ, Baggaley RC, Steyn P, Temmerman M. HIV and contraception – complex issues for safe choice: the latest recommendations from the World Health Organization (WHO). 20th International AIDS Conference, Melbourne, abstract THAC0505LB, 2014.

[91] Clark JT, Clark MR, Shelke NB, Johnson TJ, Smith EM, Andreasen AK, Nebeker JS, Fabian J, Friend DR, Kiser PF. Engineering a segmented dual-reservoir polyurethane intravaginal ring for simultaneous prevention of HIV transmission and unwanted pregnancy. PLoS One 2014; 9(3): e88509.

[92] Johnson TJ, Clark MR, Albright TH, Nebeker JS, Tuitupou AL, Clark JT, Fabian J, McCabe RT, Chandra N, Doncel GF, Friend DR, Kiser PF. A 90-day Tenofovir reservoir intravaginal ring for mucosal HIV prophylaxis. Antimicrobial Agents and Chemotherapy 2012; 56(12): 6272–6283.

[93] Scarsi K et al. Efavirenz, but not nevirapine antiretroviral therapy, decreases exposure tolevonorgestrel released from a sub-dermal contraceptive implant. Journal of the International AIDS Society 2014; 17(3): 4, abstract 0131.

[94] Chen MCP, Kwok C, Bernholc A, Low N. For the HC-HIV IPD meta-analysis study group hormonal contraception and HIV infection: results from a large individual participant data meta-analysis. 20th International AIDS Conference, Melbourne, abstract THAC0503, 2014.

[95] Kilembe WKW, Naw HK, Brill I, Vwalika B, Chomba E, Johnson B, Haddad L, Tichacek A, Allen S. Weighing 17 years of evidence: does hormonal contraception increase HIV acquisition risk among Zambian women in discordant couples? 20th International AIDS Conference, Melbourne, abstract THAC0504, 2014.

[96] WHO, author. Traditional medicine strategy 2002–2005. World Health Organisation, Geneva, 2002.

[97] King R, Homsy J. Involving traditional healers in AIDS education and counselling in sub-Saharan Africa: a review. AIDS 1997; 11(Suppl A): S217–S225.

[98] Langlois-Klassen D, Kipp W, Jhangri GS, Rubaale T. Use of traditional herbal medicine by AIDS patients in Kabarole District, Western Uganda. The American Journal of Tropical Medicine and Hygiene 2007; 77(4): 757–763.

[99] Zhang X, Huang SZ, Gu WG, Yang LM, Chen H, Zheng CB, Zhao YX, Wan DC, Zheng YT. Wikstroelide M potently inhibits HIV replication by targeting reverse

transcriptase and integrase nuclear translocation. Chinese Journal of Natural Medicines 2014; 12(3): 186–193.

[100] Napolitano A, et al. Qualitative on-line profiling of ceramides and cerebrosides by high performance liquid chromatography coupled with electrospray ionization ion trap tandem mass spectrometry: the case of Dracontium loretense. Journal of Pharmaceutical and Biomedical Analysis 2011; 28; 55(1): 23–30.

[101] Nakamura N. Inhibitory effects of some traditional medicines on proliferation of HIV-1 and its protease. Yakugaku Zasshi 2004; 124: 519–529.

[102] Chen SX, Wan M, Loh BN.Active constituents against HIV-1 protease from Garcinia Mangostana. Planta Medica 1996; 62(4): 381–382.

[103] Sasaki H, Takei M, Kobayashi M, Pollard RB, Suzuki F. Effect of glycyrrhizin, an active component of licorice roots, on HIV replication in cultures of peripheral blood mononuclear cells from HIV-seropositive patients. Pathobiology 2002–2003; 70(4): 229–236.

[104] Otake T, Mori M, Ueba N, Sutardjo S, Kusumoto IT, Hattori M, Namba T. Screening of Indonesian plant extracts for antihuman immunodeficiency virus-type1 (HIV-1) activity. Phytotherapy Research 1995; 9: 6–10. 13.

[105] Calabrese C. A phase I trial of andrographolide in HIV positive patients and normal volunteers. Phytotherapy Research 2002; 14: 333–338.

[106] Kim HJ, Woo ER, Shin CG. A new flavonol glycoside gallate ester from Acer okamotoanum and its inhibitory activity against human immunodeficiency virus-1 (HIV-1) integrase. Journal of Natural Products 1998; 61: 145–148.

[107] Lin YM, Anderson H, Flavin MT, Pai YSH, Mata-Greenwood E, Pengsuparp T, Pezzuto JM, Schinazi RF, Hughes SH, Chen FC. In vitro anti-HIV activity of biflavonoids isolated from Rhus succedanea and Garcinia multiflora. Journal of Natural Products 1997; 60(9): 884–888.

[108] Boyd MR, Hallock YF, Cardellina II JH, Manfredi KP, Blunt, JW, McMahon JB, Buckheit RW, Bringmann G, Schaeffer M. Anti-HIV michellamines from Ancistrocladus korupensis. Journal of Medicinal Chemistry 1994; 37(12): 1740–1745.

[109] Li HY, Sun NJ, Kashiwada Y, Sun L, Snider JV, Cosentino LM, Lee KH. Anti-AIDS agents, 9. Suberosol, a new C31 lanostane-type triterpene and anti-HIV principle from Ployalthia suberosa. Journal of Natual Products 1993; 56(7): 1130–1133.

[110] Yu D, Morris-Natschke SL, Lee KH. New developments in natural products-based anti AIDS research. Medicinal Research Reviews 2007; 27(1): 108–132.

[111] Zhu, K, Cordeiro ML, Atienza J, Robinson EW, Chow S. Irreversible inhibition of human immunodeficiency virus type integrase by dicaffeoylquinic acids. Journal of Virology 1999; 73(4): 3309–3316. 23.

http://dx.doi.org/10.5772/61000

[112] Yao XJ, Wainberg MA, Parniak MA. Mechanism of inhibition of HIV-1 infection in vitro by purified extract of Prunella vulgaris. Journal of Virology 1992; 187(1): 56–62.

[113] Bessong PO, Obi CL, Andreola ML, Rojas LB, Pouysegu L, Igumbor E, Meyer JJ, Quideau S, Litvak S. Evaluation of selected South African medicinal plants for inhibitory properties against human immunodeficiency virus type 1 reverse transcriptase and integrase. Journal of Ethnopharmacology 2005; 99(1): 83–91. 34.

[114] Ahn MJ. Inhibition of HIV-1 integrase by galloyl glucoses from Terminalia chebula and flavonol glucoside gallates from Euphorbia pekinensis. Planta Medica 2002; 68: 454–457.

[115] WHO. Microbicides. http://www.who.int/hiv/topics/microbicides/microbicides/en/

[116] Miller C, Rosenberg Z, Bischofberger N. Use of topical PMPA to prevent vaginal transmission of SIV. Presented at: 9th International Conference on Antiviral Research, Japan, 19–24 May 1996.

[117] Abdool Karim Q, Abdool Karim SS, Frohlich JA, et al. Effectiveness and safety of tenofovir gel, an antiretroviral microbicide, for the prevention of HIV infection in women. Science 2010; 329(5996): 1168–1174.

[118] Cutler B, Justman J. Vaginal microbicides and the prevention of HIV transmission. Lancet Infectious Diseases 2008; 8: 685–697.

[119] Hicks DR, Martin LS, Getchell JP, Heath JL, Francis DP, McDougal JS, et al. Inactivation of HTLV-III/LAV-infected cultures of normal human lymphocytes by nonoxynol-9 *in vitro*. Lancet. 1985; 2: 1422–1423.

[120] Wyrick PB, Knight ST, Gerbig DG, Jr, Raulston JE, Davis CH, Paul TR, et al. The microbicidal agent C31G inhibits *Chlamydia trachomatis* infectivity *in vitro*. Antimicrobial Agents and Chemotherapy 1997; 41: 1335–1344.

[121] Piret J, Desormeaux A, Bergeron MG. Sodium lauryl sulfate, a microbicide effective against enveloped and nonenveloped viruses. Current Drug Targets 2002; 3: 17–30.

[122] Abdool Karim SS, Richardson BA, Ramjee G, Hoffman IF, Chirenje ZM, Taha T, et al. Safety and effectiveness of BufferGel and 0.5% PRO2000 gel for the prevention of HIV infection in women. AIDS. 2011; 25: 957–966.

[123] Tyssen D, Henderson SA, Johnson A, Sterjovski J, Moore K, La J, et al. Structure activity relationship of dendrimer microbicides with dual action antiviral activity. PLoS One 2010; 5: e12309.

[124] O'Loughlin J, Millwood IY, McDonald HM, Price CF, Kaldor JM, Paull JR. Safety, tolerability, and pharmacokinetics of SPL7013 gel (VivaGel): a dose ranging, phase I study. Sexually Transmitted Diseases 2010; 37: 100–104.

[125] Herrera C, Cranage M, McGowan I, Anton P, Shattock RJ. Reverse transcriptase inhibitors as potential colorectal microbicides. Antimicrobial Agents and Chemotherapy 2009; 53: 1797–1807.

[126] Abdool Karim Q, Abdool Karim SS, Frohlich JA, Grobler AC, Baxter C, Mansoor LE, et al. Effectiveness and safety of tenofovir gel, an antiretroviral microbicide, for the prevention of HIV infection in women. Science 2010; 329: 1168–1174.

[127] FHI and the Centre for the AIDS Programme of Research in South Africa. Factsheet: Results of the CAPRISA 004 trial on the effectiveness of tenofovir gel for HIV prevention. Research Triangle Park, NC USA, July 2010. http://pdf.usaid.gov/pdf_docs/Pnadt312.pdf

[128] Joshi SN, Katti U, Godbole S, Bharucha K, B KK, Kulkarni S, et al. Phase I safety study of Praneem polyherbal vaginal tablet use among HIV-uninfected women in Pune, India. Transactions of the Royal Society of Tropical Medicine and Hygiene 2005; 99: 769–774.

[129] Joshi SN, Dutta S, Kumar BK, Katti U, Kulkarni S, Risbud A, et al. Expanded safety study of Praneem polyherbal vaginal tablet among HIV-uninfected women in Pune, India: a phase II clinical trial report. Sexually Transmitted Infections 2008; 84: 343–347.

Chapter 2

HIV Infection — A Sociological Approach to the Prevention of the HIV Pandemic

Carmen Rodríguez Reinado and
Teresa Blasco Hernández

Additional information is available at the end of the chapter

http://dx.doi.org/10.5772/60929

1. Introduction

> "The first step [in transforming] reality is [usually] learning to see it [from] a new perspective (and being capable of showing it to others [in] this light)." *Jorge Riechmann*

Despite the fact that over three decades have passed since the first recorded case of AIDS in 1981, many questions remain unanswered regarding the HIV pandemic: how did HIV originate? When will an effective vaccine be available? How do strategies and measures for prevention need to be designed and implemented?

Currently, the prevention and elimination of HIV is one of the major challenges for public health worldwide. The HIV pandemic constitutes a social problem of great magnitude. It is a complex social phenomenon that is difficult to address. Thus, in order to study its complexity, it is necessary to adopt an interdisciplinary approach. In this sense, the sociological discipline and in particular, the sociology of health, is an important tool for the study and understanding of HIV. The general purpose of this chapter is to reveal and justify the relevance of integrating a sociological perspective to the study of HIV prevention. Firstly, the extent and magnitude of the epidemic on a global scale is described. Secondly, sociological theories and methodologies that might be usefully applied in the field of HIV prevention and treatment are presented and justified. Finally, conclusions are drawn considering a number of relevant and pertinent analytical elements that are crucial to the development of HIV prevention policies.

2. The globalization of the pandemic

At present, there is evidence that globalization has affected health care in a variety of ways. In this sense, the majority of the most prestigious institutions and organizations in the field of public health have become standard-bearers for the concept of global health. As such, the concept of global health is a consequence of the process of globalization. The definition of global health pursues equity in health matters worldwide; it is a priority objective for the international technocratic agenda [1].

The globalization process, with its multiple dimensions (economic, political, social, ecological, etc.), has had a significant impact on global health. For instance, economic globalization through the internationalization of trade and the communications revolution has resulted in the globalization of risks and of certain diseases [2]. In addition, ecological globalization, alongside the environmental and ecological changes it entails, has also had an effect on health [3]. This can be illustrated by the following: water deprivation due to scarcity implies major health risks; air pollution has caused an increase in respiratory diseases; climatic change with its ensuing extreme temperature variations affect cardiovascular diseases and the depletion of the ozone layer has increased the incidence of skin cancer [4]. On the other hand, the interdependence generated between governments and transnational problems, characteristic of political globalization, have shifted power away from the State in favour of the creation of international institutions. Thus, the World Health Organisation is today the largest exponent of health, while UNAIDS serves this purpose in the case of HIV.

Consequently, social phenomena such as health tourism, the migration of health professionals to developed countries, the existence of global risks, the resurgence of diseases that had previously been limited (such as tuberculosis) in developed countries and the global emergence of infectious diseases (avian influenza, HIV, etc.) are greatly related to the globalisation process. Specifically, globalisation has important repercussions for emerging infectious diseases: "Since the 1970s, newly emerging diseases have been identified at the unprecedented rate of one or more per year. There are now at least 40 diseases that were unknown a generation ago" [5].

In general terms, the relationship established between globalization and global health is not a positive one. However, it is worth noting that globalization has also had a positive impact on certain aspects of global health, given that it offers opportunities and provides improvements related to population health. For instance, globally, the total poverty rate has declined from 20% to 5% over the past 25 years [6]. Globalization, to the extent that it produces greater economic growth, generally involves improvements in population health. For instance, globalization has resulted in better health care conditions. This is evidenced by the success achieved in relation to children's nutritional status and mortality among breast-fed babies, as demonstrated by specific indicators, greater opportunities for health care choices (patients whose health problems cannot be treated in their own countries can explore the international health care available and choose the most convenient option), an increase in the external aid of developed countries as evidenced by the MDGs in the case of malaria, tuberculosis and HIV (the containment of the spread of AIDS in many countries through the implementation of prevention programmes) [7], and the fact that new information and communication technologies enable health professionals from anywhere in the world to access scientific evidence and improve their clinical decisions [6].

Concerning the objective of this chapter, however, the relationhip established between globalization and HIV is robust. So much so that HIV, along with other diseases such as tuberculosis and malaria, is presently termed a "global disease". To a large extent, this is the result of the movement of goods and people, which has also increased the likelihood of diseases spreading worldwide. Diseases, like goods and people, also commute across oceans and borders. For this reason, one of the main concerns of international public health is the speed, as well as the high rates, of the worldwide spread of highly contagious diseases, as illustrated recently by the alarm triggered concerning Ebola infection.

HIV is a clear exponent of transnationalization and constitutes a global epidemic that now poses one of the major threats to global health. Such has been the scope of the pandemic and the resulting consequences that today, it can be affirmed that HIV represents one of the most severe public health epidemics ever suffered by humanity. Therefore, considering the gravity of the situation, the international organism UNAIDS was created to respond to this issue.

According to an UNAIDS 2013 report, it is estimated that on a global scale, 35.3 million people were living with HIV in 2012, an increase compared to previous years [8]. This is largely due to greater accessibility to treatment. In other words, there are progressively more people in the world receiving antiretroviral therapy, which raises their life expectancy. The distribution according to population group is 31.8 million adults and 3.2 million children [8]; 2.3 million new cases of HIV infection were reported throughout the world in 2013, compared to the 3.4 million cases recorded in 2001 [8]. Consequently, these figures show that there has been a decline of approximately 33%. In the case of new infections HIV in children, 240 000 children worldwide (210 00-280 000) contracted HIV in 2013, compared to 580 000 (530 000-640 000) in 2001, signifying a decrease of 58% [8]. Similarly, the number of deaths from AIDS has also declined: 1.6 million deaths were recorded in 2012, compared to 2.3 million recorded in 2005. Specifically, 1.3 million deaths occurred among adults and 190 000 among children.

HIV indicators	2002	2012
People living with HIV (Total)	30.7 million	35.3 million
New HIV infections (Total)	3.3 million	2.3 million
AIDS-related deaths	2.1 million	1.6 million
People accessing treatment	There is no data available	12.9 million

Source: UNAIDS, 2013

Table 1. Structural indicators of HIV

Despite the progress that has been made, epidemiological data continues to show alarming figures, as reflected in Table 1. As such, there remain major obstacles in the eradication of the pandemic. According to UNAIDS' most recent report (2013), some of these challenges are [8]:

1. Reducing the sexual transmission of HIV in African countries where a decline in the use of the masculine condom has been detected.
2. Reducing HIV transmission among people who inject drugs, since data shows this remains highly prevalent, whereas HIV prevention coverage remains low.
3. Reducing new infections in children, as well as maternal mortality during pregnancy.
4. Improving the availability of and accessibility to antiretroviral therapy in low and middle-income countries.
5. Reducing the number of tuberculosis-related deaths in HIV patients.
6. Eliminating stigma, discrimination and coercive laws and practices in relation to HIV.
7. Eliminating gender inequalities, abuse and violence that cause the feminization of HIV.
8. The integration of people affected by HIV.
9. The overall lack of resources in the fight against AIDS.

HIV constitutes a clear example of social inequality in relation to health. In overall terms, the highest prevalence of the pandemic occurs in countries with low human development indicators. This increases social injustice and accentuates existing inequalities in these countries. According a UNAIDS report (2013), some of the countries that present higher prevalence rates with regard to global prevalence are [8]:

Country/ Region[1]	Prevalence of HIV (2012)
Swaziland	28.3%
Lesotho	24.7%
Botswana	24.4%
South Africa	18.4%
Zimbabwe	15.6%
Namibia	15.2%
Mozambique	12.9%
Malawi	11.4%
Equatorial Guinea	9.7%
North America	0.8%
Canada	0.3%
Western and Central Europe	0.2%

Source: UNAID, 2013

[1]Table 2 shows the existing discrepancies in the pandemic's global distribution; some countries show a higher HIV prevalence, according to a 2013 sample, while other continental regions show lower levels of prevalence.

Table 2. Prevalence rate of HIV infection in adults

Similarly, the overall distribution of AIDS-related deaths shows that the greatest incidence occurs in countries with low and moderate development rates: Nigeria (13%), South Africa

(13%), India (8%), Mozambique (5%), United Republic of Tanzania (5%), Zimbabwe (4%), Uganda (4%), Kenya (4%), Malawi (3), Ethiopia (3%), China (2%), Russian Federation (2%), Democratic Republic of the Congo (2%) and Indonesia (2%)[8]. In the aforementioned countries, the epidemic represents a major public health issue. Not only is it a medical and health care issue, but it also constitutes one of the major obstacles to economic and social development [9]. For example, the high percentage of adult AIDS-related deaths results in the loss of the youngest and most productive individuals in a society, who are vital to economic development. Economic productivity also decreases, because AIDS sufferers and their caregivers stop working. Additionally, the educational system in these countries is affected by the percentage of teachers who die from AIDS, which means the loss of a significant part of the most educated population. Furthermore, the health care expenditure generated by providing health care services for people living with HIV and AIDS entails budgetary restrictions within the public sector. This constrains investments in other sectors aimed at promoting social and economic development. Finally, the scope of the epidemic in these countries is increasing, deepening poverty and existing social inequalities, and consequently inverting the human development trend. The HIV/AIDS epidemic has therefore become a priority for public policies in these countries. As a result, the response to HIV/AIDS and the fight against poverty has become the same battle [10]. For this reason, the elimination of HIV/AIDS has been established as a Millennium Goal, the sixth MDG [11], specifying the need to: "Halt and begin to reverse the spread of HIV/AIDS by 2015". Thus, the inclusion of HIV as a Millennium Goal evidences the global acknowledgement of the destructive and generalized effects of HIV/AIDS, as well as the belief that it is possible to overcome the situation by means of greater and more intensive national and international action, as well as the active will to do so.

3. Why is a sociological perspective of the HIV pandemic pertinent?

> "Health sociology is no longer, nor should [it] be, the simple contribution of techniques to the health care service but, on the contrary, should mean methodological independence [for dealing] with health from an interdisciplinary viewpoint, in which the biomedical aspect is only an additional component, however important it may be".[1]

Currently, it is widely recognized that the study of HIV constitutes a complex social phenomenon in which there is an interrelation between multiple social, economic, political, cultural and environmental factors in those communities where the pandemic develops and spreads. For instance, although HIV is a chronic disease in some European countries, in some African countries it is a deadly disease. Therefore, insofar as the epidemic influences the lifestyles, practices and subjectivities of a population, it is necessary to study it by utilizing tools that provide a more qualitative and in-depth knowledge of the phenomenon. Consequently, social sciences have begun to study the complex connections established in relation to the HIV phenomenon with the aim of providing knowledge for its understanding and comprehension.

---

1 Cited in: Donati P. Sociology of health. Madrid: Díaz de Santos; 1994.

However, despite existing evidence, the epidemiological method has been the benchmark for most of the approaches in the study of issues concerning public health in general and HIV in particular [10]. In this respect, it is worth noting that, currently, the epidemiological method cannot cope with the complexity of the HIV phenomenon on its own. Therefore, there is a need for HIV to be studied by different disciplines in order to address the complexity of the problem. For instance, the positivist method involves the limitation of not being able to grasp the qualitative aspects of health and disease. Thus, neither the subjective aspects of the disease nor the cultural factors influencing the HIV epidemic are present in epidemiological studies. In this sense, there is a need to generate qualitative information to help guide the design of prevention policies, particularly in regions heavily affected by the epidemic, such as African countries.

Social sciences provide a wide range of research theories and methodologies that can be extremely useful for studying HIV in general and in particular, its prevention and treatment. The sociological discipline, insofar as it seeks to explain and understand collective behaviour within a social context, the meanings of actions and the multicausality of phenomena, constitutes an essential tool in the construction of knowledge for an in-depth understanding of the HIV pandemic. Therefore, sociological theories constitute fruitful ground for investigating health and disease within the current context, as will be discussed throughout this chapter.

Health sociology, as a discipline, is a pertinent tool for the study of HIV. One of the reasons for the emergence of this discipline is the crisis of medicine, not as a science, but as a model of social practice [12]. One of the basic premises on which sociology is based is the need to focus on the analysis of health and not of disease, as opposed to the biomedical model that has primarily focused on disease. Such a fundamental purpose is in accordance with the need for placing greater emphasis on HIV prevention rather than treatment, in order to eradicate the pandemic. Therefore, assumptions that involve focusing on health from a sociological perspective constitute basic assumptions for prevention when applied to the field of HIV [13]:

- Preventative action holds keeping people healthy as a central objective and is based on actively guiding willingness and ability, considering health as a process and not as a state; emphasizing the dynamic role of the subject as a pole of active reciprocity in respect of medical and health care institutions and roles.
- To expect a permanent engagement with lifestyle changes focused on health, not only on behalf of the individual, but also on behalf of the social and health care system; planning and programming to prevent the disease both at an individual and collective level.
- To expect health to be promoted and safeguarded by all social actors, firstly, by all individuals, and in all cases, not wholly delegated to specific specialized places and centres.

Below, Table 3 shows some aspects that are likely to be investigated from a sociological perspective:

As will be discussed below, the different theoretical contributions of sociology will enable public health to approach health issues from a wider perspective, providing pertinent tools

http://dx.doi.org/10.5772/60929

HIV objective issues	Theories and approaches
Perceptions and social representations of HIV	Phenomenology
Reasons for non- adherence to antiretroviral therapy	Ethnomethodology
Professional-patient relationships	Symbolic interactionism
Itineraries and satisfaction with HIV care	Phenomenology
Reasons for the adoption of preventive practices	Ethnomethodology
Stigma and HIV	Symbolic interactionism

Table 3. HIV objectives and sociological theories

for designing effective action in the fight against HIV. Additionally, sociology provides a multidimensional perspective for the study of behaviour towards HIV, the social roles that are played in professional-patient interaction, as well as the role of health care institutions and the social networks that influence the prevention of HIV. Finally, theoretical contributions of sociology are also relevant for designing and implementing health promotion programmes in relation to HIV.

4. Sociological approach to HIV research

Among the multiple sociological theories that offer a suitable approach for the study of HIV prevention, three relevant theories will be outlined: symbolic interactionism theory, ethnomethodology and phenomenological sociology. All of these are essential analytical tools for further exploring the above-mentioned aspects.

4.1. Symbolic interactionism theory

This theory focuses on explaining how people create their own identity and define themselves through their social experiences, that is, through their interaction with other people. Society is understood as a result of everyday, face-to-face, interaction among people. Through this interaction, people define and give meaning to the social world in which they live [14].

Symbolic interactionism is based on multiple premises. The most relevant and useful scenarios [15] for the study of HIV are: 1. Human beings react in one way or another depending on their perception of the object, person or situation they face, that is, the meaning they prescribe to a situation. 2. The individual (subject) adopts an active role in creating meanings. 3. Things do not have an inherent meaning; the meaning of things arises or emerges as a consequence of the social interaction established between people. 4. Meanings are handled in and modified through an interpretative process carried out by the person. 5. Common meanings make communication between human beings possible.

In summary, according to this theory, social reality is symbolically created during the course of social interaction and is therefore subject to change. Human behaviour is social and is based on communication; therefore, people create and interpret social situations and their meanings during this communicative process. It is during the course of social interaction that objects gain meaning for the person or persons. These social meanings are created and modified during the dialogue of social interation.

Thus, the symbolic interactionist perspective is especially useful in the construction of behaviour, as it gives a primary role to the concept of the interaction that occurs between the members of a social group. Furthermore, "human beings interpret or define the actions of others, without being limited to simply reacting to them. Their response is not directly elaborated as a consequence of the actions of others, but is based on the meaning they give to such actions" [15]. Therefore, in relation to health and disease, and the prevention of HIV, this theory constitutes an important theoretical perspective for studying and explaining the social conduct of people and groups of people who interact with each other on the basis of sharing symbolic meanings. In the field study of HIV, symbolic interaction theory has been extensively applied [16]. This theory is useful for studying the stigma that exists among people living with HIV. Recently, it has been published a meta-analysis about ART non-adherence. The results of the study suggest that the existence of stigma is a factor of non-adherence [17]. This systematic review identified 34 studies that applied this theory. These studies indicated existing intrapersonal, interpersonal and structural barriers as a result of stigma as factors of non-adherence [17].

The process of social interaction constitutes a fundamental aspect in the study of the doctor-patient relationship. Since communication does not have a unidirectional character, the emission and reception of messages does not occur in a passive way. Such constant feedback creates a process that influences the way in which the disease and the person's subjective experience are created. This theory has been used to study the relationship between people infected with HIV and health professionals [18]. Recently, an interesting study conducted in Spanish health services analysed the relationship between people living with HIV and physicians as it concerns interventions developed within the areas of sexuality and safe sex [19].

Hence, symbolic interaction allows for a broader view of the approach to doctor-patient interaction, because it enables an understanding of the processes of social interaction that take place during the course of the relationship (doctor-patient). Subsequently, it also allows for an analysis of the role of the patient and health professionals in their encounters throughout the disease process. Furthermore, the communicative process that is established motivates the participation of other people, the family and the community. Therefore, the meanings and the subjective experiences of HIV-positive people are created during the social interaction process, not only with health professionals, but also with other individuals and groups with whom the HIV-positive person interact in normal everyday life. In this sense, studying doctor-patient interaction is useful for identifying the potential cultural barriers that can arise from this interaction. For instance, Spain recently conducted a research study, the objective of which was to understand and analyse the experience of immigrant HIV-positive women with health professionals and treatment services [20].

The fundamental contribution of symbolic interaction to the field of social cognition is the consideration that mental processes are the product of symbolic interaction and not of internal individual processes [21]. Emotions are an example of mental processes that have been studied from a symbolic interaction approach, given that they are expressed in response to social relationships or situations, or both. Human interaction possibly plays the most important role in the activation and expression of emotions [14]. Thus, emotions are biological responses to social situations and the interaction between the people involved in such situations. From this perspective, health and disease are understood as human constructions perceived in a subjective manner by the population. It entails analysing peoples' everyday views of disease, the ideological connotations that health professionals attach to diseases, and the construction and application of medical knowledge [22]. Altogether, according to this theory, it is possible to analyse aspects that are relevant for the study of the HIV phenomenon, such as the different constructions created by people in their interaction with others, the meanings, perceptions, life experiences, beliefs, values in relation to HIV, guilt feelings for being HIV-positive, stigma, risk perception, as well as reasons for abandoning treatment.

4.2. Phenomenological sociology

The focus of analysing this theory is how meanings are created in the individual's consciousness. In other words, how life experiences influence and form part of the interrelationships established between two or more actors in everyday life and how these meanings can be revealed to an observer [23]. In the field of HIV research, this theory has been applied for studying the social about of the virus. The study of social representations of HIV has been extremely relevant to understanding the perceptions and meanings attached to the disease by the general population [24].

A series of key notions that summarize the author's thoughts and that constitute analytic tools for the study of the HIV phenomenon are described below:

- **Lifeworld (lebenswelt):** the lifeworld concept is an essential category for understanding the reality of the world of common-sense, as well as the reality of social action and interaction [25]. It refers to the intersubjective social world inhabited by the actor in daily life by applying a "natural attitude". This lifeworld is characterized as being an intersubjective and public world for the individual, and hence shared by and accessible to everyone. One of its main defining characteristics is that it is a pre-existing world. It is an intersubjective world that exists before being born and is given to the individual to experiment with and to interpret. In essence, it constitutes the horizon that embraces all possible ways of living and experiencing (where the fulfilment of humans in their human condition takes place) and of constructing a social life, transcending the vital experience of a particular actor. In the field of HIV research, this theory has been applied to the study and understanding of the different perceptions and meanings of the virus, as well as its influence on how people live and experience the disease [26].

- **Intersubjectivity:** this concept is essential for assimilating the mutual understanding that occurs between people during their interaction. It is defined by Alfred Schutz [27] as "simultaneity... for it means that I grasp the subjectivity of the alter ego at the same time as I live in my own stream of consciousness... and this grasp [of] simultaneity of the other as well as his reciprocal grasp of me, makes possible 'our' being in the world together". The foundation of this concept is based on the social world, on the lifeworld; therefore, it is an intersubjective world, not a private world, one that is common to all. However, the intersubjective world is not only composed of subjective sensitivities, that is, what is received by the senses, but also of subjects' interpretations of those sensations. Therefore, it is based on how the subject interprets his/her surrounding world, as well as on the elements that condition this surrounding world and that make it possible to change or maintain the subject's interpretations and actions.

- **Typifications and recipes:** in the social world or lifeworld, people have a store of knowledge. A great part of this knowledge comprises what are known as "typifications" and "recipes". Typifications are schemes of reference, "knowledge that the world we live in is a world of more or less well circumscribed objects with more or less definite qualities, objects among which we move, which resist us and upon which we may act" [27]. Typifications exist in society; they are socially approved and are acquired through the socialization process and throughout the course of life. In contrast, recipes concern the knowledge used to understand or control aspects of experience, in other words, aspects that are related to situations and actions in the lifeworld, whereas typifications refer to the knowledge used to understand people or objects.

- **Meanings and motives:** action constitutes a human conduct consciously projected by the actor; hence, social action is that which involves the attitudes and actions of others, and is aimed at them during the course of the action. Meanings refer to the way in which actors determine what aspects of the social world are important to them, whereas motives attempt to reveal the reasons that explain the actions of the actors.

- **Roles:** defined as the typifications of what actors are expected to do in certain social situations. In the field of HIV research, the study of gender roles, both male and female, has been used to understand the reasons for why people maintain unsafe HIV behaviours [28-30].

- **Reification:** this concept is an analytical tool used by the authors from an integral perspective of the social world. Reification is the tendency to perceive human products "as if they were something other than human products – such as facts of nature, results of cosmic laws, or manifestations of divine will" [27].

- **Legitimizations:** these centre on the knowledge of reality in order to legitimize their existence.

In short, phenomenological sociology constitutes an important conceptual tool for approaching the study of HIV. This is the case because it is a theoretical perspective that permits for capturing the subjective meanings that people attach to their actions; additionally, it serves to describe and understand interpretations of meanings within the world, as well as for gaining a sense of the actions and interactions of people who are HIV-positive.

4.3. Ethnomethodology

The primary objective of this theory is to analyse the individual's actions in daily life. Thus, it analyses how people define and construct, face-to-face (through interaction), each social situation. The traits that constitute social order are products of the activity itself. This order is "produced by the participants" and essentially carried out by means of verbalization [31]. Therefore, the study of language (the decoding of cultural meanings) acquires great importance. The study of social representations of HIV has been very relevant for understanding the perceptions and meanings related to HIV among the general population. For instance, a study recently conducted in South Africa analysed the discourse on risk perception that adolescents have in order to assess whether the contents of HIV prevention campaigns were suitable [32].

For an ethnomethodology, social reality is above all a reflexive and interactive activity that is socially constructed. According to this theoretical model, human society is the result of repeated interpretations that occur during the course of interaction. Ethnomethodologists' concern is that which Weber calls "significant behaviour" [21]. In order to understand this theoretical approach and its relevance for the study of the HIV phenomenon, it is necessary to know how it views social reality, the most significant premises in this context being the following five situations [33]:

1. Everybody, through our thoughts and actions, is immersed in a process of creating social reality. It is a process of which we are not aware.

2. The social construction of reality is constantly happening.

3. In their daily lives, people organize the world in coherent realities and this social reality depends on the participants' incessant reciprocal interaction and social construction of reality.

4. Given that this interactive and reflexive work constitutes reality, such a reality cannot be sustained without it. Therefore, each social reality is not a solid structure, but a very fragile creation that can break.

5. People live in diverse social worlds and they may move from one reality to another. Thus, behaviour that might be considered reprehensible in a certain social context may be acceptable in a different one.

Authors such as Caballero (1991) have described and analysed some basic concepts developed by ethnomethodologists, which constitute highly useful analytical tools for understanding and studying the HIV phenomenon [34], namely:

- **Explanations:** by means of the explanation process, people make sense of the world [35]. Explanations are used by actors to do things such as describing, analysing, criticizing and idealizing specific situations [36]. As such, this theory has been applied for identifying the reasons why people living with HIV leave treatment services [37]. Additionally, this theory has been applied for identifying the reasons why certain preventive practices, such as making an early diagnosis, are not acquired by certain populations [38-40].

- **Reflexive action and interaction:** the concept of reflexivity refers to how people who are interacting maintain the presumption that they are guided by a certain reality. In other words, humans interpret signals, words, gestures and information provided by other humans in a way that supports a certain view of reality. Even contradictory evidence is reflexively interpreted to maintain beliefs and knowledge.
- **Indexicality:** this term refers to phrases in which meaning varies depending on the context. It is therefore considered that all explanations must be interpreted within their specific context.

5. Research methodologies for studying the HIV pandemic

The sociological theories described in the previous section allow for investigating the phenomenon of HIV from its essential premise: HIV is a complex and dynamic social phenomenon that acquires different meanings depending on the social and cultural context of each society. These meanings, representations, perceptions, beliefs, values and life experiences will give meaning to and guide the behaviour and actions of people in relation to HIV. Furthermore, these different values and meanings influence the preventive practices that people adopt against HIV. Therefore, it is evidenced that there are qualitative aspects to the HIV phenomenon that also need to be known in order to prevent and eradicate the pandemic [10]. For this reason, most of the interventions being carried out in this field take the social dimension of HIV into consideration.

Therefore, sociological theories described in the previous section allow for grasping the qualitative aspects of HIV. However, the study of HIV using these sociological theories can only be developed from qualitative research strategies. In the scientific arena, the discipline that has traditionally investigated HIV has, however, been clinical epidemiology. For this reason, the research found in scientific literature is mostly prevalence and/or ecological studies. Consequently, in overall terms, there is a predominance of knowledge based on data that mainly describes how the epidemic is distributed among the population, depending on certain factors [10]. Furthermore, the qualitative factors that define the phenomenon of the HIV epidemic have evidenced the need for developing research methodologies that enable the study of the epidemic, transcending the simple observation of how it is quantitatively distributed within a certain population [10].

Using a qualitative methodology allows us to understand and comprehend the phenomenology of HIV from the perspective of the actors, as it focuses the way people interpret and give meaning to their experiences and the world in which they live. It approaches social reality from a holistic perspective, trying to explain, describe and understand people's discourses on a particular social phenomenon [41]. In brief, seeking the meaning of phenomena is the main function of "the so-called qualitative" [42].

A qualitative methodology is equipped with multiple data collection or production procedures that share common aspects, such as the understanding of social phenomena [43] or the centrality of discursive practices and discourse analysis [44]. However, each data collection method offers a particular type of information. Multiple procedures exist for collecting qualitative data. Some of the most representative techniques of the qualitative social research methodology perspective, which can be very useful for approaching the HIV phenomenon, are the following: qualitative interview, focus group, life history and participant observation. It is worth noting that, like the rest of the techniques for collecting and analyzing information on research, these techniques ensure the confidentiality and privacy of the respondents to the extent that the information is treated anonymously and not personalized. Such techniques are usually applied in cross-sectional studies.

5.1. The qualitative interview

The origin of qualitative interviews may be traced through the fields of anthropology, sociology, psychology and journalism. In the 19th and early 20th centuries, this approach began to be consciously applied in social research [45]. It is important to distinguish between the social research interview – in its different formats – and other types of interviews, such as those carried out by health professionals during the course of their duties. Although there are multiple differences, their objective – that is, the purpose of the social research interview – may be highlighted thus: "the research interview intends to construct [a] social sense of the individual's behaviour or of the behaviour of the individual's reference group, by gathering a set of personal data" [46].

Presenting a single concept of the qualitative interview is complicated, because both the conceptualization and the practice of the interview are determined by the different paradigmatic perspectives and positions adopted in relation to qualitative research. Therefore, the diversity of interview styles and manners is fairly heterogeneous. This heterogeneity causes some authors to talk about qualitative "interview families", as in the case of Herbert J. Rubin and Irene S. Rubin [47], who include in this category interviews that have a *semistructured* format (in reference to the focalized interviews of Merton and collaborators) and those that are *unstructured* (referring to the works of Douglas [45]. They also define a *combined modality,* present in many qualitative interviews, where there are "parts that are more structured and others that are less structured, however the balance between them varies" [45]. The different styles and forms of interviews determine if they are more or less structured. There is not only one way of interviewing a person; nonetheless, depending on the higher or lower level of flexibility of the guide, interviews will be more or less structured. They can thus be classified in the following way:

- **Structured interviews:** consist of providing structured questionnaires in which both the sequence and the formulation of the questions are predetermined.
- **Semistructured interviews:** as with the previous type, the questions are previously defined in an interview guide but their sequence, as well as their formulation, may vary depending on each interviewee. In other words, the researcher asks a series of questions (generally open at the beginning of the interview) that define the area of research, but he/she has the freedom to pursue ideas that might be relevant by asking new questions.

- **In-depth interviews:** also termed "open-ended interviews". These generally cover only one or two themes, but in greater depth. The rest of the questions that the researcher asks emerge gradually from the answers of the interviewee and focus fundamentally on the clarification of details, with the aim of delving deeper into the theme being studied.

In this sense and from a phenomenological perspective, supported by authors such as Taylor and Bogdan [43], the in-depth interview must be understood as "repeated face-to-face encounters between the researcher and informants directed toward understanding informants' perspectives on their lives, experiences or situations as expressed in their own words". According to these authors, in-depth interviews are appropriate in the following situations:

1. Where there is a wish to study events from the past, or it is not possible to have access to a particular type of setting and subsequently the settings, or the people, are not accessible in any other way.

2. The research depends on data from a wide range of people or settings.

3. When there are time constraints on research in comparison with other techniques, such as participant observation. Interviews permit for the more efficient use of time.

4. The researcher wishes to focus on the subjective human experience.

The qualitative interview is adequate for approaching people's experiences. It is a tool with a communicative character that attempts to capture the meanings mediated by the constructions that subjects build on the basis of their experience. Thus, in the case of HIV-positive people, as in the case of other social phenomena "contrasted with disease, which is a concept of biology –more specifically, of pathology– illness is a phenomenon which is apparent to the *individual* in terms of an altered state of perception of self" [41]. Therefore, the assessment carried out by a doctor is objective, differing from the subjective perspective of the ill person, because he/she is the one whose life is affected by HIV. For this reason, through the discourse that results from the interview, knowledge is generated about the life experiences, feelings, thoughts and perceptions of people that are HIV-positive. In addition, the meanings, norms and values created by people are binding on the members of a group, because they generate and condition people's behaviour. This is why the qualitative interview can help to explain the behaviour people demonstrate towards HIV and its treatments.

The qualitative interview is very useful in the field of studying the HIV phenomenon "when the hypothesis is a conflict between norms. On the one hand, there are norms which are dominant, referential, usually reproduced in discourses because they conform to what has been legitimated, what has to be said. On the other hand, there are norms in practice, reproduced in practice" [41], i.e., what is really done. Therefore, the relevance of its use in the prevention of HIV results from the knowledge provided when there is a divergence, or conflict, between social norms. For example, health professionals and the population in general point out the non-existence of stigma and discrimination of HIV-positive people in their discourses. However, they may be carrying out practices that lead to the stigmatization and discrimination against people affected by HIV. Furthermore, HIV-positive people may be acting in a way different to that which would normally be expected and might not be adopting preventive

http://dx.doi.org/10.5772/60929

practices recommended by health services (legitimated discourse). For this reason, patients make evaluations on the basis of their own direct experience. In this sense, communicating to the ill person what he or she should do facing the illness in general and in particular towards its prevention is complex, because the patient is the one who is emotionally involved in a way that no else is. Therefore, the patient evaluates their condition based in their own experience. This self-evaluation is key to overcoming the illness, important in the adaption process to the illnessand in the preventive practices put in place. Consequently, the interview technique is highly relevant for identifying "above all, what is really done, or what is really thought, as the expression of following norms which deviate from the general norm" [41].

One advantage often emphasized when applying this qualitative technique is its suitability for ensuring the confidentiality of the serostatus interviewee, as opposed to other group qualitative techniques. Another advantage, because of the atmosphere of trust and privacy created between the interviewer and the interviewee, is the degree of freedom that respondents reach when responding to questions, which leads to expressing in confidence their experiences and opinions about HIV. On the other hand, a limitation that has been noted of this approach is that to achieve a degree of saturation sampling, a larger number of interviews must be conducted as opposed to other group qualitative techniques, resulting in research that is costly both in terms of time and financial budget.

5.2. Focus group

Research studies in the health care field primarily use focus groups and to a lesser extent, discussion groups. The focus group, also called the "group interview" [49], tends to be considered as "One specific technique within the broader category of group interviewing to collect qualitative data. The hallmark of focus groups is the explicit use of group interaction to produce data and insights that would be less accessible without the interaction found in a group" [50].

The focus group is a technique that initially emerged in North American sociology as an extension of the focalized interview; coherently, its model is inquiry via questionnaire. The group modality reveals more nuances and more diverse responses than the individual interview, but always in a context of strong directivity in which a progressive logic prevails (step 1, step 2, etc., of the questionnaire). The group is constantly kept dependent on the moderator, who promotes the contrast between individuals rather than a group dynamic [49]. In this methodological practice, there is always a guide containing questions related to the research objective. The questions are aimed at the people who participate in the group, to be answered by the group. The researchers prefix the questions in the guide.

In its most extreme form, the focus group is a directive technique, because discussion among participants is non-existent if they simply respond to the moderator's questions one by one. However, in its more open form, there is the possibility of debate around explicit positions, in which the conversation is limited only to registering stated opinions [49]. It is also a structured technique, which uses the reflections of a group of people to reveal in-depth information on the theme being studied. It essentially consists of moderating a debate between a group of people who share certain experiences (possibly HIV), sociodemographic characteristics (age, socioeconomic level, etc.), with the objective of discussing and reflecting on the different viewpoints of the theme. Creating a permissive ambiance is a key element for the discussion of these different points of view [49].

Quite often, focus groups and discussion groups are confused with one another. Although they have similarities, they also exhibit multiple differences. One difference worth highlighting is that the discussion group is designed to investigate the common areas of a group of people who, when placed in a discursive situation (conversation), tend to represent discourses that are more or less typical of the social groups to which they belong. However, in the group interview, a personal point of view prevails; hence, people listen as a group but answer as single interviewees [51]. The focus group is therefore a very useful qualitative technique for designing and assessing programmes and services. For example, for assessing user needs and satisfaction, identifying obstacles for implementation, developing educational materials, or assessing the quality of services. It is also useful for researching a certain phenomenon of interest, as in the case of HIV, especially when the aim is to understand attitudes and perceptions towards risk and behaviour, or to analyse cultural beliefs and values. Finally, the focus group is useful for the development of adequate measuring instruments aimed at the target population [52].

The focus group can be used as a research and assessment method, or as a complementary measure to other qualitative and quantitative methods, and is recommended when the objective is to learn about participants' experiences and perspectives. It is highly useful for studying what participants think of the group, but is especially valuable for finding out *why* they think the way they do [53]. Through this methodological practice, we may analyse the discourses produced by a group. This is useful for identifying user needs and satisfaction, and knowing the different points of view of key people regarding a theme as conflicting as the HIV phenomenon.

An advantage of this type of group technique is the fact that it allows for obtaining a large degree of information, as it reaches its saturation sampling level with fewer groups needing to be conducted. However, it has the disadvantage –as it happens in the case of the confidentiality of HIV serostatus– that it does not preserve discretion in front of the various components of the group.

5.3. Life history

Different social research techniques are included under the heading "biographic documents" (biographies, autobiographies, diaries, letters, life histories, etc.). Although these share common assumptions, their application is very different. The choice of one over another will depend on each approach's adequacy concerning the research objective. Among biographic documents, life history has been consolidated as one of the most efficient sources for obtaining data.

The aim of the life history is to collect a person's overall life history. The person involved is considered a key informant. Due to its scope, the life history is collected over an extended period of time. It tends to be exhaustive, using other testimonies or documents to corroborate or complete data. This technique is used when an exceptionally rich biographic narrative is available and the narrative corresponds to an extremely singular subject [54]. According to Sarabia, the term, "life histories" describes both stories of an entire lifetime and partial narratives related to certain life stages or biographic moments. Furthermore, it is worth noting that the term refers not only to the narrative, but also to all information gathered about the life under study (information from school stages, health care sources, etc.) and, obviously, to the analyses carried out by the researcher or researchers [55].

The use of life history as a research technique presents both advantages and limitations. According to Valles [45], some of the primary advantages that are worth noting are:

1. The retrospective and longitudinal character of the gathered data provides in-depth knowledge on the chronology, contexts of emergence and the development of social interaction, as well as the individual's points of view.

2. Having to conduct several interviews for each case or cases being studied elicits greater robustness and quality of data.

3. The biographic method, particularly the life history, has been recognized for its great capacity to implement the articulation of methods and techniques (methodological triangulation).

4. Emphasis on the objectives of the social experience as opposed to the objectivism of the experiment; the survey and systematic observation.

Similar to the individual interview, this qualitative data collection technique can prove to be extremely appropriate, due to the privacy guaranteed to individuals, which requires preserving confidentiality and anonymity, as is the case when involving HIV-positive people.

5.4. Observation

Observation is a common activity in everyday life. This type of common and generalized observation can be transformed into a powerful social research tool, and a scientific technique for data collection, when applied in the following ways:

1. Aiming and focusing observation at a particular and previously formulated research object.

2. Systematically planning the phases, aspects, settings and people to be observed.

3. Controlling and relating observation to social propositions and theories.

4. Subjecting observation to veracity, objectivity, reliability and precision controls [43].

Participant observation may be considered the prime example for illustrating that qualitative research methods are more akin to practices than techniques [42]. There are multiple definitions of participant observation. According to Taylor and Bogdan [43], the expression "participant observation" is used to define research that involves the social interaction between the researcher and the informants within the informants' context, a process during which data collection is conducted in a systematic and non-intrusive manner. Marshall and Rossman [56] define it as "The systematic description of events, behaviours and artefacts in the social setting chosen for study" [56]. It therefore involves observing the context by means of integrating the researcher into the everyday life of the observed group, in a manner that is neither unstructured nor covert. Participant observation provides not only descriptions of people, events and interactions that occur between people, but also of the experience, life experiences and sensations of the researcher [44].

The primary use of participant observation is to be found in the study of that which falls relatively outside the norm: that which is still not understood, is incipient, relates to other cultures, half-hidden or clandestine groups, as well as that which tends to be confined to institutions (whole institutions, work centres, laboratories, etc.). In other words, in those places where what is normal is bracketed and where it is understood that things are socially different to what is considered either normal, or to what appears in the institutions' formal discourses [42]. Consequently, participant observation is especially useful for in-depth studies of the everyday life of organizations, institutions and social groups that occupy a peripheral space within society. In the area of health care, this means using it to study the everyday and organizational lives of health centres, specific professional associations, hospital wards, etc. [42]. Participant observation is adequate when seeking to reveal the practical rules of a community, group, organization or institution.

Participant observation is defined by the interaction between the observer and the observed, within the context of the observed, and therefore involves the importance of the community setting that is to be observed. Choosing the settings to be observed is of the utmost importance for the research, as not all settings allow for the presence of an observer, nor are they susceptible to being observed. The particular research determines the selection of the setting and the scenario that will be observed, and not the other way around [43].

Therefore, participant observation reveals the practical rules of people affected by HIV when in a group, of the associations of HIV-positive people, of health service organizations and of the exact representation of a given culture, among others. Furthermore, as well as bringing forth participants' discourses that are embedded in everyday practices, it enables the identification of discrepancies between discourse and behaviour. For instance, HIV-positive people undergoing antiretroviral treatment may say that they are following treatment when in fact, it is observed that treatment dropouts are frequent. Therefore, knowing the practical rules that condition the behaviour of people towards HIV is highly important for the development of intervention programmes aimed at the prevention of HIV. These programmes need to be adapted to the social and cultural rules that prevail in the different social and cultural contexts of the societies in which interventions will be undertaken.

6. Conclusions

As discussed above, HIV is a complex phenomenon in which many aspects (social, cultural, etc.), not only clinical and biological, are interrelated. Intervening factors in the HIV phenomenon include social, economic, political, cultural and environmental aspects. The HIV phenomenon interacts with lifestyles and practices, as well as with the subjectivities of the population in communities where it develops and spreads. Therefore, it is currently a fact that the epidemiological method is insufficient for providing holistic and hermeneutic knowledge on the issue. For this reason, a primary conclusion of this study is the need for applying other methodologies and theoretical tools to study the phenomenon with the aim of providing such knowledge. Furthermore, this knowledge is a key element for assuring efficient and effective HIV prevention policies and strategic planning. In this sense, sociology and in particular health sociology constitutes a pertinent conceptual and methodological tool for studying the HIV phenomenon in all its complexity. In this sense, it seeks to explain and understand the collective behaviour that occurs in a social context, the meanings of actions and the multicausality of phenomena.

The theories that have previously been explained are relevant methodological and theoretical tools for comprehending the complexity that defines HIV. Though these instruments differ, they do have certain common characteristics that should be taken into consideration. A common premise is: conceiving human action in terms of its intentionality, autonomy and reflexivity. All these characteristics share a subjective view of human behaviour, because they define its discourses. Consequently, the relevance and contribution of these theories to the study of health and disease, and specifically to the study of HIV, is now a fact. The advantages of this are multiple:

- Enabling the understanding of the health-disease-attention process and ultimately, the behaviour that results from the interaction between those involved in this process, as well as offering coherence to these conducts. In this sense, it reveals conducts towards both the diagnosis and the treatment of HIV.

- Knowing and understanding how individuals and groups participate in the construction of social representations of HIV.

- Knowing and analysing the social control mechanisms that arise in relation to people with HIV, such as stereotypes, prejudices, stigma and discrimination.

- Analysing the different meanings that exist in the construction of the HIV phenomenon; a construction that is built on perceptions, life experiences, images, ideas, representations and social control mechanisms. These meanings enable us to understand how people relate their way of thinking to their way of acting towards HIV.

These theories are relevant and pertinent for obtaining useful knowledge to guide the design of effective and efficient health promotion policies and strategies, specifically for the prevention of HIV, as they focus on the problem of how actors in different contexts create a view of reality. Finally, a series of methodological tools were discussed whose validity and pertinence for the study of HIV are currently beyond any doubt. This has been evidenced by multiple studies in the field of HIV prevention, which have been conducted using this qualitative methodology.

Acknowledgements

To Néstor Hernández Jurado and Ricardo García Castañeda for their collaboration in the translation of the manuscript. To the Institute of Health Carlos III, Spanish Research Network of Tropical Diseases (RICET; RD06/0021/0000), Ministry of Science and Innovation of Spain.

Author details

Carmen Rodríguez Reinado[1*] and Teresa Blasco Hernández[1,2]

*Address all correspondence to: carmenrr1974@yahoo.es

1 National Centre for Tropical Medicine, Health Institute Carlos III, Spain

2 Networks Collaborative Research Subdivision- ISCII, Spain

References

[1] Marchiori P. Globalization, Poverty and Health. Conference Hugh Rodman Leavel Health Collective, Buenos Aires, 2006; 3: 281-297.

[2] Valero M, Tanner M. Globalization and health: The case of tropical and neglected diseases. Rev MVZ 2008;13(1): 1252-1264.

[3] McMichael MB. Globalization, Climate Change, and Human Health. The New England Journal of Medicine 2013; 368: 1335-14.

[4] Vargas F. Health protection against new environmental risks. Rev. Environmental Health 2001; 1: 4-5.

[5] World Health Organization. A safer future. Global Public Health Security in the 21st Century. The World Health Report 2007. Geneva: World Health Organization; 2007.

[6] Guillén M. Is globalization civilizing, destructive or feeble? A critique of five key debates in the social science literature. Annual Review of Sociology 2001; 27: 235-260.

[7] Blasco T., (editor). Social dimensions of tuberculosis in immigrant population of the Community of Madrid: a qualitative study. Madrid: Teseo; 2011.

[8] United Nations Organization. Report on the global AIDS epidemic Joint program of the United Nations Geneva: United Nations; 2013.

[9] United Nations Organization. Impact of AIDS. New York: United Nations; 2004.

[10] Rodríguez C, Blasco T, Vargas A, Benito A. The Pertinence of Applying Qualitative Investigation Strategies in the Design and Evaluation of HIV Prevention Policies. In:

Yi-Wei Tang (ed.) Recent Translational Research in HIV/AIDS. USA: Intech; 2011.p550-567.

[11] Gómez C. The Millennium Development Goals and decentralized cooperation. Rev Papers 2007; 83: 1557- 1587.

[12] Baum F. Public health research: the debate on quantitative and qualitative methodologies. Reviews of Public Health 1997; 5: 175-193.

[13] Donati P., (editor). Sociology of health. Madrid: Díaz de Santos; 1994.

[14] Cockerham WC., (editor). Sociology of medicine. Madrid: Prentice Hall; 2002.

[15] Blumer H., (editor). Symbolic interactionism: perspective and method. Barcelona: Time D.L.; 1982

[16] Klunklin A, Greenwood J. Symbolic interactionism in grounded theory studies: women surviving with HIV/AIDS in rural northern Thailand. J Assoc Nurses AIDS Care 2008; 17 (5): 32-41.

[17] Katz IT, Ryu AE, Onuegbu AG, Psaros C, Weiser SD, Bangsberg DR, Tsai AC. Impact of HIV-related stigma on treatment adherence: systematic review and meta-synthesis. J Int AIDS Soc 2013; 13 (16): 18640.

[18] Porto TS, Silva CM, Vargens OM. Caring for women with HIV/AIDS: an interactionist analysis from the perspective of female healthcare professionals. Rev Gaucha Enferm 2014; 35 (2): 40-6.

[19] Villaamil F. Shared embarrassment: (not) talking about sex in HIV-related doctor-patient encounters. Med Antr Anthropol 2014; 33(4): 335-50.

[20] Guionnet A, Navaza B, Pizarro de la Fuente B, Pérez-Elías MJ, Dronda F, López-Vélez R, Pérez-Molina JA. Immigrant women living with HIV in Spain: a qualitative approach to encourage medical follow-up. BMC Public Health 2014; 14(1): 1115.

[21] Álvaro JL., (editor). Social Psychology: Theoretical and methodological perspectives. Madrid: Siglo XXI; 1995.

[22] Bleda JM. Social determinants of health and disease. Barataria 2005; 7: 149-160.

[23] Schütz A, Walhs G., (eds). Phenomenology of the social world. Comprehensive Introduction to Sociology. Barcelona: Polity Press; 1972.

[24] Brijnath B. It's about TIME: engendering AIDS in Africa. Cult Health Sex 2007; 9 (4): 371-86.

[25] Salas R. The world of life and the sociological phenomenology of Schutz notes for a philosophy of experience. Journal of Philosophy 2008; 15: 167-20.

[26] Colombini M, Mutemwa R, Kivunaga J, Stackpool L, Mayhew SH. Integra Initiative. Experiences of stigma among women living with HIV attending sexual and repro-

ductive health services in Kenya: a qualitative study. BMC Health Serv Res 2014; 20 (1): 412.

[27] Schütz A., (editor). The meaningful construction of the social world. Comprehensive Introduction to Sociology. Cambridge: Polity Press; 1993.

[28] Sherman SG, Footer K, Illangasekare S, Clark E, Pearson E, Decker MR. What makes you think you have special privileges because you are a police officer? A qualitative exploration of police's role in the risk environment of female sex workers. AIDS Care 2014; 31: 1-8.

[29] Lesia N, Miller AC, Rigodon J, Joseph JK, Furin J. Addressing gender inequity in HIV care in rural Lesotho: the 'Male Initiative'. Int Health 2013; 5(1): 72-7.

[30] Chikovore J, Hart G, Kumwenda M, Chipungu GA, Desmond N, Corbett L. Control, struggle, and emergent masculinities: a qualitative study of men's care-seeking determinants for chronic cough and tuberculosis symptoms in Blantyre, Malawi. BMC Public Health 2014; 9 (14): 1053.

[31] Schütz A, Luckmann T., (eds).The structures of the life world. London: Routledge; 1973.

[32] Myroniuk TW. Global discourses and experiential speculation: Secondary and tertiary graduate Malawians dissect the HIV/AIDS epidemic. J Int AIDS Soc 2011; 14: 47.

[33] Mehan H. Wood H., (eds). The Reality of Ethnomethodology. N. York: Wiley; 1975.

[34] Caballero JJ. Ethnomethodology: an explanation of the social construction of reality. Reis 1991; 56: 83-114.

[35] Handel W. Ethnomethodology: How People Make Sense. New York: Prentice-Hall; 1982.

[36] Bittner E. Objectivity and Realism in Sociology. In: Phenomenological Sociology: Issues and Applications, George Psathas (ed). N. York: John Wiley; 1973.p123-146.

[37] Tabatabai J, Namakhoma I, Tweya H, Phiri S, Schnitzler P, Neuhann F. Understanding reasons for treatment interruption amongst patients on antiretroviral therapy: a qualitative study at the Lighthouse Clinic, Lilongwe, Malawi. Glob Health Action 2014; 30 (7): 24795.

[38] Yamego W, Kouanda S, Berthé A, Yaya-Bocoum F, Gausset Q, Mogensen HO, Konaté B, Ky-Zerbo O. Why people delay seeking care after a positive HIV test: a qualitative study in Burkina. Med Sante Trop. 2014; 24 (1): 58-62.

[39] Sikweyiya YM, Jewkes R, Dunkle K. Impact of HIV on and the constructions of masculinities among HIV-positive men in South Africa: implications for secondary prevention programs. Glob Health Action 2014; 1 (7): 24631.

[40] Caitlin E, Amy K, Medly M, Sweat M, Reilly, K. Behavioural interventions for HIV prevention in developed countries: a systematic review and meta-analysis. WHO Bulletin 2010; 88: 561-640.

[41] Blasco T, Arribas A, Martin-Crespo, C. Research on socio-health disciplines. Madrid: Foundation for the Development of Nursing; 2012.

[42] Callejo J. Observation, interview and group discussion: silence three research practices. Rev. Esp. Public Health, 2002; 76 (5): 409-422.

[43] Taylor SJ, Bogdan R. Introduction to qualitative research methods. Barcelona: Polity Press; 1987.

[44] Dingwall R. Accounts, Interviews and Observations. In: Miller G, Dingwall. R (eds.) Context & Method in Qualitative Research. London: Sage; 1997.p23-52.

[45] Valles M.S., (editor). Qualitative interviews. Methodological Notebooks. Madrid: Ariel; 2002.

[46] Alonso L.E., (editor). The qualitative approach in Sociology. Madrid: Fundamento; 1994.

[47] Herbert J, Rubin I. Qualitative Interviewing: The Art of Hearing Data. Michigan: Sage; 2011.

[48] Coe RM., (editor). Sociology of medicine. Madrid: Alianza; 1984.

[49] Colectivo IOE. What does the discussion group. A critical review of the use of group techniques in studies of migration? Journal of Social Science Methodology 2010; 19: 73-99. Available in: http://www.colectvoioe.org/uploads/d70e92469ea5d534c31d5b25acaf48ae0c593b25.pdf.

[50] Morgan D.L. Focus groups as qualitative research. London: Sage;1988.

[51] Rodríguez C, Blasco T., (eds). Recommendations for good practice in the implementation cycle of improvement in quality of care. Guide for health professionals. Madrid: National Centre for Tropical Medicine-Health Institute Carlos III; 2013. Available in: http://gesdoc.isciii.es/gesdoccontroller?action=download&id=03/04/2014-52f00fa198.

[52] Canales M. Discussion groups. In: Delgado JM, Gutiérrez J (eds). Methods and qualitative techniques in social science research. Madrid: Síntesis; 1994. p288-311.

[53] García M, Mateo I. The focus group as a qualitative research technique in health. Design and implementation. Rev Primary Care 2010; 25(3): 181-186.

[54] Pujadas JM., (editor). The biographical method: the use of life histories in Social Sciences. Madrid: Center for Sociological Research; 1992.

[55] Sarabia B. Life stories. Spanish Journal of Sociological Research 1987; 29: 165-86.

[56] Marshall C, Rossman G., (eds). Designing qualitative research. Newbury Park, CA: Sage; 1989.

Chapter 3

Vertical Transmission of HIV — Medical Diagnosis, Therapeutic Options and Prevention Strategy

Enrique Valdés Rubio and Rodolfo Guiñez Gahona

Additional information is available at the end of the chapter

http://dx.doi.org/10.5772/61202

1. Introduction

In the eight Millennium Development Goals, the World Health Organization proposed the improvement of HIV/AIDS epidemiological rates worldwide through disease prevention and treatment as a goal to achieve in 2015. Reaching the virtual worldwide eradication of vertical transmission (prevention of mother-to-child transmission [PMTCT]) is among such goals.

This chapter will address topics related mainly to diagnostic and therapeutic aspects that have been proven to be useful in the prevention of HIV vertical transmission (VT). The aim is to provide the reader with a clinical guideline for the management of an HIV(+) pregnant woman based on levels of evidence, grading of recommendation, and experts' opinions and to individualize those healthcare strategies that have demonstrated to be effective in the reduction of HIV vertical transmission. Such achievement will highlight the importance of ordering an HIV test to all pregnant women during prenatal control visit. The latter, in case of carrier status, will help to decrease viral load in HIV(+) mothers to undetectable or almost undetectable levels. It will also enable the formulation of a management strategy based on clinical and laboratory parameters, with the use of the most adequate pharmacological management, thus decreasing exposure of the newborn of an HIV(+) mother, to blood, genital secretions, or amniotic fluid, and to identify the best opportunity to program delivery and termination of breastfeeding.

This Clinical Guideline is intended for midwives, medical students, gynecology and obstetrics fellows/residents, maternal-fetal medicine fellows/residents, obstetricians serving at level 2 and 3 hospitals, and specialists in maternal-fetal medicine, who aim at updating their knowledge on the diagnosis and management of gestations affected by HIV/AIDS.

All the aforementioned will bring insights on why healthcare strategies intended to prevent fetal infection have become a paradigm of perinatal medicine since the application of such biomedical interventions has been proven to be successful in the prevention of HIV transmission from an infected pregnant woman to her child, decreasing risk levels to 2%, as observed in the United States.

2. Developing the guide

The attempt at improving epidemiological rates of HIV/AIDS through the prevention and treatment of the disease is one of the eight Millennium Development Goals proposed by the World Health Organization. Worldwide, the virtual eradication of mother-to-child transmission is one of the goals to be accomplished [1, 2].

The present guide will be developed based on the method proposed by Harbour et al., which in turn is based on the formulation of various questions that will be answered according to levels of evidence, grading of recommendation, and experts' opinions [3].

Vertical transmission (VT) of HIV is defined as that occurring from mother to child during gestation, delivery, or breastfeeding. The VT rates range between 13% and 48%. [4-7]. Preventive strategies have been set out to lower VT rates to less than 2%. Pregnancy, delivery, and breastfeeding are the most susceptible periods for VT of HIV [8, 9]. Maternal viral load (VL) is the main independent risk factor for transmission. Certain sexually transmitted diseases (STD) also increase the risk of VT. Likewise, low maternal CD4 cell counts also constitute a risk factor for VT, which is independent from VL [10].

The prevalence of vertical transmission (VT) in the various regions of the world varies according to geographic site and specifically according to the contribution of economic resources invested by different countries worldwide in the various strategies for healthcare policies, aiming at the prevention and treatment of infected mothers [2].

In countries with low infection prevalence rates such as Chile, efforts have been targeted to the decrease of vertical transmission (VT), which is responsible for 99% of HIV infections among children younger than 13 years old [5, 11].

Mother-to-child transmission as route of exposure has decreased, from rates of approximately 30% in 1996, prior to the first VT prevention protocol (ACTG 076), to 0.7% for HIV and 0.6% for AIDS, during the 2006-2010 period [4, 12-14].

To optimize prevention of VT, the clinical approach to a seropositive pregnant woman must be based on a thorough assessment of her initial health status, with a full physical examination, focusing particularly on those signs that point toward an opportunistic infectious condition and evaluating her current immune status.

The strategy for prevention of VT has been based on the continuous review of the pooled evidence and has followed the impact factor of such evidence to suggest valid recommendations from expert opinions. It is of key importance to further evaluate new behaviors tending to identify, among other aspects: the eventual induction of resistance and toxicity of antivirals both in the pregnant mother as well as in the newborn, and their potential effect on subsequent quality of life, the use of micronutrients and the identification of their impact on VT decrease, and the evaluation of vaginal delivery as an option in pregnant women with a low viral load [2, 14-20].

Once the effectiveness of biomedical patient benefits in VT prevention has been demonstrated, it is important to ensure the collection of epidemiological history in order to generate an adequate means of notification, which constitutes data required for reassessing the design and the effectiveness of preventive programs. To attain such goals, it is key to maintain and improve diagnosis and primary prevention of infection in women in childbearing age. Furthermore, it is important to avoid the high rate of unwanted pregnancies and abortions, which represent indirect indicators of risk behaviors in such population. Likewise, one should aim at reaching 100% of screening during the first trimester, at the possibility of repeating such screening during the third trimester and at training maternity staff in rapid testing for the detection of carrier status during labor for pregnant women not having previously undergone such screening [2].

3. Medical diagnosis

3.1. Early diagnosis

Most women discover their carrier status or disease during pregnancy or after delivery upon the detection of the infection in the newborn. With regard to the latter, and despite the fact that there is no consensus on the recommendation of universal screening to all women upon their pre- and/or postconception visit, the American College of Obstetricians and Gynecologists and the Royal College of Obstetricians and Gynecologists United kingdom recommend performing the test on a routine basis, a behavior commonly adopted in many countries worldwide [21, 22]. In fact, most of such countries have also integrated a mandatory pretest counseling, the need for an informed consent, and the willfulness of people upon deciding to undergo the testing. Thus, sample collection requires the participation of staff trained in "counseling". The latter has reinforced the decision of women to undergo the test and has resulted in a significant rise of adhesion to preventive behaviors and therapy (Uganda and Rwanda) [23, 29, 30].

The recommended test for screening is the fourth-generation ELISA. Such laboratory examination enables the simultaneous detection of Ag p24 and its respective antibodies, and therefore the window period is reduced to approximately 30 days with a sensitivity of 99.9% and a specificity of 99.5%. Despite the latter, it is important to stress that the positive predictive value of such test during pregnancy is approximately 50%, as a result of being applied on a low prevalence population. Thus, a confirmation test is required, and therefore patients with positive ELISA test should undergo a confirmatory test with Western blot. The confirmatory Western blot technique is carried out with a nitrocellulose strip onto which HIV envelope proteins have been added. When patient serum is transferred to the strips, any antibody against the virus present in serum will bind to the respective specific antigen on the strip. Western blot results are interpreted by observing the colored bands that are identified according to their position and particular characteristics. When results are indeterminate, a new sample must be ordered after 3 months to reevaluate eventual positivity [2, 31, 32, 36].

Furthermore, for pregnant patients with unknown serological status that seek healthcare because of labor initiation or medical situations in which pregnancy interruption is imminent, health services should be equipped with rapid diagnostic techniques (visual or instrumental). Despite their nonoptimal specificity and sensitivity, in the event of being positive, such techniques would enable the recommendation of peripartum preventive measures, with prior provision of the informed consent by the patient. Such emergency evaluations may be performed even by individuals lacking a specific training when other human resources are unavailable [33-36].

3.2. HIV detection test requisition among pregnant women: who is eligible?

With regard to the indication of universal HIV testing for women at their preconception consultation and/or at the beginning of their antenatal follow-up visit, the American College of Obstetricians and Gynecologists recommends that it is carried out on a routine basis, as it is the common practice in many countries of the world. In fact, most women are aware of their carrier status during pregnancy or during the puerperium upon screening for neonatal infection. As for the latter, it has been demonstrated that ordering the test together with pre- and posttest counseling improves awareness on the disease, adherence to therapy, and development of behaviors in the carrier to prevent transmission to her individual environment [22-27]. With regard to pre- and postconception counseling, defined as a "confidential conversation between a patient and a counselor that aims at the acquisition by the former of skills to face the stress related to an eventual carrier status, at achieving HIV/AIDS-related decision making during pregnancy, and learning of strategies for the prevention of vertical transmission," it is advisable to address the following topics:

- Information about basic aspects of HIV/AIDS transmission and prevention
- Signature of the informed consent or statement of declination of the test
- Evaluation of the HIV detection test final result, with posttest counseling
- Reinforcement of preventive strategies for HIV and other STD during pregnancy
- Supply of emotional support in the case the result of one or both tests is reactive or positive
- Provision of information on pregnancy control and/or follow-up procedures at the specialties level and consequent referral in cases with reactive or positive test results
- Support to therapy adherence, exams, and periodic follow-up if applicable
- Record of the activity in the pertaining documents

The trend worldwide regarding HIV test ordering has progressed toward mandatory programs. These are more efficient and less harmful than those that are voluntary or the routine programs with implicit but revocable consent. International organizations (WHO/UNAIDS) recommend guidelines regarding avoidance of compulsoriness of HIV testing and prioritization of guidance, education, and advise for its performance [25, 27, 28]. The recommendations/ guidelines should be undertaken regardless of seropositivity prevalence in the population. Such management protocols would enable an adequate control of mother-to-child transmission at the population health level, while protecting mother rights and preventing stigmatization and discrimination. To the WHO, national policies and practices regarding compulsoriness of HIV testing should be reviewed to eliminate any testing that is not voluntary. Mandatory testing or testing under coercion on individuals belonging to vulnerable groups or groups with high risk of infection such as pregnant women should not be performed. Voluntary testing amplification and counseling must include a better protection of risk behavior and seropositivity related stigma and discrimination. Additionally, more support for bonding and connection to prevention, treatment, care, and support services should be provided. Despite the latter and the trends seen in both poor as well as in developed countries, there are some exceptions, such as several states at the United States of America and countries like Chile. In Chile, the HIV/AIDS law has been in force since 2005 but does not accept compulsoriness; however, the 2011 Decree of the Ministry of Health indicates that HIV testing is mandatory for pregnant women [23-27].

It is imperative, therefore, for women at the last trimester or those at due date with unknown serology for HIV antibodies to undergo an urgent HIV screening rapid test. Similarly, counseling must be offered in this case and the corresponding informed consent obtained [23-27]. Should such test be reactive, the vertical transmission prevention protocol should be applied immediately (Level 4 evidence) [19-21, 35, 36].

Based on experts' opinion, HIV testing should be offered to all pregnant women by their second control visit at the latest. Should the result of the test be negative, the latter should be repeated between 32 and 34 weeks of gestation in women under higher risk of acquiring HIV during the first trimester of pregnancy (pathological alcohol consumption, drug addiction, sex workers, multiple sexual partners, etc.), i.e., Grade D recommendation.

3.3. Medical examinations and specialty consultations that should be ordered in HIV(+) pregnant women

Every patient with confirmed serology should be referred to consultation, and immediate coordination should be implemented in order to provide the patient with assessment by a multidisciplinary team (Grade D recommendation).

Routine exams different from those performed on the nonpregnant HIV-positive women are not justified in the pregnant patient with recent positive serology, with the exception of those clinically warranted (Grade D recommendation).

Other STDs should be actively ruled out. Hepatitis B and hepatitis C serology as well as tuberculin skin testing (PPD) should also be performed (Grade D recommendation). Lymphocyte count, viral load, and viral genotyping should be ordered by the immunologist or the infectologist (Grade D recommendation).

The following are listed laboratory tests that should be routinely carried out [2]:

- Rubella serology: both IgG and IgM are evaluated to evidence current or past infection. If there is no evident immunity against rubella, postpartum vaccination is recommended.
- Urine culture: aiming at ruling out an infection of the urinary tract.
- Hepatitis B virus surface antigen: to evaluate the presence of disease, since the transmission mechanism and the risk of vertical transmission are similar, and in the event of a synergic effect in disease progression
- RPR or VDRL: these are nontreponemic tests for syphilis detection. They are highly sensitive but poorly specific. Therefore, if a positive result is obtained, it should be confirmed with a more specific test detecting antibodies against *Treponema pallidum*, such as FTA-ABS (fluorescent treponemal antibody absorption). The presence of such microorganism is associated with increased vertical transmission [9].
- Hepatitis C serology: the purpose of this test is to rule out the carrier status since it is common among HIV-infected patients. It is considered an opportunistic infection and might be patient death cause.
- PPD (purified protein derivative) testing for tuberculosis: to evaluate a tuberculosis diagnosis. In HIV-carrier patients, a cutaneous reaction measuring 5 mm is enough to be considered positive (at least 10 mm should be seen in the remainder of patients). False-positive results may exist, for instance, in patients previously vaccinated with BCG (bacillus Calmette-Guérin). This infectious association should be considered since it worsens patient prognosis.
- *Toxoplasma gondii* serology: to detect the potential opportunistic infection, mainly with encephalic involvement. In a carrier, a latent *T. gondii* infection may be reactivated as a result of a deterioration of cellular immunity in these patients.
- Cytomegalovirus cytology: CMV is the most common viral opportunistic disease in AIDS. It is associated with severe immunosuppression, and the reactivation of a latent disease is its usual form of onset. The disease usually has high mortality rates.
- Gonococcus, chlamydia, mycoplasma, and Ureaplasma cultures: since they share in common their mechanism of transmission, other sexually transmitted infections should be ruled out.

3.4. Immunological parameters

3.4.1. CD4 T-cell count and viral load assessment (PCR)

These are prognostic factors for vertical transmission, and they are determinant factors for the appropriate time to initiate ART. They are also parameters for the assessment of the therapeutic response.

3.4.2. Genotyping

Its evaluation is critical to assess resistance to antiretroviral therapy.

This information indicates that HIV(+) pregnant women should be assessed and treated by a multidisciplinary medical team (Infectologist, immunologist, pharmacist, obstetrician, and neonatologist) (Level 4 evidence) [16-21]. Additionally, as previously mentioned, screening for various STDs found to be related with increased VT is of key importance. Such screening should include herpes simplex virus 2 and *T. pallidum* (Level 2+ evidence [2-9].

4. Pre- and postnatal treatment

4.1. Therapeutic options

In pregnant HIV carriers, the transmission of the infection to the fetus can occur mainly during delivery (65%), but also during pregnancy and breastfeeding with approximate rates of 35% and 15%, respectively. Such risk for transmission increases with certain factors such as maternal primary infection during pregnancy, intercurrent sexually transmitted infections, decreased CD4 counts, and high viral loads (27). In relation with the latter, and despite the fact that viral loads lower than 1000 copies/ml present a significantly lower risk for vertical transmission, there is no viral load exemption from VT risk. Thus, triple-drug highly active antiretroviral therapy (HAART) regimens have been proven to reach the goal of undetectable viral load levels with a reasonable risk versus benefit quotient, especially during the peripartum period where the risk of infection of the product of conception is higher. It is during that same period that it is advised to incorporate zidovudine to the regimen, since it has demonstrated its efficacy in abbreviated regimens prescribed during the intrapartum and postpartum periods [2, 37-50].

Moreover, the study of the teratogenic risks entailed by the different drugs used in ART regimens has not evidenced a higher incidence of congenital defects than that observed in general population. Likewise the APRI (Antiretroviral Pregnancy Registry International) study on the prevalence of congenital defects was 2.2 per 100 live births when assessing the use of ART at any stage of pregnancy and was 3% when therapy was used during the first trimester. With the exception of efavirenz, which is categorized by the FDA as D, because of its association with neural tube defects, the rest of ARV is categorized as B or C [2]. There are reports in which AZT might be related to an increase of hypospadia rates among the exposed human population, and others where delavirdine might be associated with increased cardiac septal defects in animals [46-49].

The following drugs or combinations should not be indicated during pregnancy: efavirenz, nelfinavir, and the association of d4T (stavudine) and ddI (didanosine). They all share teratogenicity and the risk of toxicity to the mother-child binomial [46-51]. Finally, to optimize the update in side effects, it is essential to fully and continuously report to the competent organizations such as APRI about the possible secondary teratogenic effects and to comply strictly with regulations on the indication for therapy initiation and drug choice according to the stage of pregnancy [46-49, 51].

Although it is true that the first attempt to control VT with a successful pharmacological regime was achieved by the protocol known as ACTG 076, a protocol attaining a decrease in VT from

29% to 5.6% in 2001, new evidence has demonstrated that triple ART was more effective than monotherapy or bitherapy in VT prevention [14, 42-45]. Thus, a protocol that associated biomedical preventive measures (cesarean section and elimination of breastfeeding) with the indication of a combination of three antiretroviral drugs (nucleosidic and nonnucleosidic inhibitors of reverse transcriptase and protease inhibitors, regimens known together as Highly Active Antiretroviral Therapy or HAART) was designed [14, 42-45].

4.2. Antiretroviral therapy during pregnancy

The purpose of pharmacological therapy during pregnancy is to prevent vertical transmission through the reduction of the viral load in the mother to undetectable levels without resulting in teratogenic effects on the fetus. There are currently 14 commonly prescribed antiretroviral drugs (Table 1) that should be used to customize regimens in which selection is based on the eventual prior treatment of the pregnancy, the status of the disease, the viral load, CD4 cell counts, and the associated toxic and teratogenic effects according to FDA (Tables 1 and 2). Despite other drugs having been demonstrated efficacious in preventing vertical transmission, it is advisable to include the use of zidovudine within the antiretroviral scheme since it is the only drug that has proven efficacy and, most of the times, to be innocuous to the fetus in protocolized regimens (AIDS Clinical Protocol 076-ACTG 076) [2].

Generic name	FDA category
Nucleoside reverse transcriptase inhibitors	
Abacavir	C
Didanosine (ddl)	B
Lamivudine (3TC)	C
Lamivudine + zidovudine (Combivir)	C
Stavudine (d4T zalcitabine)	C
Zidovudine (ZDV, AZT)	C
Nonnucleoside reverse transcriptase inhibitors	
Delavirdine	C
Evavirenz	X
Nevirapine	C
Protease inhibitors	
Amprenavir	X
Indinavir	C
Nelfinavir	X
Ritonavir	B
Saquinavir	B

Table 1. Antiretroviral agent categories according to FDA

Category	Interpretation
A	Controlled studies fail to demonstrate risk
B	No evidence of risk for humans
C	The existence of risk cannot be ruled out; should only be used when potential benefits justify potential risk to the fetus
D	Proven risk
X	Contraindicated in pregnancy

Table 2. FDA pregnancy categories

4.2.1. ART toxicity and side effects

One of the aspects that need to be assessed for the selection of a pharmacological therapy is the eventual toxic effect of such medications on the mother-child binomial. Thus, studies have reported that approximately 80% of treated pregnant women developed certain side effects such as anemia, nausea, vomiting, abnormal liver enzyme results, or hyperglycemia [44-49]. As a consequence of the aforementioned, it is essential to know the side and toxic effects of the drugs generally used (Table 3) in order to identify them and act accordingly in the event of using them.

4.2.2. Protease inhibitors

In the general population, protease inhibitors have been linked to the induction of variable degrees of carbohydrate intolerance. The latter should be considered when prescribing the patient such drugs to the pregnant woman since they might trigger the development of gestational diabetes [44-49].

4.2.3. Nucleoside—reverse transcriptase inhibitors

There is evidence that nucleoside reverse transcriptase inhibitors may induce mitochondrial dysfunction by virtue of their high affinity for gamma DNA-polymerase found in mitochondria. Among the drugs of such family that are more intensely related to such adverse effect are d4T (stavudine) and ddI (didanosine) and, to a lesser extent, ZDV (Zidovudine), 3TC (lamivudine), ABC (abacavir), and TDF (tenofir). The association between such type of drugs and lactic acidosis with or without concomitant liver steatosis is also known. Such conditions are more commonly seen in association with the use of d4T (stavudine) (0.8%-1.2%) [44-49]. The clinical picture resulting from such entity is similar to Hellp syndrome, a condition that may or may not be associated to polyneuropathies, fatty liver, myopathies, cardiopathies, and lactic acidosis. Finally, there are literature reports on children from mothers exposed to zidovudine or zidovudine/lamivudine (AZT/3TC) who developed mitochondrial dysfunction-related symptoms, a finding that was not observed in the cohort of patients following the ACTG/076 protocol [2].

AR	Main toxicity	Other toxicities
AZT	Anemia - Neutropenia	Gastrointestinal-headache-rash
d4T	Polyneuropathy, lipoatrophy, lactic acidosis	Pancreatitis, hepatic steatosis
3TC	-	Gastrointestinal-headache
ddl	Pancreatitis, polyneuropathy	Gastrointestinal, Hyperuricemia
Abacavir	Hypersensitivity reaction	Gastrointestinal
Tenofovir	-	Gastrointestinal, Renal
Efavirenz	CNS: Vertigo, Psychosis	Rash, hepatotoxicity, dyslipidemia
Nevirapine	Rash, Hepatotoxicity	
PI (except for Atanazavir)	Lipodystrophy, dyslipidemia, diabetes	Liver toxicity, gastrointestinal, osteonecrosis
Indinavir	Metabolic, hyperbilirubinemia, kidney stones	Gastrointestinal
Atanazavir	Hyperbilirubinemia, rash	Gastrointestinal

Table 3. Antiretroviral agent toxicity

4.3. Opportunity for ART initiation in pregnancy

Several cohort studies show that the late initiation of ART is associated both with higher VT as well as with longer duration of VT. The latter is based on the fact that when therapy duration was 9.5 weeks, VT was significantly higher than when therapy duration was 16 weeks ($P <$ 0.001) [21]. Conversely, in a study conducted at the United Kingdom and Ireland VT was significantly higher among patients with a delayed initiation of therapy (25 + 6 vs. 30 + 1 weeks, <0.001; level of evidence: 2++) [2, 14]. Conditions of ART initiation during pregnancy are listed as follows:

- A pregnant woman without prior therapy should initiate ART from 20 weeks of gestation (Grade B recommendation).
- When VL is higher than 100,000 copies/ml, ART should be initiated by week 14 (Grade B recommendation).
- If the pregnant woman has clinical or immunological criteria for ART initiation, or if seroconversion occurs during gestation, ART must be initiated immediately (Grade B recommendation).
- A low frequency of VT (5%) has been observed during the second trimester of pregnancy. Thirty-four percent of VT occurs during the antepartum and 66% occurs during delivery [2, 7, 10, 12]. However, placental transmission may occur from 13 weeks (Level 2++ evidence C).

4.4. Choice of drugs to start ART

Triple ART or HAART (highly active antiretroviral therapy) is the preferred choice. The use of zidovudine (AZT) in association with lamivudine (3TC) 600 and 300 mg per day, respectively, is recommended for the prevention of HIV vertical transmission. A preparation including both drugs in a fixed drug combination of 300 mg AZT and 150 mg 3TC is commercially available (grade of recommendation: A). Lopinavir/ritonavir (800/200 mg daily) or saquinavir/ritonavir (2000/200 mg daily) are recommended as a third drug (Grade C recommendation). The use of nevirapine (NVP) as a third drug may be considered in patients with CD4 T-cell counts lower than 250 cells/mm^3 (200-400 mg daily) (Grade C recommendation).

A higher incidence of malformations failed to be demonstrated on 3,000 pregnancies exposed to AZT and 3TC. The 3TC+AZT combination has evidenced a higher efficacy in the prevention of VT than AZT as monotherapy. Cohort studies have reported a reduction in HIV mortality and transmission with the use of AZT+3TC (Level 2+ evidence). There is not enough comparative evidence of the efficacy of other ARV combinations on VT prevention (Level 2+ evidence) [19, 20, 43, 45].

The use of NVP in pregnant women with CD4 T-cell counts between 250 and 350 cells/mm^3 failed to confirm an increase of the risk of suffering severe adverse effects. The benefits of using NVP in pregnant women outweigh the risks (Level 2+ evidence) [19, 20, 43, 45].

4.5. Procedures for monitoring ART during pregnancy

Efficacy of ART is measured through the decrease of viral load. ART is effective if the decrease is near 1 log of VL 2 weeks after the initiation of therapy and 1.5 log at 4 weeks. Achieving a decrease of 2 logs between 28 and 34 weeks of gestation is also considered effective [19]. The viral load should be assessed upon the first control visit. Viral load should be controlled 2 and 4 weeks after the initiation of therapy or after a change in therapy. Subsequently, VL should be controlled on a monthly basis until becoming undetectable. At gestation weeks 34-36, a VL assessment should be performed to define the route of delivery, eventual additional ART, and to plan ART for the newborn (Grade D recommendation).

In patients starting ART before week 24, a VL every 2 months (8 weeks) and at week 34 is recommended (Grade D recommendation).

Several clinical guidelines propose such management based on expert recommendations (Level 4 evidence) [15-17, 19-21].

4.6. What are the best moment and the recommended route for delivery?

A cesarean section should be indicated at 38 weeks of gestation in women with HIV infection without ART during pregnancy, in women without a VL result at gestation week 34, or in cases of VL >1,000 copies/ml (Grade B recommendation).

A vaginal delivery may be allowed in mothers under ART from 24 weeks of gestation or earlier, with VL <1,000 copies/ml at week 34, CD4 T-cell counts above 250, and that additionally meet the following conditions:

- Gestational age greater than 37 weeks
- Single fetus in cephalic presentation
- Favorable obstetric conditions

- Care provided by specialist physician
- Informed consent from the patient

Invasive maneuvers (amniocentesis, chorionic villus biopsy, internal monitoring, artificial rupture of membranes) and instrumental delivery (forceps, spatulas) should be avoided (Grade D recommendation) though oxytocin may be used for labor guidance. The use of methylergonovine for the management of uterine inertia should be avoided if the patient is using protease inhibitors.

Elective cesarean section at 38 weeks of gestation, before an eventual rupture of membranes or initiation of spontaneous labor, substantially reduces the risk of HIV transmission. On its own, elective cesarean section reduces the risk of HIV transmission in 50%. Cesarean section together with antiretroviral therapy during the antenatal period, during delivery and administered to the newborn with the addition of termination of breastfeeding, achieves decreases close to 90% with final vertical transmission rates under 2% (Level 2++ evidence) [52-57].

Studies with large patient numbers have failed to show benefits in favor of cesarean section in women undergoing ART with VL <1,000 copies/ml. Shapiro showed transmission rates for vaginal delivery of 0.8 v/s 0.5 for cesarean section (OR 1.4 (0.2-6.4)) in patients with viral load lower than 1,000 copies/ml. (Level 2+ evidence) [53]. Moreover, cesarean section has been seen to cause 7-10-fold increases in morbidity, mainly infectious, as compared to vaginal delivery (Level 2+ evidence) [57]. Obstetric procedures that increase the risk of fetal exposure to maternal blood such as amniocentesis, villus biopsy, and invasive monitoring have been implicated by some researchers as transmission risk factors (Level 2+ evidence) [30]. The use of oxytocin is not contraindicated; however, ergot derivatives accumulate in patients receiving protease inhibitors because of the inhibitory action of the latter on cytochrome 3A4, and exaggerated vasoconstriction and ischemia have been described in relation with their use in association (Level 4 evidence) [15-20].

4.7. Antiretroviral drugs used during delivery or cesarean section

Intrapartum intravenous AZT shall be used in the indicated dose, regardless of the chosen route for delivery (Grade B recommendation), as follows:

- Loading dose: 2 mg/kg, infused over 1 h (in case of cesarean, 4 h prior to surgery)
- Maintenance dose: 1 mg/kg/h during cesarean section (to run 3 h after the loading dose) or during labor, until the cord is clamped
- In case AZT 200 mg is unavailable, the oral administration of AZT/3TC upon the initiation of labor or 4 h prior to scheduled cesarean section is recommended

Nevirapine 200 mg single dose before cesarean section shall be added in any of the following settings (Grade B recommendation):

- The late initiation of the protocol (later than 34 weeks and patients that failed to complete 4 weeks of ART upon delivery)

- VL week 34 >1,000 copies/ml
- Intrapartum HIV (+) diagnosis that did not receive ART

When NVP is used intrapartum, AZT/3TC should be added for 7 days postpartum to decrease the risk of developing resistance to NVP (Grade B recommendation).

The use of IV AZT during delivery enables reaching effective fetal plasma levels thus generating a preexposure prophylaxis. The latter, together with the oral administration of AZT suspension to the newborn for 6 weeks, enables a postexposure prophylaxis that as a whole has an impact on VT regardless of the patient having received AZT within her ART regimen during pregnancy or even, in the case of an eventual resistance to AZT (Level 2++ evidence) [53-55].

4.8. Breastfeeding management

Pharmacological cessation of breastfeeding shall proceed in all HIV(+) women even if such result is just from the rapid intrapartum test (Grade B recommendation). Based on four studies in which mothers acquired HIV-1 after birth, the estimated risk of transmission is 29% (95% CI 16-42%). The analysis of five studies showed that when the mother became infected before delivery, the additional risk of transmission through breastfeeding, beyond *in utero* or intrapartum transmission, is 14% (95% CI 7-22%) (Level 2+ evidence) [56, 57].

5. Special situations

5.1. What to do with HIV(+) pregnant women who received previous ART and are currently without ART?

A CD4 T-cell count, a VL, and a viral genotyping study are recommended in women previously exposed to ART and who discontinued therapy. The latter will enable designing the therapeutic regimen based on patient history and current genotype. Viral load should be assessed after 4 to 6 weeks of the initiation of ART, and a new genotyping study should be performed in case of failure, for adjustment of the latter. Zidovudine should be included in the ART regimen when possible (Grade D recommendation).

Several clinical guidelines propose such management based on expert recommendations (Level 4 evidence) [15-20].

5.2. What to do with HIV(+) women undergoing ART who become pregnant?

Women undergoing ART who become pregnant are recommended to maintain ART if their VL is undetectable. If the regimen includes drugs that increase toxicity (D4T) or contains Efavirenz, these should be withdrawn and replaced with lopinavir/ritonavir or by saquinavir/ritonavir, including, when possible, AZT in the regimen (Grade D recommendation). The WHO guidelines do not recommend the use of the antiretroviral medication efavirenz (EFV) during the first trimester of pregnancy because of its potential fetal teratogenic effects, mostly involving defects of neural tube closure. Nevertheless, there are no categorical studies supporting such recommendation (Level 3 evidence). Likewise, the use of the ddl/d4T combination should be terminated [15-21].

The genotyping study should be performed on pregnant women undergoing ART with VL >1,000 copies/ml, particularly in pregnancies that have not achieved such goal at 34 weeks of gestation. Moreover, the addition of a single dose of nevirapine at the moment of delivery is suggested (Grade D recommendation).

Several clinical guidelines propose such management based on expert recommendations (Level 4 evidence) [15-21].

5.3. What to do with HIV(+) pregnant women who reach 32 weeks of gestation without ART?

In pregnant women reaching the 32nd week of gestation or more without ART, it is recommended to assess CD4 T-cell levels and VL and to initiate immediately ART with AZT/3TC coformulated, together with a protease inhibitor (PI). Nevirapine (NVP) can be used instead of a reinforced PI when CD4 T-cell counts are lower than 250 cells/mm^3 (Grade D recommendation).

There is wide experience on the use of NVP during pregnancy. The drug has a risk of severe hepatotoxicity with CD4 >250 cells/mm^3, especially in coinfection with HBV and HCV. Several clinical guidelines propose such management based on expert recommendations. When NVP is used during delivery, AZT/3TC needs to be used subsequently to prevent drug resistance induced by NVP (Level 4 evidence) [15-21].

5.4. What to do with HIV(+) pregnant women close to delivery date without prior ART?

The following are to be observed:

- Ideally assess CD4 T cells and VL.
- Intravenous zidovudine as per regimen.
- Single dose of nevirapine.
- Resolution of delivery through cesarean section.
- Use AZT/3TC for 1 week, add PI, until evaluating the best regimen to continue therapy (Grade D recommendation).

Several clinical guidelines propose such management based on expert recommendations (Level 4 evidence) [15-21].

5.5. What to do with HIV(+) pregnant women who have been treated with ribavirin?

Because of the potential teratogenesis of ribavirin, its preconception withdrawal for at least 4 months in women and at least for 7 months in case the couple had received such drug should be counseled. In case of an eventual use during pregnancy, it should be immediately withdrawn, and a consultation visit should be arranged to assess maternal liver function.

5.6. What to do with HIV(+) pregnant women with threat of premature delivery?

The administration of IV AZT 2 mg/kg/h, together with tocolytic therapy, during the first hour followed by 1 mg/kg/h until dynamics ease up, according to ART administration policy during delivery, is recommended in the presence of regular uterine dynamics, despite cervical modifications being scarce. If unable to slow down the situation and if delivery is triggered and/or rupture of membranes ensues, a cesarean section shall be performed sufficiently in advance (Grade C recommendation).

Premature delivery constitutes a risk factor for perinatal transmission of the virus: a maternal viral load (VL) of <400 c/ml in a delivery occurring before 34 weeks was related to an 8-fold increase in the risk of transmission as compared to term delivery (Level 2+ evidence) [58].

5.7. What to do with HIV(+) pregnant women with premature rupture of membranes?

All patients should receive ART and undergo the usual control and therapeutic measures such as the administration of prophylactic antibiotics, steroids, and eventually the use of magnesium sulfate as neuroprotector. In case of a suspected infection or loss of fetal well-being, pregnancy interruption must be carried out. The recommended delivery route is cesarean section. The management of each case depends on the gestational age (Grade D recommendation).

In pregnancies of less than 26 weeks, a conservative therapy is recommended in view of the risk of severe sequels as a result of prematurity and high neonatal mortality (Grade D recommendation). Between weeks 26 and 30, each case shall be evaluated according to maternal and fetal status, the virological status of the mother, if she has been administered a therapy or not, and the neonatal outcomes of the center (Grade D recommendation). Between 30 and 34 weeks, the general behavior that is recommended is to terminate pregnancy. In view of the higher tendency to an increase of reported VT in premature deliveries with PROM even while receiving ART, the preferred route for delivery shall be cesarean section (Grade D recommendation)

There is a clear difference in the risk of severe sequels between gestational ages (61.5% at week 23 and 10% at week 28). In view of the higher risk of VT in preterms, a cesarean section shall be considered (Level 2+ evidence) [21, 56, 58].

Before the use of ART during pregnancy, several studies found a relationship between the duration of the rupture of membranes and the VT, particularly if such duration was greater than 4 h. In women with less than 24 h since the rupture of membranes, for every hour that elapses after the rupture, the risk of vertical transmission rises in 2%. Because the risk of fetal infection in patients with PROM and very low plasmatic viral load and/or under ART is unknown, treatment of PROM has not been fully clarified. Several clinical guidelines propose such management based on expert recommendations (Level 4 evidence) [15-21].

6. Conclusion

Recommendations and protocols discussed above are easy to implement in countries with adequate resources, consolidated healthcare systems, and proven functional system with trained healthcare personnel and high literate population. Countries must strategically choose their models for the provision of services, taking into consideration the type of epidemics, cost-effectiveness, equity in access, and available resources. The WHO at present collaborates with poor countries, proposing a "Health Systems Platform for HIV/AIDS." Such idea comprises the following areas that are considered as crucial: (1) labor systems that ensure the availability of a sufficient number of trained healthcare providers that work in an adequate facility and in safe conditions, (2) systems to purchase and distribute medications and other supplies, (3) fair funding systems to prevent people from being pushed into poverty when they become ill, and (4) healthcare information systems to alert the administrators of healthcare assistance and those in charge of elaborating policies addressing risks for persons in situations that might severely worsen. Of all these necessities, the most urgent is the availability of a sufficient number of health professionals. Nevertheless, there are some experiences gained through the participation of untrained personnel in some stages of the process; for instance, in the diagnosis of the condition of HIV carrier, this should not be de-emphasized.

Author details

Enrique Valdés Rubio* and Rodolfo Guiñez Gahona

*Address all correspondence to: evaldes@vtr.net

Departamento de Obstetricia y Ginecología, Hospital Clínico Universidad de Chile, Unidad de Medicina Materno Fetal, Chile

References

[1] The Millennium Development Goals. (2012). Eight goals for 2015. Available at http://www.who.int/topics/millennium_development_goals/diseases/es/index.html Accessed June 30, 2012.

[2] Valdés E. HIV/AIDS: vertical transmission: In: Current Perspectives in HIV Infection, Shailendra K. Saxena (Ed.), 2013, ISBN: 978-953-51-1057-6, InTech. DOI: 10.5772/53204. Available at: http://www.intechopen.com/books/current-perspectives-in-hiv-infection/hiv-aids-vertical-transmission.

[3] Harbour R, Miller J. A new system for grading recommendations in evidence based guidelines. BMJ 2001; 323: 334-6.

[4] Connor EM, Sperling RS, and Gelber R. Reduction of maternal-infant transmission of human immunodeficiency virus type 1 with zidovudine treatment. N Engl J Med 1994, 331(18), 1173-80.

[5] Valdés E. VIH-SIDA y embarazo: actualización y realidad en Chile. Rev Chil Obstet Ginecol 2002; 67(2): 160-6.

[6] Abarzúa F. VIH y Embarazo. Capítulo 21, pp. 413-423. Available at www.acog.cl/educación.php?sort=dd. Accessed June 30, 2012.

[7] The European Collaborative Study. Maternal viral load and vertical transmission of HIV-1: an important factor but not the only one. AIDS 1999; 13: 1377-85.

[8] Bollen LJ, Whitehead SJ, Mock PA, et al. Maternal herpes simplex virus type 2 coinfection increases the risk of perinatal HIV transmission: possibility to further decrease transmission? AIDS 2008; 22: 1169-76.

[9] Mwapasa V, Rogerson S, Kwiek JJ, Wilson PE, Milner D. Maternal syphilis infection is associated with increased risk of mother-to-child transmission of HIV in Malawi. AIDS 2006; 20: 1869-77.

[10] Magder LS, Mofenson L, Paul ME, Zorrilla CD, Blattner WA, Tuomala RE, LaRussa P, Landesman S, Rich KC. Risk factors for in utero and intrapartum transmission of HIV. J Acquir Immune Defic Syndr 2005 Jan 1; 38(1): 87-95.

[11] García M, and Olea A. Evolución y situación epidemiológica de la infección por virus de inmunodeficiencia humana y síndrome de inmunodeficiencia adquirida en Chile. Rev Chil Infectol 2008; 25: 162-70.

[12] Valdés E. In VIH-SIDA y embarazo: Urgencias y complicaciones en Obstetricia Chapter. M García Huidobro. J Hasbún. Editorial Mediterráneo, 2006; 447.

[13] Joint United Nations Programme on HIV/AIDS (UNAIDS)/WHO/UNICEF. A guide on indicators for the monitoring and reporting on the health sector response to HIV/AIDS. Geneva, World Health Organization, 2011. Available at: http://www.who.int/hiv/data/UA2011_indicator_guide_en.pdf. Accessed October 15, 2011.

[14] Townsend CL, Cortina-Borja M, Peckham CS, de Ruiter A, Lyall H, Tookey PA. Low rates of mother-to-child transmission of HIV following effective pregnancy interventions in the United Kingdom and Ireland, 2000-2006. AIDS 2008; 22: 973-81.

[15] BHIVA guidelines for the management of HIV infection in pregnant women 2012. HIV Med 2012; 13(Suppl. 2), 87-157.

[16] Protocolo Infección por VIH y Gestación. Unidad de Infecciones Perinatales. Servicio de Medicina Materno-Fetal Instituto Clínico de Ginecologia, Obstetricia y Neonatologia (ICGON), Hospital Clínic de Barcelona. Update 2011.

[17] Documento de consenso para el seguimiento de la infección por el VIH en relación con la reproducción, embarazo, parto y profilaxis de la transmisión vertical del niño

expuesto. Grupo de expertos de la Secretaría del Plan Nacional sobre el Sida (SPNS), Grupo de Estudio de Sida (GeSIDA)/Sociedad, Española de Ginecología y Obstetricia (SEGO) y Sociedad Española de Infectología Pediátrica (SEIP).

[18] Panel on Treatment of HIV-Infected Pregnant Women and Prevention of Perinatal Transmission. Recommendations for Use of Antiretroviral Drugs in Pregnant HIV-1-Infected Women for Maternal Health and Interventions to Reduce Perinatal HIV Transmission in the United States. Available at: http://aidsinfo.nih.gov/contentfiles/lvguidelines/PerinatalGL. Accessed February 20, 2014.

[19] Norma General Técnica No. 0141 del 2012. Norma Conjunta de Prevención de la Transmisión Vertical del VIH y Sífilis. Minsal 2012.

[20] Guía Clínica 2010 Sindrome de Inmunodeficiencia Adquirida VIH/SIDA. Minsal 2010.

[21] Royal College of Obstetricians and Gynaecologists. (2010). Management of HIV in pregnancy. Green-top Guideline No. 39 June. Available at: http://www.rcog.org.uk/Womens-health/clinical-guidance/management-hiv-pregnancy-green-top-39. Accessed June 30, 2012.

[22] Routine human immunodeficiency virus screening. Committee Opinion No. 596. American College of Obstetricians and Gynecologists. Obstet Gynecol 2014; 123: 1137-9.

[23] De Bruyn M, Paxton S. HIV testing of pregnant women-what is needed to protect positive women's needs and rights? Sex Health 2005; 2: 143-51.

[24] Dhai A, Noble R. Ethical issues in HIV. Best Pract Res Clin Obstet Gynaecol 2005; 19: 255-67.

[25] Bowden FJ. Reconsidering HIV testing-consent is still the key. Sex Health 2005; 2: 165-7.

[26] Chou R, Smits AK, Huffman LH, Fu R, Korthuis PT; US Preventive Services Task Force. Prenatal screening for HIV: a review of the evidence for the U.S. Preventive Services Task Force. Ann Intern Med 2005; 143: 38-54.

[27] Campos-Outcalt D. Time to revise your HIV testing routine. J Fam Pract 2007; 56: 283-4.

[28] Service delivery approaches to HIV testing and counseling (HTC): a strategic HTC policy framework. World Health Organization, 2012. ISBN 978-92-4-159387-7.

[29] Kottow M. Detección de seropositividad VIH en embarazadas: consideraciones bioéticas. Rev Chil Salud Pública 2011; 15(3): 165-70.

[30] Rujumba J, et al. Pregnant women's experiences of routine counseling and testing for HIV in Eastern Uganda: a qualitative study. BMC Health Services Research 2013; 13: 189.

[31] ShafieeH, Wang S, Inci F, Toy M, Henrich TJ, Kuritzkes DR, and Demirci U. Emerging technologies for point-of-care management of HIV Infection. Review in advance first posted online on November 12, 2014. (Changes may still occur before final publication online and in print.)

[32] Buttó S, Suligoi B, Fanales-Belasio E, and Raimondo M. Laboratory diagnostics for HIV infection. Ann Ist Super Sanità 2010; 46(1): 24-33.

[33] Smith CB, Battin MP, Francis LP, and Jacobson JA. Should rapid tests for HIV infection now be mandatory during pregnancy? Global differences in scarcity and a dilemma of technological advance. Dev World Bioeth 2007; 7(2): 86-103.

[34] Lim Y, Kim JY, Rich M, Stulac S, Niyonzima JB, et al. Improving prevention of mother-to-child transmission of HIV care and related services in Eastern Rwanda. PLoS Med 2010; 7(7): e1000302.

[35] Galli RA, et al. Evaluation of the accuracy and ease of use of a rapid HIV-1 antibody test performed by untrained operators at the point of care. J Clin Virol 2013; 58S: e65-9.

[36] Melvin Z, Alarcon AJ, Velasquez JC, et al. Rapid HIV type 1 testing of women presenting in late pregnancy with unknown HIV status in Lima, Peru. AIDS Res Hum Retroviruses 2004; 20(10): 1046-52.

[37] Eshleman SH, Mracna M, Guay LA, Deseyve M, Cunningham S, Mirochnick M, Musoke P, Fleming T, Glenn Fowler M, Mofenson LM, Mmiro F, Jackson JB. Selection and fading of resistance mutations in women and infants receiving nevirapine to prevent HIV-1 vertical transmission (HIVNET 012). AIDS 2001; 15(15): 1951-7.

[38] Menson EN, Walker AS, Sharland M, et al. Underdosing of antiretrovirals in UK and Irish children with HIV as an example of problems in prescribing medicines to children, 1997-2005: cohort study. BMJ 2006; 332(7551): 1183-7.

[39] Gras L, Kesselring A, Griffin J, van Sighem A, Fraser C, Ghani A, et al. ATHENA Cohort Study. CD4 cell counts of 800 cells/mm^3 or greater after 7 years of highly active antiretroviral therapy are feasible in most patients starting with 350 cells/mm^3 or greater. J Acquir Immune Defic Syndr. 2007; 45: 183-92.

[40] Palella F, Deloria-Knoll M, Chmiel J, Moorman A, Wood K, Greenberg A, et al. Survival benefit of initiating antiretroviral therapy in HIV-infected persons in different CD4+ cell strata. Ann Intern Med. 2003; 138: 620-6.

[41] Tai JH, Udoji MA, Barkanic G, Byrne DW, Rebeiro PF, Byram BR, et al. Pregnancy and HIV disease progression during the era of highly active antiretroviral therapy. J Infect Dis 2007; 196(7): 1044-52.

[42] Cooper ER, Charurat M, Mofenson L, Hanson IC, Pitt J, Diaz C, Hayani K, Handelsman E, Smeriglio V, Hoff R, Blattner W; Women and Infants' Transmission Study Group. Combination antiretroviral strategies for the treatment of pregnant HIV-1-in-

fected women and prevention of perinatal HIV-1 transmission. J Acquir Immune Defic Syndr. 2002 Apr 15; 29(5): 484-94

[43] Tuomala RE, Watts DH, Li D, Vajaranant M, Pitt J, Hammill H, et al. Improved obstetric outcomes and few maternal toxicities are associated with antiretroviral therapy, including highly active antiretroviral therapy during pregnancy. J Acquir Immune Defic Syndr 2005; 38(4): 449-473.

[44] Siegfried N, van der Merwe L, Brocklehurst P, Sint TT. Antiretrovirals for reducing the risk of mother-to-child transmission of HIV infection. Cochrane Database Syst Rev 2011; (7): CD003510.

[45] Recommendations from the GESIDA/Spanish AIDS Plan regarding antiretroviral treatment in adults with human immunodeficiency virus infection. Enferm Infecc Microbiol Clin 2007; 25(1): 32-53.

[46] El Beitune P, Duarte G, Quintana SM, Figueiro-Filho EA, Marcolin AC, and Abduch R. Antiretroviral therapy during pregnancy and early neonatal life: consequences for HIV-exposed uninfected children. Braz J Infect Dis 2004; 8: 140-50.

[47] Poirier MC, Olivero OA, Walker DM, and Walker VE. Perinatal genotoxicity and carcinogenicity of anti-retroviral nucleoside analog drugs. Toxicol Appl Pharmacol 2004; 199(2): 151- Accessed January 21, 2014.61.

[48] Brogly SB, Ylitalo N, Mofenson LM, Oleske J, Van Dyke R, Crain MJ, Abzug MJ, Brady M, Jean-Philippe P, Hughes MD, and Seage GR 3rd. In utero nucleoside reverse transcriptase inhibitor exposure and signs of possible mitochondrial dysfunction in HIV-uninfected children. AIDS 2007; 21: 929-38.

[49] Lorenzini P, Spicher VM, Laubereau B, Hirschel B, Kind C, Rudin C, et al. Antiretroviral therapies in pregnancy: maternal, fetal and neonatal effects. Swiss HIV Cohort Study, the Swiss Collaborative HIV and Pregnancy study, and the Swiss Neonatal AHIV study. AIDS 1998; 12(18): F241-7.

[50] Directrices unificadas sobre el uso de los antirretrovirales en el tratamiento y la prevención de la infección por VIH: recomendaciones para un enfoque de salud pública, junio de 2013. Organización Mundial de la Salud. ISBN 978 92 4 350572 5.

[51] Safety and Toxicity of Individual Antiretroviral Agents in Pregnancy. Available at: http://img.thebody.com/hivatis/pdfs/pregnancy_guide.pdf. Accessed January 21, 2014.

[52] Warszawaski J, Tubiana R, Le Chenadec J, et al. Mother-to-child HIV transmission despite antiretroviral therapy in the ANRS French Perinatal Cohort. AIDS 2008; 22: 289-299.

[53] Shapiro D, Tuomala R. Mother to child HIV transmission risk according to ART, mode of delivery, and viral load in 2895 US women (PACTG 367). Oral presentation

at the 11th Conference on retroviruses and opportunistic infections. San Francisco CA, February 2004 (abstract 99).

[54] Read JS, Newell ML. Efficacy and safety of cesarean delivery for prevention of mother-to-child transmission of HIV-1. Cochrane Database Syst Rev 2005, Issue 4. Art. No.: CD005479. DOI: 10.1002/14651858.CD005479.

[55] Jamieson DJ, Read JS, Kourtis AP, Durant TM, Lampe MA, Dominguez KL. Cesarean delivery for HIV-infected women: recommendations and controversies. Am J Obstet Gynecol 2007; 197(3): S96-100.

[56] European Collaborative Study. Mode of delivery in HIV-infected pregnant women and prevention of mother-to-child transmission: changing practices in Western Europe. HIV Med 2010; 11: 368-378.

[57] Dunn DT, Newell ML, Ades AE, Peckham CS. Risk of human immunodeficiency virus type 1 transmission through breastfeeding. Lancet 1992; 340(8819): 585-8.

[58] Mirpuri J, Jain L. Issues of prematurity and HIV infection. Clin Perinatol 2010; 37: 887-905.

Section 2

Replication, Resistance, Treatment Options and Therapy Responses

Chapter 4

Inhibition of HIV Replication by Host Cellular Factors

J.M. Azevedo-Pereira, Pedro Canhão, Marta Calado,
Quirina Santos-Costa and Pedro Barroca

Additional information is available at the end of the chapter

http://dx.doi.org/10.5772/60795

1. Introduction

Human immunodeficiency viruses 1 and 2 (HIV-1 and HIV-2) infection leads to immunological failure and Acquired Immunodeficiency Syndrome (AIDS). During transmission and dissemination within a new host, HIV must overcome several cellular mechanisms aiming to inhibit or restrict its infection and its spread to other host cells. Not surprisingly, as a well-adapted human pathogen, HIV has evolved in order to counteract and subvert these cellular inhibitory factors. Defining how viral and cellular proteins interact remains a critical area of research with direct implications in the knowledge of transmission, pathogenic mechanisms, vaccine design and molecular targets for therapeutic intervention.

In this chapter, the mechanisms involved in the inhibitory activity of some cellular proteins and the way HIV evades those host cell restrictions will be focused on. Particular attention will be given to the tripartite motif 5 (TRIM5) protein family, involved in viral uncoating; the retroviral protection factors, apolipoprotein B mRNA-editing enzyme catalytic polypeptide-like (APOBEC) and Tetherin, involved in the reverse transcription and viral release respectively; and to the sterile alpha motif [SAM] and histidine/aspartic acid [HD] domain-containing protein 1 (SAMHD1), which mediates the restriction of HIV-1 replication in dendritic cells. This review will also delve into the mechanisms of two recently described factors: MxB, which restricts HIV nuclear import and integration, and cholesterol-25-hydroxylase that converts cholesterol to a soluble antiviral factor (25-hydroxycholesterol) that blocks HIV fusion with target cells.

2. Brief overview on HIV replication cycle

The replication cycle of HIV can be divided into five major steps: (i) virus-receptor interactions and fusion; (ii) reverse transcription and proviral integration; (iii) HIV genomic DNA transcription; (iv) HIV mRNA splicing, nuclear export and translation; and (v) viral assembly, release and maturation (Figure 1).

The first step of the cycle begins with the binding of the virion gp120 surface subunit (SU glycoprotein) to CD4 receptor present in T-cells, macrophages and dendritic cells. The SU glycoprotein and the gp41 transmembrane subunit (TM glycoprotein) remain associated by non-covalent binding. Both SU and TM are proteolytically cleaved from the envelope (Env) precursor protein by a cellular convertase, furin, within the endoplasmatic reticulum (ER). The SU glycoprotein allows viral binding to cellular receptors – CD4 and a coreceptor belonging to the chemokine receptor's family – while the TM protein is involved in the fusion between the viral envelope and the host cell membrane [1]. After initial binding to CD4, SU undergoes structural changes that lead to the exposure (or formation) of the coreceptor-binding site. Although several chemokine receptors were identified as mediators of HIV entry *in vitro*, CCR5 and CXCR4 seem to be the two major coreceptors [2, 3]. After SU glycoprotein binding to co-receptor additional conformational changes are observed, exposing the N-terminal region of TM (dubbed the "fusion peptide"), which mediates the fusion between the viral and host membranes (reviewed in [4, 5]). This viral fusion process may occur through a direct pH-independent fusion mechanism with plasma membrane [6], or via endocytosis and fusion with endosomes [7].

After viral fusion, the viral capsid enters the cytoplasm and the viral RNA is converted to double-stranded DNA, a reaction mediated by the viral reverse transcriptase (RT), that occurs in a cytoplasmic complex named the reverse transcriptase complex (RTC). RT has three essential activities for virus replication: RNA-dependent DNA polymerase (i.e. reverse transcriptase), RNase H activity that cleaves the genomic RNA in RNA/ DNA hybrids during cDNA synthesis, and DNA-dependent DNA polymerase activity (for synthesis of the second strand of the proviral DNA). The result is a double-stranded DNA replica of the original genomic RNA. The double-stranded viral DNA, as part of the preintegration complex (PIC), penetrates the host cell nucleus through the pores in the nuclear membrane. Another viral enzyme, integrase, inserts the double-stranded viral DNA in the host cell chromosomal DNA (reviewed in [8]). The PIC is composed of several cellular and viral components, e.g. viral DNA, RT, integrase (IN), capsid (CA), matrix (MA) and Vpr proteins. In activated cells, the proviral DNA is transcribed, acting as a template for mRNA synthesis. The viral mRNA exists as three distinct classes: multiply spliced (~2kb), single-spliced (4-5kb) and unspliced (9kb). The multiply spliced transcripts are the first to accumulate soon after infection and encode the regulatory proteins Tat, Rev and Nef. The accumulation of Rev protein enables the efficient nuclear export of single-spliced and unspliced mRNA and to an increase in the levels of these mRNAs (reviewed in [9]).

http://dx.doi.org/10.5772/60795

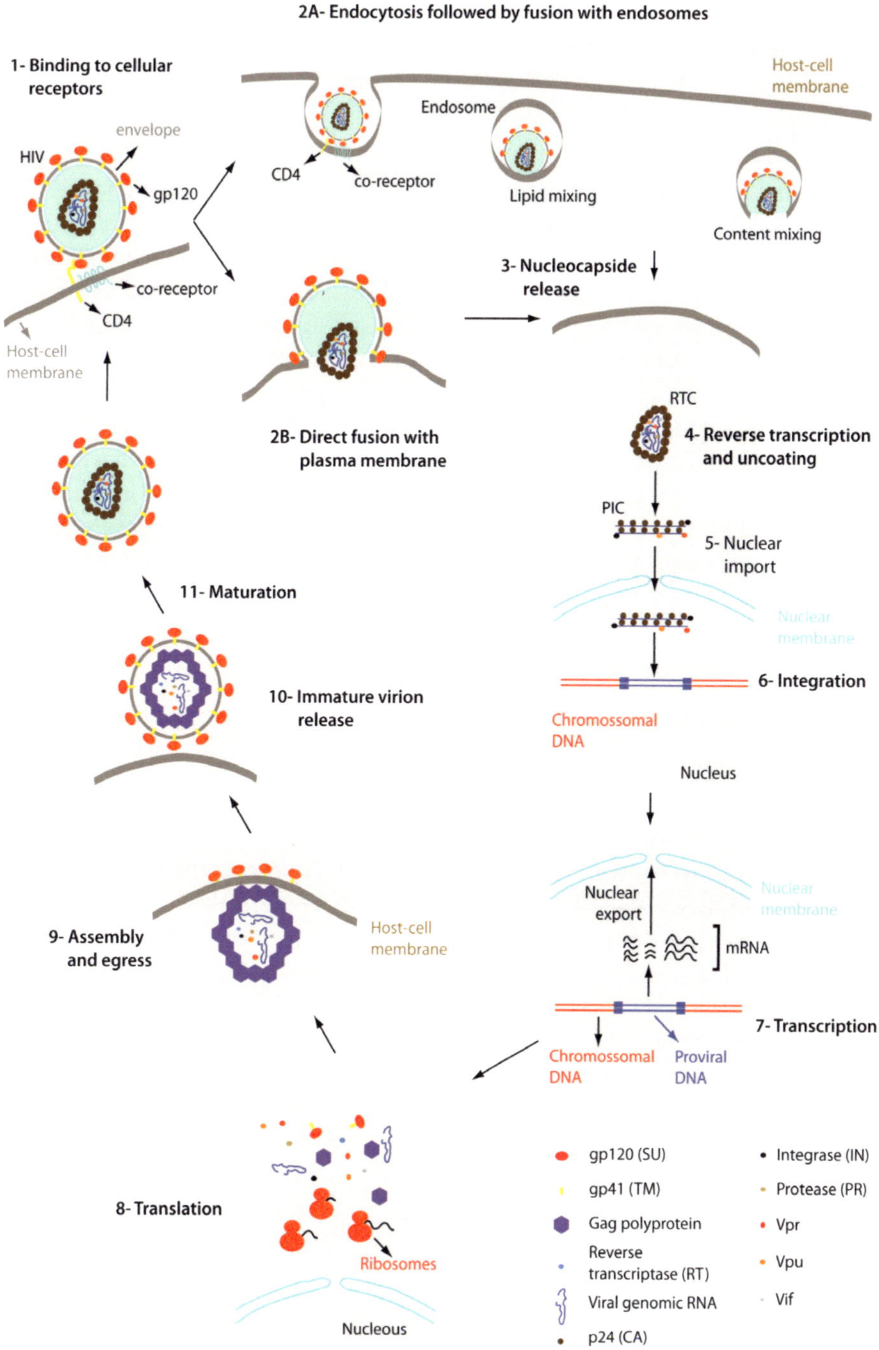

Figure 1. Schematic representation of HIV replication cycle. HIV initiates infection by attaching (1) to cellular receptors: CD4 and a chemokine receptor (co-receptor). The interactions with both receptors trigger the fusion between viral envelope with cellular membrane, either after endocytosis (2A) or by direct fusion with plasma membrane (2B). The release of viral nucleocapside into the cytoplasm (3) precedes the formation of the reverse transcriptase complex (RTC)

where the reverse transcription takes place (4). The RTC transforms to the preintegration complex (PIC), composed by several cellular and viral components, that is imported to the nucleus where viral DNA is integrated into cellular chromosomal DNA (5 and 6). The proviral DNA is then transcribed (7) and mRNA migrates to the cytoplasm and translated to viral proteins (8). Assembly of different components of viral particles occurs at plasma membrane (9). After egress and release of immature virions (10), the proteolytical cleavage of Gag polyprotein takes place leading to mature virions (11).

After replication, transcription and translation, the viral genome information is ready to proceed to the final step: the viral assembly, the release and maturation of recently formed virions. The nucleocapsid assembly occurs through protein-protein interactions mediated by the uncleaved Gag polyprotein – through the capsid (CA) domain [10] – that also recruits the viral genomic RNA, through the interaction between the nucleocapsid (NC) domain and the RNA packaging signal (*Psi* sequence) [11]. The NC domain also mediates the formation of the RNA dimer via a palindromic sequence in the dimer linkage structure (DLS) sequence, which is located in the *Psi* sequence. In addition, specific cellular tRNAs are packaged. The assembly of the virus particle, which final steps occur at the plasma membrane (reviewed in [12]), is partly regulated by the Vpu and Vif proteins, which play an important role in the assembly of the virus. At the cell membrane, the immature viruses are released and maturation takes place through polypeptide cleavage mediated by the viral protease. The mature virus is now able to infect other cells.

3. Organization of viral genome

The majority of replication competent retroviruses depend on three genes: "group specific-antigen" (*gag*), "polymerase" (*pol*) and "envelope"(*env*) genes. The “classic” structure of a retroviral genome is: 5'LTR-*gag*-*pol*-*env*-LTR 3 ' (Figure 2). The non-coding LTR ('long terminal repeat") represents the two ends of the viral genome and they are linked to host cell DNA after integration. The *gag* and *env* genes encode the core and the viral envelope glycoproteins respectively. The *pol* gene encodes for the RT, IN and protease [13]. In addition, HIV contains in its 9.749 kb RNA, six additional genes: *vif, vpu* (only in HIV-1), *vpr, vpx* (only in HIV-2), *tat, rev, and nef*) which contribute to their genetic complexity and helps virus in several steps during replication cycle [14].

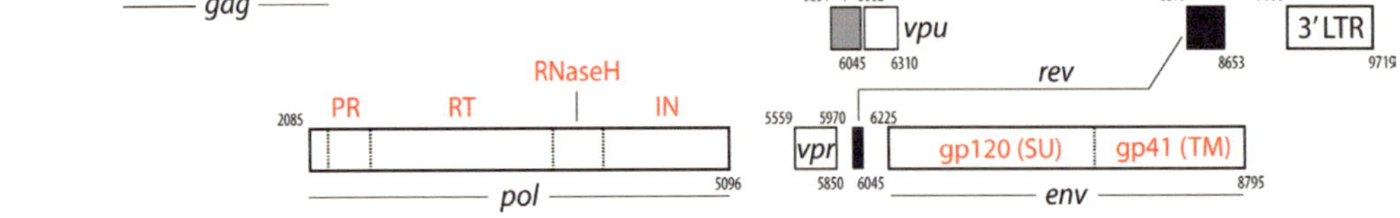

Figure 2. HIV-1 genome organization. The major viral proteins encoded by *gag*, *pol* and *env* genes are indicated in red. Numbers indicate the beginning and ending of each gene according to nucleotide numbering of HXB2CG HIV-1 strain (GenBank accession number: K03455).

http://dx.doi.org/10.5772/60795

The *vif* gene codes for Vif, a protein that increases the infectivity of the HIV particle. This protein is found inside HIV-infected cells, and its main function is to interfere with one of the innate immune system's defenses - a cellular protein called APOBEC3G [15].

The "Viral protein U", (coded by *vpu* gene), enhances the release of new viral particles, helping them to bud from the host cell. Vpu also works within the infected cell to enhance the degradation of CD4 protein. This has the effect of reducing the amount of CD4 present in plasma membrane, therefore reducing the likelihood of superinfection [16].

The "Viral protein R", (coded by *vpr* gene), is incorporated into viral particles through a specific interaction with Gag proteins. It has several functions during intracellular steps of viral replication. For instance, Vpr is present in the PIC and has been shown to influence the reverse transcription and the nuclear import of viral DNA; it also modulates cell cycle progression and apoptosis of infected cell [17].

Tat and Rev are regulatory proteins coded by *tat* and *rev* genes. They are present in the nucleus of infected cells and bind to defined regions of the viral DNA and RNA. These proteins enhances the transcription of proviral DNA into mRNA, promote the RNA elongation, stimulate the transport of HIV-1 mRNA from the nucleus to the cytoplasm and also are essential for translation [9].

Tat is a regulatory transactivator protein, which enhances the activation of HIV long terminal repeat (LTR) increasing the efficiency of HIV genomic transcription. This enhancement is also the result of additional interaction between Tat and cellular transcription factors such as NF-κB and SP-1. Furthermore, Tat also plays a crucial role in AIDS pathogenesis, especially in the development of HIV-associated dementia, dysregulation of cytokine expression and induction of apoptosis [9]. As referred earlier in this chapter, Rev facilitates the nuclear export of single-spliced and unspliced viral mRNAs (~4 kb and ~9 kb mRNAs respectively). The molecular mechanism underlying Rev activity involves a direct interaction between Rev protein and a *cis*-acting sequence-specific target named RRE (Rev-responsive element). RRE is found within the *env* gene in all incompletely spliced mRNAs [9, 18]. It has been shown that Nef protein has several functions. It induces down-regulation of CD4 [19] and the HLA class I and II molecules from the surface of HIV infected cells [20], which may represent an important escape mechanism for the virus to avoid recognition by CD4+ T cells. Nef may also interfere with T cell activation, as a result of selective binding to various proteins that are involved in intracellular signaling [21].

4. Cellular factors with inhibitory activity on HIV replication and implications in viral pathogenesis

Innate immunity had evolved as a mechanism to defend eukaryotes from bacterial and viral infections. These mechanisms rely on different cellular restriction factors that suppress the replication of the pathogens, namely retroviruses [22].

During HIV-1 infection, incoming viral RNA triggers a TLR7/8-mediated innate immune response, resulting in the production of type I interferon (IFN). In particular IFNα has been shown to be up-regulated after TLR sensing during acute infection with HIV-1 or SIV [23-25]. Accordingly, initial observations *in vitro* revealed that pre-treatment of macrophages with type-I IFN inhibited the replication of HIV-1, indicating that potent inhibitory factors were induced after IFN exposure [26, 27]. Most of them are still uncharacterized.

The identification of cellular restriction factors and the viral proteins that antagonize those restrictions have stimulated an active area of research that explores crucial mechanisms underlying HIV interference with cellular restriction factors and innate immunity. In this subchapter specific cellular factors with inhibitory activity on HIV replication are discussed including how viral-encoded proteins counteract these factors.

4.1. TRIM5α

The search for the mechanisms underlying the innate cellular resistance to retroviral infections shown by different non-human primate species, has led to the identification of a cytoplasmic factor that prevented infection of Old World monkeys by HIV-1 [28]. This factor – TRIM5α – was identified as a member of the tripartite motif (TRIM) family of proteins, a large family of cellular proteins with distinct biological activities including innate immune signaling [29]. After its initial identification in rhesus macaques (rhTRIM5α) [28] and owl monkeys (TRIM-Cyp) [30], TRIM5α was also identified as a retroviral restriction factor in humans [31, 32] that is induced by both type I and type II IFN [33].

Different models have been proposed for retroviral inhibition mediated by TRIM5 proteins [34]. They suggest that these proteins mediate restriction by directly binding to specific determinants in the viral CA protein, blocking HIV replication soon after viral release in host cell cytoplasm. The TRIM proteins family is defined by three domains (RING, B-Box2, and Coiled- Coil), which are present in all members of this family. The N-terminal RING domain possesses E3 ubiquitin ligase activity that is crucial for retrovirus restriction [35, 36]. The B-Box2 and Coiled Coil (CC) domains are thought to contribute to the higher and low order multimerization of TRIM5α, respectively. The TRIM5α also possesses a C-terminal capsid binding domain that mediates specific recognition and restriction of certain retroviruses [37]. The recognition of viral capsid determinants (CA protein) relies on three variable regions present in the C-terminal domain of TRIM5α, and apparently they are equally involved in retrovirus recognition and restriction [38-41].

Several studies have addressed the mechanisms by which TRIM5α protein prevents viral infection and different models have been proposed to explain this restriction. The "accelerated uncoating" model was based on the observation that cytosolic CA protein was specifically dissociated in rhTRIM5α-expressing cells [42] leading to the proposal of a "proteasome independent capsid degradation" mechanism. This model suggests that the stripping of capsid protein prevents viral RTC to proceed to subsequent steps in infectious replication cycle, namely the reverse transcription and nuclear import [42]. An alternative model was primarily based on the observation that proteasome inhibitors allows reverse transcription and integration, without affecting the TRIM5α-mediated restriction [43, 44]. Accordingly, a "two-step restriction mechanism" was proposed, suggesting that restriction activity of TRIM5α occurs by both proteasome-dependent and -independent pathways. The relative contribution of each pathway is apparently dependent on host cells-viruses combinations [45].

4.2. APOBEC3

One important form of intrinsic immunity against retroviral infections is provided by apolipoprotein B mRNA-editing enzyme catalytic polypeptide-like (APOBEC) family proteins, and particularly by human APOBEC3G (A3G) and APOBEC3F (A3F) [46-49]. These two proteins are cellular antiretroviral factors that possess inhibitory activity against HIV-1 replication [22, 48, 50].

APOBEC proteins act on single-stranded DNA or RNA substrates and their main function is to induce alterations in the nucleotide sequence through cytidine deamination, converting cytidines to uridines (C to U) or deoxycytidines (dC) to deoxyuridines (dU).

The A3G protein, which expression seems to be regulated at a transcriptional level through NFAT and IRF binding to specific sites located in A3G promoter region [51, 52], is packed inside newly formed HIV-1 virions by a specific interaction with the amino-terminal region of NC domain of HIV-1 Gag polyprotein [53-57]. As expected due to the interaction with NC, A3G is present in viral core as a ribonucleoprotein complex together with genomic RNA, NC, IN and Vpr [58]. Interestingly, binding of A3G to HIV genomic RNA led to inactivation of deaminase activity, while the action of HIV RNase H, which degrades the RNA chain during reverse transcription activates its enzymatic activity [58]. After viral entry into a new cell and during reverse transcription, the released A3G targets the minus-strand DNA product and induces a dC to dU deamination resulting in a dG to dA hypermutation in the HIV-1 double-stranded DNA genome of the replicating virus. This hypermutation activity ultimately introduces mutations and stop codons that disrupt the normal expression and function of viral proteins [46, 59]. A3G can also interfere directly with viral reverse transcriptase preventing RT-dependent cDNA elongation independently of deaminase activity [60]. Finally there is also evidence suggesting that A3G reduces the integration of HIV-1 DNA by interfering with PIC functions [61, 62]. In addition to A3G, also A3F seems to exhibit inhibitory activity against HIV-1 replication [47, 49, 63, 64].

Despite their ability to hinder HIV replication, these proteins only show their potent inhibitory effect with HIV-1 mutants lacking a functional *vif* gene, since the Vif protein expressed by wild-type HIV-1 blocks the function of these host cell proteins [50, 65-70]. Basically, Vif binds to A3G in the cytoplasm of infected cell and directs it for polyubiquitination and proteasomal degradation, preventing its inclusion into the newly formed virions thus overcoming the inhibition of viral replication mediated by A3G [67-69, 71]. A cellular E3 ubiquitin ligase complex consisting of cullin5, elonginB, elonginC and RING finger proteins that binds an E2 ubiquitin-conjugated enzyme, induces the polyubiquitination of A3G. This complex is recruited by Vif that connects it to its substrate inducing the polyubiquitination of A3G [67-69, 71-73]. Additionally, Vif also interferes with the translation of A3G mRNA, reducing its intracellular pool [72, 74].

Besides A3G and A3F proteins, the human genome also contains genes encoding five others members of the APOBEC3 family. However, of these five additional genes, apparently only three (APOBEC3A, APOBEC3B and APOBEC3C) are expressed in human cells. Recent data shows that APOBEC3A is recruited at post-entry HIV-1 replication complexes [75-79]. Its expression is induced in monocyte-derived macrophages (MDM) by interferon-alpha (IFN-α) and it seems to promote resistance to HIV-1 infection in MDM [75]. The APOBEC3C protein is a weak inhibitor of wild-type or *vif*-deficient HIV-1 [63, 64, 80] although it was described, together with APOBEC3B, as a potent inhibitor of simian immunodeficiency virus (SIV) replication [81]. As for A3G, the APOBEC3B protein is also packed inside HIV-1 virions due to a specific interaction with the NC protein. It induces a potent inhibition of HIV-1 replication and it seems to be resistant to HIV-1 Vif protein [82]. However, APOBEC3B is expressed at very low levels in human tissues, in contrast to A3G and A3F [82].

4.3. Tetherin/ BST-2

In early 2008, an additional restriction factor dubbed Tetherin, previously referred to as BST-2, CD317 or HM1.24, was described [83, 84]. The main function of this IFN-induced protein [85, 86] remained elusive until it was identified as an intrinsic antiviral factor that restricts the egress of HIV and other enveloped viruses by tethering mature virions to the host cell membrane [83, 84, 87-91]. Tetherin is a type II membrane protein highly expressed at the plasma membrane of B cells at all differentiation stages, bone-marrow CD34+ cells and T-cells [92]. It has an unusual topology consisting of an amino-terminal cytoplasmic tail (CT), followed by a transmembrane region that anchors tetherin to the plasma membrane and a coiled-coil extracellular domain that is also linked to the plasma membrane by a carboxy-terminal glycophosphatidylinositol (GPI) anchor [93, 94]. Due to the presence of this GPI anchor, tetherin is mainly located in cholesterol-rich microdomains also referred as "lipid rafts". Tetherin is involved (through the CT domain) in the organization of subapical actin cytoskeleton in polarized epithelial cells [95] and unlike other GPI-anchored proteins, is endocytosed from lipid rafts in a clathrin-mediated pathway [96].

Coincident with the identification of tetherin as an antiviral factor, it was also found that it was the target of the HIV-1 accessory protein Vpu, providing a plausible mechanism for the well-established but ill-defined, virus-release function of Vpu [83]. The Vpu is a small transmembrane (TM) protein encoded by the *vpu* gene present in the genomes of HIV-1 and some SIV strains, but absent in HIV-2. It is anchored to the plasma membrane of the infected cell by its amino-terminal region. Initial studies showed that Vpu protein besides its ability to degrade CD4 protein [97], was also required for efficient replication of HIV-1 in some cell types and that the restriction factor counteracted by Vpu was a protein located at cell surface [16, 98-101]. This factor was found to be IFNα-inducible and showed the ability to block the release of Vpu-defective virions by directly tethering them to the plasma membrane of virus-producer cells. The trapped virions are subsequently internalized by endocytosis and probably degraded in lysosomes [83, 85]. Remarkably, the lipid rafts localization of tetherin is coincident with the preferential site for budding and egress of enveloped viruses [102, 103], providing further explanation for the mechanism by which tetherin blocks virion release. Several aspects of the Vpu-mediated antagonism of tetherin are still controversial. It was initially proposed that Vpu impairs the transport of newly synthetized tetherin by sequestering it within the trans-Golgi network [104-106]. Additionally, Vpu might block the recycling of tetherin after its internalization from the lipid rafts [104, 106, 107]. Finally, it was also proposed that Vpu might directly internalize tetherin from cell membrane [108-110]. Interestingly, it was observed that treatment with proteasomal inhibitors lead to increased levels of tetherin and loss of Vpu-mediated enhancement of HIV-1 release. These results suggest that the Vpu-induced down-regulation of tetherin might at least in part involve proteasomal degradation of the restriction factor [111-113]. The exact mechanisms of tetherin down-modulation from cell surface, intracellular sequestration or degradation remain to be determined. These three distinct mechanisms may act cooperatively counteracting tetherin to varying degrees in different cellular contexts. Regardless the model that is preferentially observed, binding of Vpu to tetherin through TM-TM interaction seems to be crucial for Vpu antagonism of the restriction factor [108, 111, 114, 115].

Despite the wide cellular distribution of tetherin and the need to counteract its viral restriction action, most primate lentiviruses do not contain a *vpu* gene. Some (e.g. SIVsmm, SIVmac, and SIVagm) use their Nef proteins to antagonize tetherin function [116-118]. This is not surprising since Nef protein - a myristoylated protein coded by *nef* gene essential for HIV replication *in vivo* - is known to act as an adaptor protein interacting with different cellular proteins. Through these interactions Nef manipulates cellular trafficking, signal transduction and gene expression in HIV infected cells (reviewed in [119]). Apparently, Nef targets the cytoplasmic tail of tetherin reducing its expression at host cell membrane [116, 118]. In alternative to Nef, HIV-2 relies on its envelope glycoprotein Env to antagonize tetherin. The proposed mechanism suggests that Env interacts directly with the ectodomain of tetherin, sequestering it away from sites of virus budding and targeting it to clathrin-mediated endocytosis [120].

Besides the referred lentiviruses, the antiviral activity of tetherin was also demonstrated against a broad range of unrelated viruses, such as filoviruses [87, 88], arenaviruses [88] and herpesviruses [121, 122]. For some of these viruses specific viral encoded antagonists has been described. For example, human herpesviruses 8 (HHV-8, also known as Kaposi's Sarcoma herpesvirus) uses K5/MIR2 - a viral protein belonging to the membrane-associated RING-CH ubiquitin ligase family - to ubiquitinate tetherin and target it for degradation [121]. In Ebola virus - a filovirus associated with hemorrhagic fever outbreaks - the tetherin-mediated restriction is counteracted by viral envelope glycoprotein [123] in a process similar to the described sequestration of tetherin by HIV-2 Env.

4.4. SAMHD1

Myeloid-lineage cells, including monocytes, dendritic cells (DCs) and macrophages, play a multifaceted role in HIV-1 initial infection and viral dissemination during acute infection. In particular, the interactions between HIV and DCs are connected with all aspects of HIV infection *in vivo*, including transmission, pathogenesis and immune control (recently reviewed in [124]). DCs exposed to HIV during sexual transmission help viral dissemination and systemic infection by two distinct mechanisms: by becoming productively infected or by transferring HIV to CD4+ T cells during immunologic synapse (IS), even in the absence of DCs infection [125-127].

Although DCs can be infected, HIV replication is generally less productive compared with CD4+ T cells. Nevertheless, extensive viral replication takes place once DCs come into contact with CD4+ T cells in lymphoid tissue in the context of IS [128]. This implies that HIV must be able to evade DC's innate immune sensing and endolysosomal degradation and then make use of DC maturation and migration to draining lymph nodes to be transmitted to highly susceptible T cells during antigen presentation process within lymph nodes (reviewed in [129]).

Infection by DNA or RNA viruses triggers innate immune responses when host recognizes specific viral molecular structures (e.g. nucleic acid and surface glycoprotein), called pattern-associated molecular patterns (PAMPs) [130-132]. These PAMPs are recognized by pattern-recognition receptors (PRRs), such as Toll-like receptors (TLRs), RIG-I-like helicases (RLH), and cytosolic DNA sensor proteins. Inside the cytoplasm, viral nucleic acid can be detected by different PRRs depending on the cell type. For example, TLR7 and TLR9 are responsible for detection of viral RNA and DNA, respectively, in plasmacytoid dendritic cells (pDCs), whereas RLHs detect viral RNA in conventional DCs, macrophages and fibroblasts [133, 134]. The recognition of PAMPs by the PRRs activates several transcription factors, namely nuclear factor-κappa binding (NF-κB) and IFN regulatory factors (IRFs). This activation leads to the production of pro-inflammatory cytokines and type-I IFNs (IFN-α and IFN-β), respectively (reviewed in [130]). The production of type-I IFNs induces the expression of hundreds of interferon-stimulated genes (ISGs) [135], providing crucial mechanisms of antiviral defense by inhibiting viral replication and spread. For example, during HIV Infection, viral single-stranded RNA (ssRNA) is recognized by TLR7/8 initiating anti-HIV immune response by inducing type I IFN. However, as a well-adapted human pathogen HIV must be able to avoid – at least in part – these cell sensing mechanisms in order to evade host innate immunity.

Sterile alpha motif (SAM) and histidine/aspartic acid (HD) domain-containing protein 1 (SAMHD1), an analogue of the murine IFN-y-induced gene Mg11 [136], was identified as a HIV-1 restriction factor that blocks early-stage virus replication in DCs and other myeloid cells [137, 138]. It acts by depleting the intracellular pool of deoxynucleoside triphosphates (dNTP), thus impairing HIV-1 reverse transcription and productive infection [139-141]. The expected lower replication in DCs may enable HIV-1 to avoid intracellular viral sensor that would otherwise trigger IFN-mediated antiviral immunity [142, 143]. It seems that while SAMHD1 effectively renders DCs less permissive to HIV-1 infection, it is somewhat paradoxically responsible for the HIV-1 evasion of immune sensing and subsequent poor priming of adaptive immunity.

HIV-2 brings in a new and interesting element: Vpx (an accessory protein encoded by *vpx* gene, present in SIVsm/SIVmac and HIV-2), that is believed to have originated by duplication of the common *vpr* gene present in primate lentiviruses [144], possibly to compensate for a theorised low HIV-2 RT affinity for dNTPs [145, 146]. This accessory protein antagonizes the effect of SAMHD1 by targeting it for proteasomal degradation using the host cell E3 ubiquitin ligase complex, in which Vpx interacts with the DCAF1 subunit of the CUL4A/DDB1 ubiquitin ligase to degrade SAMHD1 via the proteasome [137, 139, 147, 148]. The degradation of SAMHD1 renders HIV-2-infected DCs much more permissive to productive infection and viral replication, allowing faster accumulation of full length viral DNA [148]. This results in a widely positive DC-specific effect in the innate immune sensing of HIV-2 infection [143, 146, 148, 149] and it may be related to the lower viral load and slower progression to AIDS that is characteristic of HIV-2 infection (reviewed in [150]). The immunologically positive effects of Vpx was also demonstrated in monocyte-derived DCs (MMDCs) infected with HIV-1 where an increased type I IFN production and up-regulation of CD86 was only observed in the presence of Vpx [146]. Hence, by avoiding productive infection of MDDCs through preservation of SAMHD1 function, HIV-1 may also control viral antigen presentation, resulting in qualitatively or quantitatively minor CD8+ and CD4+ responses [146, 149, 151]. Furthermore, individuals with low SAMHD1 activity or silenced SAMHD1, present an enhanced immune response to HIV-1 infection, as previously hypothesised [139, 143] [139, 143] and demonstrated [146].

4.5. MxB

The myxovirus resistance (Mx) genes were discovered in the 1960s when it was observed that wild mice were resistant to influenza viruses, whereas inbred mice were susceptible [152]. This trait was later mapped to a locus on mouse chromosome 16 [153-156]. Mx family proteins are found in almost all vertebrates, demonstrating their evolutionary importance for host organisms [157]. Humans Mx gene resides on chromossome 21 [158] and encodes two proteins, called MxA and MxB, that belong to the family of dynamin-like large GTPases. The MxA protein has been recognized as a potent cell restriction factor with antiviral activity against pathogenic DNA and RNA viruses [159].

The X-ray crystal structure of human MxA showed that this protein can be divided into a globular GTPase head, a largely C-terminal α-helical stalk domain and a series of α-helices found in sequences adjacent to these domains which fold in the protein tertiary structure to form the bundle signaling element (BSE) [160]. On the basis of sequence homology and computer modeling the predicted structure of MxB is almost superimposable with that of MxA, having 63% amino acid sequence identity.

In contrast to human MxA protein that inhibits a variety of viruses [161], MxB was initially described as lacking antiviral activity against influenza or vesicular stomatitis virus [162]. Instead, MxB was solely related to cellular functions, such as regulating nuclear import and cell-cycle progression [163, 164].

This view was challenged in 2011, when Schoggings and collaborators addressed an overexpression screening to test the antiviral activity of more than 380 human interferon stimulated gene (ISGs) products against a panel of viruses, where they first uncovered an antiviral activity of human MxB against HIV-1 [165].

More recently, three additional studies [166-168] showed that MxB overexpression potently reduces the permissiveness of the cells in a single-cycle HV-1 infection assay. They also demonstrate that silencing MxB expression reduced the inhibitory potency of the interferon-α demonstrating its importancc in the interferon-mediated response against the early steps of HIV-1 infection.

The next step was to understand which specific post-entry event of the HIV replication cycle was affected by MxB expression. Recent studies agreed that MxB expression potently inhibited HIV-1 infection after reverse transcription but before integration [166-168]. So MxB might be interfering with one or more of the following processes: 1) HIV-1 uncoating; 2) nuclear import of the HIV-1 PIC; or 3) nuclear maturation of the PIC.

Fricke and colleagues [169] suggested a model in which MxB binds to the HIV-1 core in the cytoplasm of the cell and prevents the uncoating process of HIV-1 through stabilization of incoming viral capsides. In addition, they demonstrated that MxB requires capsid binding and oligomerization for effective restriction.

More recently, Matreyek et al. [170] observed that MxB restricts HIV-1 after DNA synthesis at steps that are coincident with PIC nuclear import and integration.

HIV-1 RNA is reverse transcribed into double stranded linear DNA and carries a fraction of the viron CA protein [171, 172]. HIV-1 CA protein is known to play a central role in mediating physical interactions with several host proteins involved in the post-entry step of infection. Some identified residues of CA involved in binding to cyclophilin A (CypA), TRIM5α, TNP03, CPSF6, NUP153 and NUP358/RanBP2 are also critical for the sensitivity of HIV-1 to the antiviral action of MxB. Results obtained by Liu and colleagues indicate that both silencing of CypA expression or disruption of the CA-CypA interaction by addition of cyclosporine A abrogated the antiviral activity of MxB, thus CypA binding to the HIV-1 CA appears to be required for MXB restriction. Furthermore, results obtained by diverse groups indicate that CA mutations counteracted MxB restriction [165-168, 170].

The viral integrase (IN) protein processes the long terminal repeat (LTR) ends of the viral DNA to yield the integration-competent PIC, which subsequently transports the viral DNA into the nucleus for IN-mediated integration [173]. Matreyek and collaborators [170] found evidence for an additional block in the formation of 2-LTR circular viral DNA (that are only present in the nucleus, and thus have been utilized as a marker of nuclear entry of viral DNA [174]). In contrast, results obtained by Liu and collaborators [167] showed that MxB reduces the levels of integrated HIV-1 DNA, though it does not affect the amount of 2-LTR circles. They concluded that MxB impairs the integration step and spares the nuclear entry of viral DNA.

Apparently, MxB antiviral activity is independent of its GTPase active site residues or stalk domain Loop4 (both previously shown to be necessary for MxA function) that confer functional oligomerization to related dynamin family proteins [166, 168]. There are two locations in MxB that exhibit the greatest sequence dissimilarity with MxA. The first one is Loop4 that is not critical for MxB antiviral activity but is important for the MxA inhibition of Influenza A and Thogotovirus infection [170, 175]. The other part of MxB with greatest dissimilarity to MxA is the N-terminal region. The specific particular functions conferred by this region are particularly important for MxB activity and consequent HIV-1 restriction [170].

In a global perspective, the post-entry step of HIV-1 replication cycle appears to be quite vulnerable to the actions of IFN-inducible restriction factors: TRIM5α, APOBEC3 proteins, SAMHD1 and, more recently, MxB use distinct mechanisms to prevent integration of this pathogenic virus in host genome. Certainly it will continue to be of interest to the scientific community the study of restriction factors of viral infection by antiviral host factors due to its impact in many areas. These findings raises hope as a potential clinical and epidemiological relevant approach which could be exploited to control HIV infections and AIDS.

4.6. Cholesterol-25-hydroxylase

Recently, a new antiviral IFN-induced protein (cholesterol 25-hydroxilase; CH25H) was identified as being able to block the fusion between viral envelope and target cell membrane. It exhibits a broadly antiviral activity against several enveloped virus including HIV, Ebola virus (Zaire strain), vesicular stomatitis virus, herpes simplex virus I, Rift Valley fever virus, Nipah virus, Influenza A (H1N1) virus and varicella zoster virus [176, 177]. It also revealed antiviral effect against poliovirus [178], a non-enveloped virus. The IFN-induced cholesterol-25-hydroxylase (*Ch25h*) gene encodes an endoplasmic-reticulum-associated enzyme (CH25H) that mediates the oxidation of cholesterol, by the addition of an extra hydroxyl group at position 25, converting it to 25-hydroxycholesterol (25HC). 25HC belongs to a large class of endogenous cholesterol derivatives named oxysterols. In addition to their involvement in basic metabolic processes, e.g. bile acids production in the liver [179], oxysterols also play a key role in several signaling pathways that influence the activation of macrophages, T-cells and B-cells, and thus the regulation of inflammatory response [177, 180-188].

Although several antiviral mechanisms have been suggested for CH25H and 25HC, they seem to inhibited HIV-1 replication by blocking the virus-cell fusion step [176]. One possible mechanism underlying this effect is the induction of cellular membrane changes affecting the topology and permissiveness for fusion of host cell membrane. There is extensive evidence that the lipid composition of target cell membrane influences HIV-1 fusion and entry. In fact, though the fusion event is triggered by HIV envelope glycoproteins, lipids also play a key role in virus-cell membrane fusion by themselves, directly affecting the viral receptor accessibility and distribution in lipid rafts domains of the plasma membrane, or the membrane fluidity and curvature [189]. The modifications in cellular membrane architecture induced by 25HC (considerably more hydrophilic than cholesterol [190]) would be of outstanding importance in the complex protein-lipid interplay required for successful virus-cell fusion events [176].

5. Conclusion

The pathogenesis of HIV infection is a highly complex network of interconnected processes. It likely borrows much of its complexity from the co-evolution with several mammalian species that HIV and predecessors lentiviruses have enjoyed over an unknown, but rather long period of time. During the complex interplay between HIV and host cell, different intrinsic cell factors are involved that mitigate or restrict HIV replication and spread as shown in Figure 3. Some of these host restrictions factors that have been identified inhibit early steps of replication cycle. In fact, the post-entry step of HIV-1 replication cycle appears to be quite vulnerable to the actions of IFN-inducible restriction factors: TRIM5α, APOBEC3 proteins, SAMHD1 and, more recently, MxB and cholesterol 25-hydroxylase, all of them use distinct mechanisms to prevent integration of viral DNA into host genome. The best characterized of these are the TRIM5α and the APOBEC3 proteins. APOBEC3 interacts with the nascent DNA during reverse transcription while TRIM5α interacts with incoming viral capsids resulting in premature disassembly. SAMHD1 protein acts prior to integration, by depleting the intracellular pool of deoxynucleoside triphosphates (dNTP), therefore impairing HIV-1 reverse transcription and accumulation of HIV double stranded DNA. Another restriction factor, Tetherin (BST- 2/

CD317), acts in late steps of viral replication cycle, by preventing viruses from leaving the cell during budding and release of viral particles. The recently described factors MxB and cholesterol 25-hydroxylase seem to inhibit the nuclear import/integration of viral DNA and the viral fusion events, respectively. Remarkably, despite this array of restriction factors, HIV had created viral proteins to subdue these restrictions emphasizing how well adapted this virus is to human host.

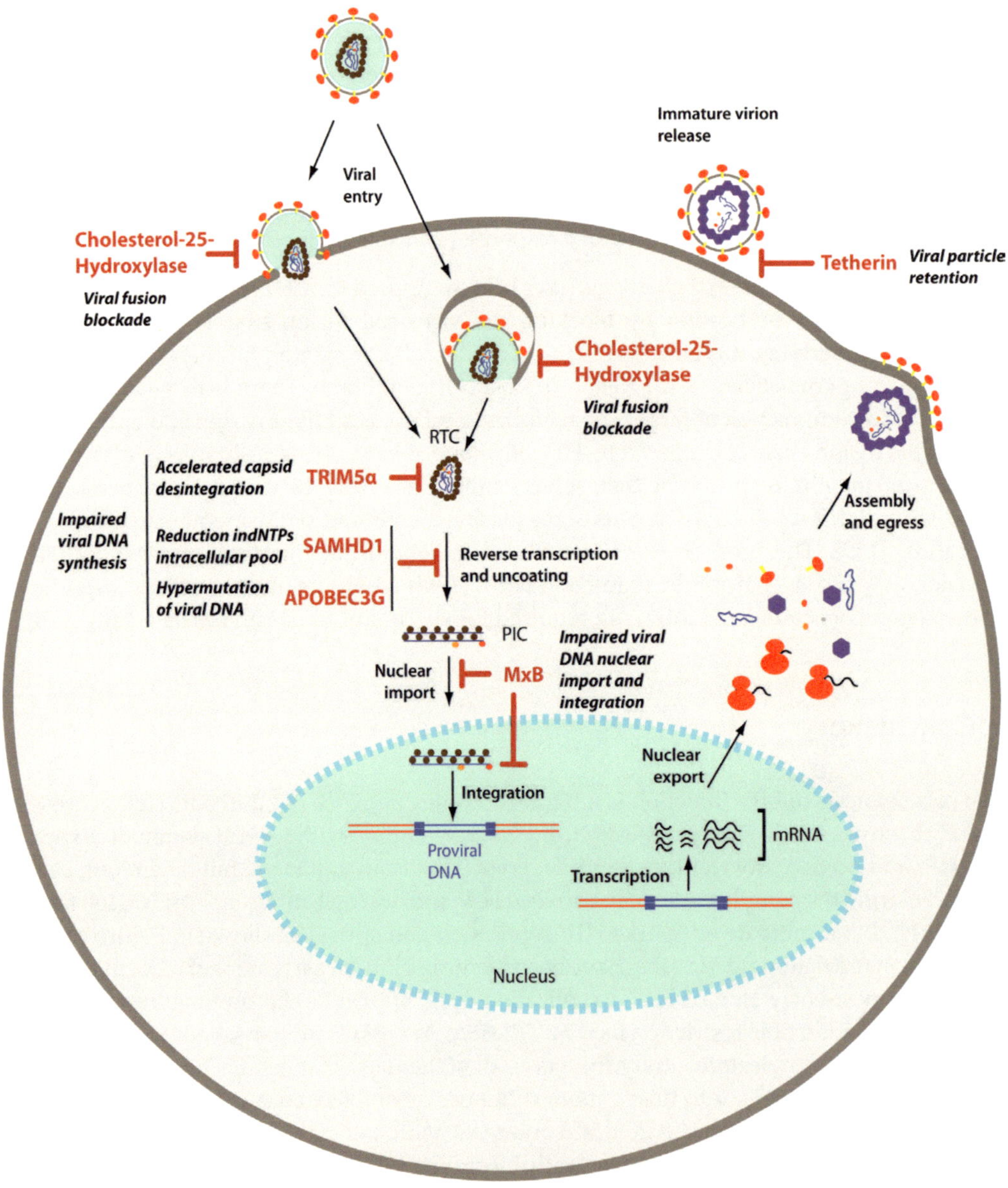

Figure 3. Schematic representation of a simplified replication cycle of HIV and the different steps that are blocked by cellular restriction factors. The cholesterol-25-hydroxylase blocks viral fusion with target cell membrane; TRIM5α, SAMHD1 and APOBEC3G impair viral DNA synthesis either by accelerating capsid disintegration, reducing dNTPs

intracellular pool or by introducing mutations in nascent chain of viral DNA; MxB impairs the nuclear import and/or the integration step; and finally, Tetherin induces virion retention at the host-cell membrane.

Finally, the identification of cellular restriction factors, such as those referred in this chapter, and the disclosure of the mechanisms by which they impede viral replication, also enabled the identification of new promising targets for therapeutic intervention. In fact, it is increasingly clear that the most successful treatment and/or prevention strategies will likely be derived from the modulation of human cell functions rather than acting directly upon viral mechanisms.

Acknowledgements

This work was supported by grants from Fundação para a Ciência e Tecnologia and Ministério da Saúde de Portugal (VIH/SAU/0006/2011) and from Gilead Sciences Portugal (Programa Gilead Génese).

Author details

J.M. Azevedo-Pereira[1,2*], Pedro Canhão[3], Marta Calado[1,2], Quirina Santos-Costa[1,2] and Pedro Barroca[4]

*Address all correspondence to: miguel.pereira@ff.ul.pt

1 Host-Pathogen Interaction Unit, Research Institute for Medicines (iMed.ULisboa), Faculty of Pharmacy, University of Lisbon (Faculdade de Famácia, Universidade de Lisboa), Lisboa, Portugal

2 Institute for Molecular Medicine (IMM). Faculty of Pharmacy, University of Lisbon (Faculdade de Farmácia, Universidade de Lisboa), Lisboa, Portugal

3 Technophage SA, Lisboa, Portugal

4 National Pharmacies Association (Associação Nacional de Farmácias), Lisboa, Portugal

References

[1] Melikyan GB. HIV entry: a game of hide-and-fuse? Current Opinion in Virology 2014;4:1–7.

[2] Alkhatib G, Combadiere C, Broder CC, Feng Y, Kennedy PE, Murphy PM, et al. CC CKR5: a RANTES, MIP-1alpha, MIP-1beta receptor as a fusion cofactor for macrophage-tropic HIV-1. Science 1996;272:1955–8.

[3] Feng Y, Broder CC, Kennedy PE, Berger EA. HIV-1 entry cofactor: functional cDNA cloning of a seven-transmembrane, G protein-coupled receptor. Science 1996;272:872–7.

[4] Clapham PR, McKnight A. Cell surface receptors, virus entry and tropism of primate lentiviruses. The Journal of General Virology 2002;83:1809–29.

[5] Doms RW, Trono D. The plasma membrane as a combat zone in the HIV battlefield. Genes & Development 2000;14:2677–88.

[6] Marsh M, Helenius A. Virus entry: open sesame. Cell 2006;124:729–40.

[7] Miyauchi K, Kim Y, Latinovic O, Morozov V, Melikyan GB. HIV enters cells via endocytosis and dynamin-dependent fusion with endosomes. Cell 2009;137:433–44.

[8] Suzuki Y, Craigie R. The road to chromatin - nuclear entry of retroviruses. Nature Reviews Microbiology 2007;5:187–96.

[9] Strebel K. Virus-host interactions: role of HIV proteins Vif, Tat, and Rev. Aids 2003;17 Suppl 4:S25–34.

[10] Gelderblom HR. Assembly and morphology of HIV: potential effect of structure on viral function. Aids 1991;5:617–37.

[11] Zhang Y, Qian H, Love Z, Barklis E. Analysis of the assembly function of the human immunodeficiency virus type 1 gag protein nucleocapsid domain. Journal of Virology 1998;72:1782–9.

[12] Meng B, Lever AM. Wrapping up the bad news - HIV assembly and release. Retrovirology 2013;10:5.

[13] Frankel AD, Young JAT. HIV-1: Fifteen Proteins and an RNA. Annual Review of Biochemistry 1998;67:1–25.

[14] Strebel K. HIV accessory proteins versus host restriction factors. Current Opinion in Virology 2013;3:692–9.

[15] Desimmie BA, Delviks-Frankenberrry KA, Burdick RC, Qi D, Izumi T, Pathak VK. Multiple APOBEC3 restriction factors for HIV-1 and one Vif to rule them all. Journal of Molecular Biology 2014;426:1220–45.

[16] Dubé M, Bego MG, Paquay C, Cohen EA. Modulation of HIV-1-host interaction: role of the Vpu accessory protein. Retrovirology 2010;7:114.

[17] Guenzel CA, Hérate C, Benichou S. HIV-1 Vpr-a still "enigmatic multitasker." Frontiers in Microbiology 2014;5:127.

[18] Pollard VW, Malim MH. The HIV-1 Rev protein. Annual Review of Microbiology 1998;52:491–532.

[19] Aiken C, Konner J, Landau NR, Lenburg ME, Trono D. Nef induces CD4 endocytosis: requirement for a critical dileucine motif in the membrane-proximal CD4 cytoplasmic domain. Cell 1994;76:853–64.

[20] Collins KL, Chen BK, Kalams SA, Walker BD, Baltimore D. HIV-1 Nef protein protects infected primary cells against killing by cytotoxic T lymphocytes. Nature 1998;391:397–401.

[21] Kirchhoff F, Schindler M, Specht A, Arhel N, Munch J. Role of Nef in primate lentiviral immunopathogenesis. Cellular and Molecular Life Sciences : CMLS 2008;65:2621–36.

[22] Bieniasz PD. Intrinsic immunity: a front-line defense against viral attack. Nature Immunology 2004;5:1109–15.

[23] Pitha PM. Innate antiviral response: role in HIV-1 infection. Viruses 2011;3:1179–203.

[24] Stacey AR, Norris PJ, Qin L, Haygreen EA, Taylor E, Heitman J, et al. Induction of a striking systemic cytokine cascade prior to peak viremia in acute human immunodeficiency virus type 1 infection, in contrast to more modest and delayed responses in acute hepatitis B and C virus infections. Journal of Virology 2009;83:3719–33.

[25] Malleret B, Manéglier B, Karlsson I, Lebon P, Nascimbeni M, Perié L, et al. Primary infection with simian immunodeficiency virus: plasmacytoid dendritic cell homing to lymph nodes, type I interferon, and immune suppression. Blood 2008;112:4598–608.

[26] Kornbluth RS, Oh PS, Munis JR, Cleveland PH, Richman DD. Interferons and bacterial lipopolysaccharide protect macrophages from productive infection by human immunodeficiency virus in vitro. The Journal of Experimental Medicine 1989;169:1137–51.

[27] Meylan PR, Guatelli JC, Munis JR, Richman DD, Kornbluth RS. Mechanisms for the inhibition of HIV replication by interferons-alpha, -beta, and -gamma in primary human macrophages. Virology 1993;193:138–48.

[28] Stremlau M, Owens CM, Perron MJ, Kiessling M, Autissier P, Sodroski JG. The cytoplasmic body component TRIM5alpha restricts HIV-1 infection in Old World monkeys. Nature 2004;427:848–53.

[29] Grütter MG, Luban J. TRIM5 structure, HIV-1 capsid recognition, and innate immune signaling. Current Opinion in Virology 2012;2:142–50.

[30] Sayah DM, Sokolskaja E, Berthoux L, Luban J. Cyclophilin A retrotransposition into TRIM5 explains owl monkey resistance to HIV-1. Nature 2004;430:569–73.

[31] Keckesova Z, Ylinen LMJ, Towers GJ. The human and African green monkey TRIM5alpha genes encode Ref1 and Lv1 retroviral restriction factor activities. Pro-

ceedings of the National Academy of Sciences of the United States of America 2004;101:10780–5.

[32] Perez-Caballero D, Hatziioannou T, Yang A, Cowan S, Bieniasz PD. Human tripartite motif 5alpha domains responsible for retrovirus restriction activity and specificity. Journal of Virology 2005;79:8969–78.

[33] Asaoka K, Ikeda K, Hishinuma T, Horie-Inoue K, Takeda S, Inoue S. A retrovirus restriction factor TRIM5alpha is transcriptionally regulated by interferons. Biochemical and Biophysical Research Communications 2005;338:1950–6.

[34] Sastri J, Campbell EM. Recent Insights into the Mechanism and Consequences of TRIM5α Retroviral Restriction. AIDS Research and Human Retroviruses 2011;27:231–8.

[35] Yamauchi K, Wada K, Tanji K, Tanaka M, Kamitani T. Ubiquitination of E3 ubiquitin ligase TRIM5 alpha and its potential role. The FEBS Journal 2008;275:1540–55.

[36] Lienlaf M, Hayashi F, Di Nunzio F, Tochio N, Kigawa T, Yokoyama S, et al. Contribution of E3-ubiquitin ligase activity to HIV-1 restriction by TRIM5alpha(rh): structure of the RING domain of TRIM5alpha. Journal of Virology 2011;85:8725–37.

[37] Diaz-Griffero F, Qin X-R, Hayashi F, Kigawa T, Finzi A, Sarnak Z, et al. A B-box 2 surface patch important for TRIM5alpha self-association, capsid binding avidity, and retrovirus restriction. Journal of Virology 2009;83:10737–51.

[38] Sawyer SL, Wu LI, Emerman M, Malik HS. Positive selection of primate TRIM5alpha identifies a critical species-specific retroviral restriction domain. Proceedings of the National Academy of Sciences of the United States of America 2005;102:2832–7.

[39] Song B, Gold B, O'Huigin C, Javanbakht H, Li X, Stremlau M, et al. The B30.2(SPRY) domain of the retroviral restriction factor TRIM5alpha exhibits lineage-specific length and sequence variation in primates. Journal of Virology 2005;79:6111–21.

[40] Stremlau M, Perron M, Welikala S, Sodroski JG. Species-specific variation in the B30.2(SPRY) domain of TRIM5alpha determines the potency of human immunodeficiency virus restriction. Journal of Virology 2005;79:3139–45.

[41] Ohkura S, Yap MW, Sheldon T, Stoye JP. All three variable regions of the TRIM5alpha B30.2 domain can contribute to the specificity of retrovirus restriction. Journal of Virology 2006;80:8554–65.

[42] Chatterji U, Bobardt MD, Gaskill P, Sheeter D, Fox H, Gallay PA. Trim5alpha accelerates degradation of cytosolic capsid associated with productive HIV-1 entry. The Journal of Biological Chemistry 2006;281:37025–33.

[43] Anderson JL, Campbell EM, Wu X, Vandegraaff N, Engelman A, Hope TJ. Proteasome inhibition reveals that a functional preintegration complex intermediate can be

generated during restriction by diverse TRIM5 proteins. Journal of Virology 2006;80:9754–60.

[44] Wu X, Anderson JL, Campbell EM, Joseph AM, Hope TJ. Proteasome inhibitors uncouple rhesus TRIM5alpha restriction of HIV-1 reverse transcription and infection. Proceedings of the National Academy of Sciences of the United States of America 2006;103:7465–70.

[45] Maegawa H, Miyamoto T, Sakuragi J-I, Shioda T, Nakayama EE. Contribution of RING domain to retrovirus restriction by TRIM5alpha... - PubMed - NCBI. Virology 2010;399:212–20.

[46] Harris RS, Bishop KN, Sheehy AM, Craig HM, Petersen-Mahrt SK, Watt IN, et al. DNA deamination mediates innate immunity to retroviral infection. Cell 2003;113:803–9.

[47] Liddament MT, Brown WL, Schumacher AJ, Harris RS. APOBEC3F properties and hypermutation preferences indicate activity against HIV-1 in vivo. Current Biology : CB 2004;14:1385–91.

[48] Wiegand HL, Doehle BP, Bogerd HP, Cullen BR. A second human antiretroviral factor, APOBEC3F, is suppressed by the HIV-1 and HIV-2 Vif proteins. The EMBO Journal 2004;23:2451–8.

[49] Zheng Y-H, Irwin D, Kurosu T, Tokunaga K, Sata T, Peterlin BM. Human APOBEC3F is another host factor that blocks human immunodeficiency virus type 1 replication. Journal of Virology 2004;78:6073–6.

[50] Sheehy AM, Gaddis NC, Choi JD, Malim MH. Isolation of a human gene that inhibits HIV-1 infection and is suppressed by the viral Vif protein. Nature 2002;418:646–50.

[51] Farrow MA, Kim E-Y, Wolinsky SM, Sheehy AM. NFAT and IRF proteins regulate transcription of the anti-HIV gene, APOBEC3G. The Journal of Biological Chemistry 2011;286:2567–77.

[52] Rose KM, Marin M, Kozak SL, Kabat D. Transcriptional regulation of APOBEC3G, a cytidine deaminase that hypermutates human immunodeficiency virus. The Journal of Biological Chemistry 2004;279:41744–9.

[53] Alce TM, Popik W. APOBEC3G is incorporated into virus-like particles by a direct interaction with HIV-1 Gag nucleocapsid protein. The Journal of Biological Chemistry 2004;279:34083–6.

[54] Cen S, Guo F, Niu M, Saadatmand J, Deflassieux J, Kleiman L. The interaction between HIV-1 Gag and APOBEC3G. The Journal of Biological Chemistry 2004;279:33177–84.

[55] Schäfer A, Bogerd HP, Cullen BR. Specific packaging of APOBEC3G into HIV-1 virions is mediated by the nucleocapsid domain of the gag polyprotein precursor. Virology 2004;328:163–8.

[56] Zennou V, Perez-Caballero D, Göttlinger H, Bieniasz PD. APOBEC3G incorporation into human immunodeficiency virus type 1 particles. Journal of Virology 2004;78:12058–61.

[57] Luo K, Liu B, Xiao Z, Yu Y, Yu X, Gorelick R, et al. Amino-terminal region of the human immunodeficiency virus type 1 nucleocapsid is required for human APOBEC3G packaging. Journal of Virology 2004;78:11841–52.

[58] Soros VB, Yonemoto W, Greene WC. Newly synthesized APOBEC3G is incorporated into HIV virions, inhibited by HIV RNA, and subsequently activated by RNase H. PLoS Pathogens 2007;3:e15.

[59] Lecossier D, Bouchonnet F, Clavel F, Hance AJ. Hypermutation of HIV-1 DNA in the absence of the Vif protein. Science 2003;300:1112–2.

[60] Iwatani Y, Chan DSB, Wang F, Maynard KS, Sugiura W, Gronenborn AM, et al. Deaminase-independent inhibition of HIV-1 reverse transcription by APOBEC3G. Nucleic Acids Research 2007;35:7096–108.

[61] Mbisa JL, Barr R, Thomas JA, Vandegraaff N, Dorweiler IJ, Svarovskaia ES, et al. Human immunodeficiency virus type 1 cDNAs produced in the presence of APOBEC3G exhibit defects in plus-strand DNA transfer and integration. Journal of Virology 2007;81:7099–110.

[62] Luo K, Wang T, Liu B, Tian C, Xiao Z, Kappes J, et al. Cytidine deaminases APOBEC3G and APOBEC3F interact with human immunodeficiency virus type 1 integrase and inhibit proviral DNA formation. Journal of Virology 2007;81:7238–48.

[63] Bishop KN, Holmes RK, Sheehy AM, Davidson NO, Cho S-J, Malim MH. Cytidine deamination of retroviral DNA by diverse APOBEC proteins. Current Biology : CB 2004;14:1392–6.

[64] Langlois M-A, Beale RCL, Conticello SG, Neuberger MS. Mutational comparison of the single-domained APOBEC3C and double-domained APOBEC3F/G anti-retroviral cytidine deaminases provides insight into their DNA target site specificities. Nucleic Acids Research 2005;33:1913–23.

[65] Mariani R, Chen D, Schrofelbauer B, Navarro F, Konig R, Bollman B, et al. Species-specific exclusion of APOBEC3G from HIV-1 virions by Vif. Cell 2003;114:21–31.

[66] Madani N, Kabat D. An endogenous inhibitor of human immunodeficiency virus in human lymphocytes is overcome by the viral Vif protein. Journal of Virology 1998;72:10251–5.

[67] Sheehy AM, Gaddis NC, Malim MH. The antiretroviral enzyme APOBEC3G is degraded by the proteasome in response to HIV-1 Vif. Nature Medicine 2003;9:1404–7.

[68] Marin M, Rose KM, Kozak SL, Kabat D. HIV-1 Vif protein binds the editing enzyme APOBEC3G and induces its degradation. Nature Medicine 2003;9:1398–403.

[69] Mehle A, Strack B, Ancuta P, Zhang C, McPike M, Gabuzda D. Vif overcomes the innate antiviral activity of APOBEC3G by promoting its degradation in the ubiquitin-proteasome pathway. The Journal of Biological Chemistry 2004;279:7792–8.

[70] Simon JH, Miller DL, Fouchier RA, Soares MA, Peden KW, Malim MH. The regulation of primate immunodeficiency virus infectivity by Vif is cell species restricted: a role for Vif in determining virus host range and cross-species transmission. The EMBO Journal 1998;17:1259–67.

[71] Yu X, Yu Y, Liu B, Luo K, Kong W, Mao P, et al. Induction of APOBEC3G ubiquitination and degradation by an HIV-1 Vif-Cul5-SCF complex. Science 2003;302:1056–60.

[72] Stopak K, de Noronha C, Yonemoto W, Greene WC. HIV-1 Vif blocks the antiviral activity of APOBEC3G by impairing both its translation and intracellular stability. Molecular Cell 2003;12:591–601.

[73] Kobayashi M, Takaori-Kondo A, Miyauchi Y, Iwai K, Uchiyama T. Ubiquitination of APOBEC3G by an HIV-1 Vif-Cullin5-Elongin B-Elongin C complex is essential for Vif function. The Journal of Biological Chemistry 2005;280:18573–8.

[74] Kao S, Khan MA, Miyagi E, Plishka R, Buckler-White A, Strebel K. The human immunodeficiency virus type 1 Vif protein reduces intracellular expression and inhibits packaging of APOBEC3G (CEM15), a cellular inhibitor of virus infectivity. Journal of Virology 2003;77:11398–407.

[75] Koning FA, Goujon C, Bauby H, Malim MH. Target Cell-Mediated Editing of HIV-1 cDNA by APOBEC3 Proteins in Human Macrophages. Journal of Virology 2011;85:13448–52.

[76] Doitsh G, Cavrois M, Lassen KG, Zepeda O, Yang Z, Santiago ML, et al. Abortive HIV infection mediates CD4 T cell depletion and inflammation in human lymphoid tissue. Cell 2010;143:789–801.

[77] Lee K, Ambrose Z, Martin TD, Oztop I, Mulky A, Julias JG, et al. Flexible use of nuclear import pathways by HIV-1. Cell Host & Microbe 2010;7:221–33.

[78] Swanson CM, Malim MH. SnapShot: HIV-1 proteins. Cell 2008;133:742, 742.e1.

[79] Yan N, Cherepanov P, Daigle JE, Engelman A, Lieberman J. The SET complex acts as a barrier to autointegration of HIV-1. PLoS Pathogens 2009;5:e1000327.

[80] Doehle BP, Schäfer A, Wiegand HL, Bogerd HP, Cullen BR. Differential sensitivity of murine leukemia virus to APOBEC3-mediated inhibition is governed by virion exclusion. Journal of Virology 2005;79:8201–7.

[81] Yu Q, Chen D, König R, Mariani R, Unutmaz D, Landau NR. APOBEC3B and APOBEC3C are potent inhibitors of simian immunodeficiency virus replication. The Journal of Biological Chemistry 2004;279:53379–86.

[82] Doehle BP, Schäfer A, Cullen BR. Human APOBEC3B is a potent inhibitor of HIV-1 infectivity and is resistant to HIV-1 Vif. Virology 2005;339:281–8.

[83] Neil SJD, Zang T, Bieniasz PD. Tetherin inhibits retrovirus release and is antagonized by HIV-1 Vpu. Nature 2008;451:425–30.

[84] Van Damme N, Goff D, Katsura C, Jorgenson RL, Mitchell R, Johnson MC, et al. The interferon-induced protein BST-2 restricts HIV-1 release and is downregulated from the cell surface by the viral Vpu protein. Cell Host & Microbe 2008;3:245–52.

[85] Neil SJD, Sandrin V, Sundquist WI, Bieniasz PD. An interferon-alpha-induced tethering mechanism inhibits HIV-1 and Ebola virus particle release but is counteracted by the HIV-1 Vpu protein. Cell Host & Microbe 2007;2:193–203.

[86] Blasius AL, Giurisato E, Cella M, Schreiber RD, Shaw AS, Colonna M. Bone marrow stromal cell antigen 2 is a specific marker of type I IFN-producing cells in the naive mouse, but a promiscuous cell surface antigen following IFN stimulation. Journal of Immunology 2006;177:3260–5.

[87] Jouvenet N, Neil SJD, Zhadina M, Zang T, Kratovac Z, Lee Y, et al. Broad-spectrum inhibition of retroviral and filoviral particle release by tetherin. Journal of Virology 2009;83:1837–44.

[88] Sakuma T, Noda T, Urata S, Kawaoka Y, Yasuda J. Inhibition of Lassa and Marburg virus production by tetherin. Journal of Virology 2009;83:2382–5.

[89] Groom HCT, Yap MW, Galão RP, Neil SJD, Bishop KN. Susceptibility of xenotropic murine leukemia virus-related virus (XMRV) to retroviral restriction factors. Proceedings of the National Academy of Sciences of the United States of America 2010;107:5166–71.

[90] Arnaud F, Black SG, Murphy L, Griffiths DJ, Neil SJ, Spencer TE, et al. Interplay between ovine bone marrow stromal cell antigen 2/tetherin and endogenous retroviruses. Journal of Virology 2010;84:4415–25.

[91] Mattiuzzo G, Ivol S, Takeuchi Y. Regulation of porcine endogenous retrovirus release by porcine and human tetherins. Journal of Virology 2010;84:2618–22.

[92] Vidal-Laliena M, Romero X, March S, Requena V, Petriz J, Engel P. Characterization of antibodies submitted to the B cell section of the 8th Human Leukocyte Differentiation Antigens Workshop by flow cytometry and immunohistochemistry. Cellular Immunology 2005;236:6–16.

[93] Zheng Y-H, Jeang KT, Tokunaga K. Host restriction factors in retroviral infection: promises in virus-host interaction. Retrovirology 2012;9:112.

[94] Kupzig S, Korolchuk V, Rollason R, Sugden A, Wilde A, Banting G. Bst-2/HM1.24 is a raft-associated apical membrane protein with an unusual topology. Traffic 2003;4:694–709.

[95] Rollason R, Korolchuk V, Hamilton C, Jepson M, Banting G. A CD317/tetherin-RICH2 complex plays a critical role in the organization of the subapical actin cytoskeleton in polarized epithelial cells. The Journal of Cell Biology 2009;184:721–36.

[96] Masuyama N, Kuronita T, Tanaka R, Muto T, Hirota Y, Takigawa A, et al. HM1.24 is internalized from lipid rafts by clathrin-mediated endocytosis through interaction with alpha-adaptin. The Journal of Biological Chemistry 2009;284:15927–41.

[97] Willey RL, Maldarelli F, Martin MA, Strebel K. Human immunodeficiency virus type 1 Vpu protein regulates the formation of intracellular gp160-CD4 complexes. Journal of Virology 1992;66:226–34.

[98] Sakai H, Tokunaga K, Kawamura M, Adachi A. Function of human immunodeficiency virus type 1 Vpu protein in various cell types. The Journal of General Virology 1995;76 (Pt 11):2717–22.

[99] Geraghty RJ, Talbot KJ, Callahan M, Harper W, Panganiban AT. Cell type-dependence for Vpu function. Journal of Medical Primatology 1994;23:146–50.

[100] Varthakavi V, Smith RM, Bour SP, Strebel K, Spearman P. Viral protein U counteracts a human host cell restriction that inhibits HIV-1 particle production. Proceedings of the National Academy of Sciences 2003;100:15154–9.

[101] Neil SJD, Eastman SW, Jouvenet N, Bieniasz PD. HIV-1 Vpu promotes release and prevents endocytosis of nascent retrovirus particles from the plasma membrane. PLoS Pathogens 2006;2:e39.

[102] Aloia RC, Tian H, Jensen FC. Lipid composition and fluidity of the human immunodeficiency virus envelope and host cell plasma membranes. Proceedings of the National Academy of Sciences of the United States of America 1993;90:5181–5.

[103] Panchal RG, Ruthel G, Kenny TA, Kallstrom GH, Lane D, Badie SS, et al. In vivo oligomerization and raft localization of Ebola virus protein VP40 during vesicular budding. Proceedings of the National Academy of Sciences 2003;100:15936–41.

[104] Dubé M, Roy BB, Guiot-Guillain P, Binette J, Mercier J, Chiasson A, et al. Antagonism of tetherin restriction of HIV-1 release by Vpu involves binding and sequestration of the restriction factor in a perinuclear compartment. PLoS Pathogens 2010;6:e1000856.

[105] Andrew AJ, Miyagi E, Strebel K. Differential effects of human immunodeficiency virus type 1 Vpu on the stability of BST-2/tetherin. Journal of Virology 2011;85:2611–9.

[106] Lau D, Kwan W, Guatelli J. Role of the endocytic pathway in the counteraction of BST-2 by human lentiviral pathogens. Journal of Virology 2011;85:9834–46.

[107] Mitchell RS, Katsura C, Skasko MA, Fitzpatrick K, Lau D, Ruiz A, et al. Vpu antagonizes BST-2-mediated restriction of HIV-1 release via beta-TrCP and endo-lysosomal trafficking. PLoS Pathogens 2009;5:e1000450.

[108] Iwabu Y, Fujita H, Kinomoto M, Kaneko K, Ishizaka Y, Tanaka Y, et al. HIV-1 accessory protein Vpu internalizes cell-surface BST-2/tetherin through transmembrane interactions leading to lysosomes. The Journal of Biological Chemistry 2009;284:35060–72.

[109] Iwabu Y, Fujita H, Tanaka Y, Sata T, Tokunaga K. Direct internalization of cell-surface BST-2/tetherin by the HIV-1 accessory protein Vpu. Communicative & Integrative Biology 2010;3:366–9.

[110] Janvier K, Pelchen-Matthews A, Renaud J-B, Caillet M, Marsh M, Berlioz-Torrent C. The ESCRT-0 component HRS is required for HIV-1 Vpu-mediated BST-2/tetherin down-regulation. PLoS Pathogens 2011;7:e1001265.

[111] Gupta RK, Hué S, Schaller T, Verschoor E, Pillay D, Towers GJ. Mutation of a single residue renders human tetherin resistant to HIV-1 Vpu-mediated depletion. PLoS Pathogens 2009;5:e1000443.

[112] Goffinet C, Allespach I, Homann S, Tervo H-M, Habermann A, Rupp D, et al. HIV-1 antagonism of CD317 is species specific and involves Vpu-mediated proteasomal degradation of the restriction factor. Cell Host & Microbe 2009;5:285–97.

[113] Mangeat B, Gers-Huber G, Lehmann M, Zufferey M, Luban J, Piguet V. HIV-1 Vpu Neutralizes the Antiviral Factor Tetherin/BST-2 by Binding It and Directing Its Beta-TrCP2-Dependent Degradation. PLoS Pathogens 2009;5:e1000574.

[114] McNatt MW, Zang T, Hatziioannou T, Bartlett M, Fofana IB, Johnson WE, et al. Species-specific activity of HIV-1 Vpu and positive selection of tetherin transmembrane domain variants. PLoS Pathogens 2009;5:e1000300.

[115] Rong L, Zhang J, Lu J, Pan Q, Lorgeoux R-P, Aloysius C, et al. The transmembrane domain of BST-2 determines its sensitivity to down-modulation by human immunodeficiency virus type 1 Vpu. Journal of Virology 2009;83:7536–46.

[116] Jia B, Serra-Moreno R, Neidermyer W, Rahmberg A, Mackey J, Fofana IB, et al. Species-specific activity of SIV Nef and HIV-1 Vpu in overcoming restriction by tetherin/BST2. PLoS Pathogens 2009;5:e1000429.

[117] Sauter D, Schindler M, Specht A, Landford WN, Munch J, Kim K-A, et al. Tetherin-driven adaptation of Vpu and Nef function and the evolution of pandemic and non-pandemic HIV-1 strains. Cell Host & Microbe 2009;6:409–21.

[118] Zhang F, Wilson SJ, Landford WC, Virgen B, Gregory D, Johnson MC, et al. Nef proteins from simian immunodeficiency viruses are tetherin antagonists. Cell Host & Microbe 2009;6:54–67.

[119] Basmaciogullari S, Pizzato M. The activity of Nef on HIV-1 infectivity. Frontiers in Microbiology 2014;5:232.

[120] Le Tortorec A, Neil SJD. Antagonism to and intracellular sequestration of human tetherin by the human immunodeficiency virus type 2 envelope glycoprotein. Journal of Virology 2009;83:11966–78.

[121] Mansouri M, Viswanathan K, Douglas JL, Hines J, Gustin J, Moses AV, et al. Molecular mechanism of BST2/tetherin downregulation by K5/MIR2 of Kaposi's sarcoma-associated herpesvirus. Journal of Virology 2009;83:9672–81.

[122] Pardieu C, Vigan R, Wilson SJ, Calvi A, Zang T, Bieniasz P, et al. The RING-CH ligase K5 antagonizes restriction of KSHV and HIV-1 particle release by mediating ubiquitin-dependent endosomal degradation of tetherin. PLoS Pathogens 2010;6:e1000843.

[123] Kaletsky RL, Francica JR, Agrawal-Gamse C, Bates P. Tetherin-mediated restriction of filovirus budding is antagonized by the Ebola glycoprotein. Proceedings of the National Academy of Sciences of the United States of America 2009;106:2886–91.

[124] Barroca P, Calado M, Azevedo-Pereira JM. HIV/dendritic cell interaction: consequences in the pathogenesis of HIV infection. AIDS Reviews 2014;16:223–35.

[125] Cameron PU, Freudenthal PS, Barker JM, Gezelter S, Inaba K, Steinman RM. Dendritic cells exposed to human immunodeficiency virus type-1 transmit a vigorous cytopathic infection to CD4+ T cells. Science 1992;257:383–7.

[126] Pope M, Betjes MG, Romani N, Hirmand H, Cameron PU, Hoffman L, et al. Conjugates of dendritic cells and memory T lymphocytes from skin facilitate productive infection with HIV-1. Cell 1994;78:389–98.

[127] Pope M, Gezelter S, Gallo N, Hoffman L, Steinman RM. Low levels of HIV-1 infection in cutaneous dendritic cells promote extensive viral replication upon binding to memory CD4+ T cells. The Journal of Experimental Medicine 1995;182:2045–56.

[128] Granelli-Piperno A, Finkel V, Delgado E, Steinman RM. Virus replication begins in dendritic cells during the transmission of HIV-1 from mature dendritic cells to T cells. Current Biology : CB 1999;9:21–9.

[129] Wu L, KewalRamani VN. Dendritic-cell interactions with HIV: infection and viral dissemination. Nature Reviews Immunology 2006;6:859–68.

[130] Akira S, Uematsu S, Takeuchi O. Pathogen recognition and innate immunity. Cell 2006;124:783–801.

[131] Pichlmair A, Reis e Sousa C. Innate recognition of viruses. Immunity 2007;27:370–83.

[132] Bowie AG, Unterholzner L. Viral evasion and subversion of pattern-recognition receptor signalling. Nature Reviews Immunology 2008;8:911–22.

[133] Kato H, Sato S, Yoneyama M, Yamamoto M, Uematsu S, Matsui K, et al. Cell type-specific involvement of RIG-I in antiviral response. Immunity 2005;23:19–28.

[134] Kumagai Y, Takeuchi O, Kato H, Kumar H, Matsui K, Morii E, et al. Alveolar macrophages are the primary interferon-alpha producer in pulmonary infection with RNA viruses. Immunity 2007;27:240–52.

[135] Samarajiwa SA, Forster S, Auchettl K, Hertzog PJ. INTERFEROME: the database of interferon regulated genes. Nucleic Acids Research 2009;37:D852–7.

[136] Li N, Zhang W, Cao X. Identification of human homologue of mouse IFN-gamma induced protein from human dendritic cells. Immunology Letters 2000;74:221–4.

[137] Laguette N, Sobhian B, Casartelli N, Ringeard M, Chable-Bessia C, Ségéral E, et al. SAMHD1 is the dendritic- and myeloid-cell-specific HIV-1 restriction factor counteracted by Vpx. Nature 2011;474:654–7.

[138] Hrecka K, Hao C, Gierszewska M, Swanson SK, Kesik-Brodacka M, Srivastava S, et al. Vpx relieves inhibition of HIV-1 infection of macrophages mediated by the SAMHD1 protein. Nature 2011;474:658–61.

[139] Goldstone DC, Ennis-Adeniran V, Hedden JJ, Groom HCT, Rice GI, Christodoulou E, et al. HIV-1 restriction factor SAMHD1 is a deoxynucleoside triphosphate triphosphohydrolase. Nature 2011;480:379–82.

[140] Lahouassa H, Daddacha W, Hofmann H, Ayinde D, Logue EC, Dragin L, et al. SAMHD1 restricts the replication of human immunodeficiency virus type 1 by depleting the intracellular pool of deoxynucleoside triphosphates. Nature Immunology 2012;13:223–8.

[141] Kim B, Nguyen LA, Daddacha W, Hollenbaugh JA. Tight interplay among SAMHD1 protein level, cellular dNTP levels, and HIV-1 proviral DNA synthesis kinetics in human primary monocyte-derived macrophages. The Journal of Biological Chemistry 2012;287:21570–4.

[142] Yan N, Lieberman J. Gaining a foothold: how HIV avoids innate immune recognition. Current Opinion in Immunology 2011;23:21–8.

[143] Manel N, Hogstad B, Wang Y, Levy DE, Unutmaz D, Littman DR. A cryptic sensor for HIV-1 activates antiviral innate immunity in dendritic cells. Nature 2010;467:214–7.

[144] Tristem M, Marshall C, Karpas A, Petrik J, Hill F. Origin of vpx in lentiviruses. Nature 1990;347:341–2.

[145] Fujita M, Nomaguchi M, Adachi A, Otsuka M. SAMHD1-Dependent and -Independent Functions of HIV-2/SIV Vpx Protein. Frontiers in Microbiology 2012;3:297.

[146] Puigdomènech I, Casartelli N, Porrot F, Schwartz O. SAMHD1 Restricts HIV-1 Cell-to-Cell Transmission and Limits Immune Detection in Monocyte-Derived Dendritic Cells. Journal of Virology 2013;87:2846–56.

[147] Kaushik R, Zhu X, Stranska R, Wu Y, Stevenson M. A cellular restriction dictates the permissivity of nondividing monocytes/macrophages to lentivirus and gammaretrovirus infection. Cell Host & Microbe 2009;6:68–80.

[148] Goujon C, Rivière L, Jarrosson-Wuilleme L, Bernaud J, Rigal D, Darlix J-L, et al. SIVSM/HIV-2 Vpx proteins promote retroviral escape from a proteasome-dependent restriction pathway present in human dendritic cells. Retrovirology 2007;4:2.

[149] Silvin A, Manel N. Interactions between HIV-1 and innate immunity in dendritic cells. Advances in Experimental Medicine and Biology 2013;762:183–200.

[150] Azevedo-Pereira JM. HIV-2 Interaction with Target Cell Receptors, or Why HIV-2 is Less Pathogenic than HIV-1. In: Saxena SK, editor. Current Perspectives in HIV Infection, Croatia: InTech; 2013, pp. 411–45.

[151] Manel N, Littman DR. Hiding in plain sight: how HIV evades innate immune responses. Cell 2011;147:271–4.

[152] Lindenmann J. Resistance of mice to mouse-adapted influenza A virus. Virology 1962;16:203–4.

[153] Haller O, Acklin M, Staeheli P. Influenza virus resistance of wild mice: wild-type and mutant Mx alleles occur at comparable frequencies. Journal of Interferon Research 1987;7:647–56.

[154] Reeves RH, O'Hara BF, Pavan WJ, Gearhart JD, Haller O. Genetic mapping of the Mx influenza virus resistance gene within the region of mouse chromosome 16 that is homologous to human chromosome 21. Journal of Virology 1988;62:4372–5.

[155] Staeheli P, Pravtcheva D, Lundin LG, Acklin M, Ruddle F, Lindenmann J, et al. Interferon-regulated influenza virus resistance gene Mx is localized on mouse chromosome 16. Journal of Virology 1986;58:967–9.

[156] Staeheli P, Sutcliffe JG. Identification of a second interferon-regulated murine Mx gene. Molecular and Cellular Biology 1988;8:4524–8.

[157] Verhelst J, Hulpiau P, Saelens X. Mx proteins: antiviral gatekeepers that restrain the uninvited. Microbiology and Molecular Biology Reviews : MMBR 2013;77:551–66.

[158] Aebi M, Fäh J, Hurt N, Samuel CE, Thomis D, Bazzigher L, et al. cDNA structures and regulation of two interferon-induced human Mx proteins. Molecular and Cellular Biology 1989;9:5062–72.

[159] Mänz B, Dornfeld D, Götz V, Zell R, Zimmermann P, Haller O, et al. Pandemic influenza A viruses escape from restriction by human MxA through adaptive mutations in the nucleoprotein. PLoS Pathogens 2013;9:e1003279.

[160] Gao S, Malsburg von der A, Dick A, Faelber K, Schröder GF, Haller O, et al. Structure of myxovirus resistance protein a reveals intra- and intermolecular domain interactions required for the antiviral function. Immunity 2011;35:514–25.

[161] Haller O, Kochs G. Human MxA protein: an interferon-induced dynamin-like GTPase with broad antiviral activity. Journal of Interferon and Cytokine Research 2011;31:79–87.

[162] Pavlovic J, Zürcher T, Haller O, Staeheli P. Resistance to influenza virus and vesicular stomatitis virus conferred by expression of human MxA protein. Journal of Virology 1990;64:3370–5.

[163] King MC, Raposo G, Lemmon MA. Inhibition of nuclear import and cell-cycle progression by mutated forms of the dynamin-like GTPase MxB. Proceedings of the National Academy of Sciences 2004;101:8957–62.

[164] Melén K, Keskinen P, Ronni T, Sareneva T, Lounatmaa K, Julkunen I. Human MxB protein, an interferon-alpha-inducible GTPase, contains a nuclear targeting signal and is localized in the heterochromatin region beneath the nuclear envelope. The Journal of Biological Chemistry 1996;271:23478–86.

[165] Schoggins JW, Wilson SJ, Panis M, Murphy MY, Jones CT, Bieniasz P, et al. A diverse range of gene products are effectors of the type I interferon antiviral response. Nature 2011;472:481–5.

[166] Goujon C, Moncorgé O, Bauby H, Doyle T, Ward CC, Schaller T, et al. Human MX2 is an interferon-induced post-entry inhibitor of HIV-1 infection. Nature 2013;502:559–62.

[167] Liu Z, Pan Q, Ding S, Qian J, Xu F, Zhou J, et al. The interferon-inducible MxB protein inhibits HIV-1 infection. Cell Host & Microbe 2013;14:398–410.

[168] Kane M, Yadav SS, Bitzegeio J, Kutluay SB, Zang T, Wilson SJ, et al. MX2 is an interferon-induced inhibitor of HIV-1 infection. Nature 2013;502:563–6.

[169] Fricke T, White TE, Schulte B, de Souza Aranha Vieira DA, Dharan A, Campbell EM, et al. MxB binds to the HIV-1 core and prevents the uncoating process of HIV-1. Retrovirology 2014;11:68.

[170] Matreyek KA, Wang W, Serrao E, Singh P, Levin HL, Engelman A. Host and viral determinants for MxB restriction of HIV-1 infection. Retrovirology 2014;11:90.

[171] Fassati A, Goff SP. Characterization of intracellular reverse transcription complexes of human immunodeficiency virus type 1. Journal of Virology 2001;75:3626–35.

[172] McDonald D, Vodicka MA, Lucero G, Svitkina TM, Borisy GG, Emerman M, et al. Visualization of the intracellular behavior of HIV in living cells. The Journal of Cell Biology 2002;159:441–52.

[173] Craigie R, Bushman FD. HIV DNA integration. Cold Spring Harbor Perspectives in Medicine 2012;2:a006890–0.

[174] Bukrinsky MI, Sharova N, Dempsey MP, Stanwick TL, Bukrinskaya AG, Haggerty S, et al. Active nuclear import of human immunodeficiency virus type 1 preintegration complexes. Proceedings of the National Academy of Sciences 1992;89:6580–4.

[175] Mitchell PS, Patzina C, Emerman M, Haller O, Malik HS, Kochs G. Evolution-guided identification of antiviral specificity determinants in the broadly acting interferon-induced innate immunity factor MxA. Cell Host & Microbe 2012;12:598–604.

[176] Liu S-Y, Aliyari R, Chikere K, Li G, Marsden MD, Smith JK, et al. Interferon-inducible cholesterol-25-hydroxylase broadly inhibits viral entry by production of 25-hydroxycholesterol. Immunity 2013;38:92–105.

[177] Blanc M, Hsieh WY, Robertson KA, Kropp KA, Forster T, Shui G, et al. The transcription factor STAT-1 couples macrophage synthesis of 25-hydroxycholesterol to the interferon antiviral response. Immunity 2013;38:106–18.

[178] Arita M, Kojima H, Nagano T, Okabe T, Wakita T, Shimizu H. Oxysterol-binding protein family I is the target of minor enviroxime-like compounds. Journal of Virology 2013;87:4252–60.

[179] Schwarz M, Lund EG, Russell DW. Two 7 alpha-hydroxylase enzymes in bile acid biosynthesis. Current Opinion in Lipidology 1998;9:113–8.

[180] Cuthbert JA, Lipsky PE. Sterol metabolism and lymphocyte responsiveness: inhibition of endogenous sterol synthesis prevents mitogen-induced human T cell proliferation. The Journal of Immunology 1981;126:2093–9.

[181] Bauman DR, Bitmansour AD, McDonald JG, Thompson BM, Liang G, Russell DW. 25-Hydroxycholesterol secreted by macrophages in response to Toll-like receptor activation suppresses immunoglobulin A production. Proceedings of the National Academy of Sciences of the United States of America 2009;106:16764–9.

[182] Bensinger SJ, Bradley MN, Joseph SB, Zelcer N, Janssen EM, Hausner MA, et al. LXR signaling couples sterol metabolism to proliferation in the acquired immune response. Cell 2008;134:97–111.

[183] Joseph SB, Bradley MN, Castrillo A, Bruhn KW, Mak PA, Pei L, et al. LXR-dependent gene expression is important for macrophage survival and the innate immune response. Cell 2004;119:299–309.

[184] Castrillo A, Joseph SB, Vaidya SA, Haberland M, Fogelman AM, Cheng G, et al. Crosstalk between LXR and toll-like receptor signaling mediates bacterial and viral antagonism of cholesterol metabolism. Molecular Cell 2003;12:805–16.

[185] Park K, Scott AL. Cholesterol 25-hydroxylase production by dendritic cells and macrophages is regulated by type I interferons. Journal of Leukocyte Biology 2010;88:1081–7.

[186] Gold ES, Diercks AH, Podolsky I, Podyminogin RL, Askovich PS, Treuting PM, et al. 25-Hydroxycholesterol acts as an amplifier of inflammatory signaling. - PubMed - NCBI. Proceedings of the National Academy of Sciences 2014;111:10666–71.

[187] Cyster JG, Dang EV, Reboldi A, Yi T. 25-Hydroxycholesterols in innate and adaptive immunity. Nature Reviews Immunology 2014;14:731–43.

[188] Reboldi A, Dang EV, McDonald JG, Liang G, Russell DW, Cyster JG. Inflammation. 25-Hydroxycholesterol suppresses interleukin-1-driven inflammation downstream of type I interferon. Science 2014;345:679–84.

[189] Teissier E, Pécheur E-I. Lipids as modulators of membrane fusion mediated by viral fusion proteins. European Biophysics Journal : EBJ 2007;36:887–99.

[190] Russell DW. Oxysterol biosynthetic enzymes. Biochimica Et Biophysica Acta 2000;1529:126–35.

Chapter 5

Immunological and Haematological Changes in HIV Infection

Wan Majdiah Wan Mohamad, Wan Suriana Wan Ab Rahman, Suhair Abbas Ahmed Al-Salih and Che Maraina Che Hussin

Additional information is available at the end of the chapter

http://dx.doi.org/10.5772/61259

1. Introduction

HIV is known to be associated with a wide range of immunological and haematological changes.The immunological changes include depletion in CD4+ T cell, cytokine dysregulation and immune dysfunction. The dominant immunologic feature of HIV infection is progressive depletion of the helper T cell (CD4+ T cell), which reverses the normal CD4:CD8 ratio and subsequently lead to immunodeficiency. CD4+ T cells interact with antigen presenting cells (APCs), B cells, cytotoxic T cells (CD8+ T cells) as well as natural killer cells. Thus, infection and depletion of CD4+ T cell population could induce profound immunodeficiency in such patients.

The haematological changes occur mainly due to several factors such as marrow defects and immune cytopenias. It is caused by HIV infection, either directly to the bone marrow, opportunistic infections, development of lymphoma as a secondary neoplasm and side effects of the drugs used for the treatment or drugs used for the complicating infection or lymphoma. In order to further understand the immunological and haematological changes that occur in HIV infection, the chapter begins with the review of immune system as well as normal haematopoiesis. It further highlights the importance of changes associated with clinical symptoms in patients with HIV.

2. The human immune system

The immune system plays an important role to protect the host from infectious agents such as bacteria, viruses, fungi and parasites. In addition, it is also important in the identification and elimination of tumor cells as well as in response to injury and trauma. Thus, an effective and efficient immune system is essential as a host defense mechanism against infectious diseases and cancer. The immune system can be further subdivided into innate and acquired or adaptive immunity (Table 1).

	Innate immunity	Acquired immunity
Physico-chemical barriers	Skin	Cutaneous and mucosal immune systems
	Mucosal membranes	Antibodies in mucosal secretions
	Lysozyme	
	Stomach acid	
	Commensal bacteria in gut	
Circulating molecules	Complement	Antibodies
Immune Cells	Granulocytes	B lymphocytes
	Monocytes/macrophages	T lymphocytes
	Natural killer cells	
Soluble mediators	Macrophage-derived cytokines	Lymphocyte-derived cytokines

Table 1. Components of the innate and acquired immune systems [1].

2.1. Innate immunity

Innate immunity is the first line of defense mechanism against the invading agents present at birth. The innate immune system includes physico-chemical barriers, circulating molecules, immune cells as well as soluble mediators [1, 2]. As compared to acquired immunity, innate immunity has no memory, poor specificity and has immediate response with lower potency.

2.2. Acquired immunity

The acquired or adaptive immune response is the second line of defense mechanism which offer better protection against re-exposure to the same pathogen [2]. The acquired immune system is further subclassified into humoral mediated immunity which involves antibody production by B lymphocytes and cell mediated immunity comprising CD4+ and CD8+T lymphocytes. Acquired immunity has immunological memory and it is highly specific. The specificity occurs because each lymphocyte carries surface receptors for a single antigen [1]. When compared to innate immunity, it has slower response, however it is much more potent and robust and the response varies among individuals.

Innate and adaptive immune systems as well as complement counteract each other to produce an effective function and mechanism of eliminating the invading agents.

http://dx.doi.org/10.5772/61259

2.2.1. *B lymphocytes*

B lymphocytes are known by their ability to produce antibodies (immunoglobulins), which are specific for particular antigen [1]. Antibodies work in several ways to combat invading pathogens. Some pathogens, particularly viruses and some bacteria as well, infect individuals by entering cells. Some of these pathogens escape humoral immunity and later on will be encountered by cell-mediated immunity, which is conferred by T lymphocytes.

2.2.2. *T lymphocytes*

Mature T lymphocytes express T-cell receptors on their surface. They are able to recognize only those antigens which are associated with the protein termed major histocompatibility complex (MHC): in humans the MHC is known as human leukocyte antigen (HLA) [2] that are presented to them on a cell surface by antigen presenting cells (APCs) [2]. When an APC (e.g. macrophage) encounter an antigen or pathogen, it will engulf, process and present the pathogen to the T cell [2].

T lymphocytes can be further subdivided into CD4+ T cells (Helper T cells) and CD8+ T cells (Cytotoxic T cells). CD4+ T cells are further subclassified into Th1 (T helper 1) and Th2 (T helper 2). Th1 is important for eliminating intracellular pathogen whereas Th2 is important for immunity against extracellular pathogen [2].

The regulation of the immune response is shown in Figure 1. The Th1 cells are involved in cell-mediated immunity against intracellular pathogens. They produce cytokines such as interleukin-2 (IL-2), interferon-gamma (IFN-gamma) and interleukin-10 (IL-10) [2]. IL-2 promotes proliferation of T lymphocytes [2] while IFN-gamma activates the cells involved in the elimination of pathogens and cells with tumour properties (e.g. monocytes, macrophages, cytotoxic T lymphocytes, natural killer cells) [1]. By contrast, the Th2 cells are mainly involved in humoral immunity and immunity against helminthic infection [2]. They produce cytokines such as IL-4, IL-5, IL-10 and IL-13. It is known that IL-4 stimulates proliferation of B lymphocytes while IL-5 promotes activation of eosinophils [2]. IL-10 has inhibitory effect while IL-13 involves in allergic reaction and helminthic infection [2]. Thus, both Th1 and Th2 cells and their cytokines counteract with each other to regulate the immune response [1].

The communication within the acquired immune system and between innate and acquired immunity involves cell surface proteins (e.g. adhesion molecules) and the soluble molecules which can produce signals from one cell to another, that is called cytokines [1].

2.3. Cytokines

Cytokines are a diverse group of intercellular signaling peptides and glycoproteins with molecular weight between 6000 and 60,000. They are produced by a variety of tissues and cells in response to stimuli [2]. Cytokines have diverse and pleiotropic effects [4]. Their binding to specific receptors on the cell surface leads to changes in growth, development or activity of the target cells. They do not only regulate immune and inflammatory responses but also involve in wound healing, haematopoiesis, angiogenesis as well as other biologic processes [2, 4].

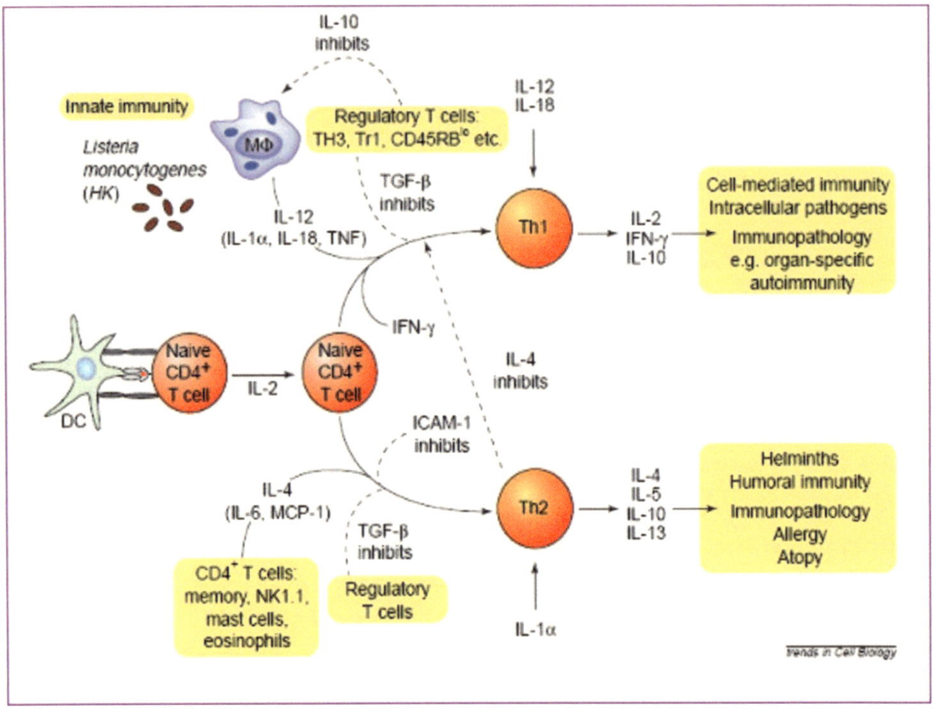

The diagram shows the mechanism of regulation of immune response. Th1 is mainly involved in cell-mediated immunity and offers protection against intracellular pathogens while Th2 is important in humoral immunity, protection against helminthic infection as well as allergic or atopic diseases such as allergic rhinitis, asthma etc.

Figure 1. The regulation of immune response [3]

3. Immunological aspects of HIV infection

3.1. Clinical features of HIV infection

In primary infection of HIV-1, patients may be asymptomatic though sometimes the disease is self-limiting. Within the incubation period of about 6 weeks, patients can present with a mononucleosis-like syndrome, which is characterized by fever, cough, painful swallowing, myalgias, arthralgias, diarrhea as well as maculopapular rash and lymphadenopathy [5]. In most circumstances, the symptoms are usually mild as contrasted to severe cases, where pneumonitis, oropharyngeal and esophageal ulcers may occur. Encephalitis, meningitis, neuropathy, radiculopathy and myelopathy are not common sickneses in HIV infection. Although the true incidence of this syndrome is not precisely known, it may also depend on the degree of exposure to the virus, it may be as high as over 50% in persons who acquire HIV-1 infection [5].

World Health Organization [6] categorized an adult or adolescent (aged > 12 years) as having AIDS in presence of at least two of the major signs in combination with one of the minor signs (Table 2).

Major signs	Minor signs
· Weight loss of more than 10% bodyweight	· Persistent cough for more than 1 month*
· Chronic diarrhea for more than 1 month	· Generalised pruritic dermatitis
· Prolonged fever for more than 1 month (intermittent or constant)	· History of herpers zoster
	· Oropharyngeal candidiasis
	· Chronic progressive or disseminated herpes · simplex infection
	· Generalised lymphadenopathy

* Persistent cough for more than 1 month should be considered as a minor sign in patients with tuberculosis

Table 2. Major and minor signs of HIV infection [6].

3.2. The classification of HIV disease

The staging and classification of HIV disease are standard tools for monitoring HIV epidemic and also serve as a guide for clinicians in managing HIV patients. It provides important information for patients and clinicians regarding the staging of HIV disease and clinical management. Currently, two major classification are used: World Health Organization (WHO) Clinical Staging and Disease Classification System and the United State Centers for Disease Control and Prevention (CDC) Classification System.

The WHO Clinical Staging and Disease Classification System (revised in 2007) is usually used in resource-constrained settings without access to CD4 cell count measurements or other diagnostic and laboratory methods [7] The system classifies the HIV disease based on the clinical manifestations of patients. By contrast, the CDC classification system assesses the HIV disease severity by CD4 cell count as well as by the presence of specific HIV-related conditions [7]. This classification system is usually beneficial in the clinical as well as epidemiologic research.

3.2.1. WHO clinical staging of HIV/AIDS and case definition

The clinical staging and case definition of HIV was developed by WHO in 1990 and revised in 2007. It is based on the clinical findings rather than CD4 cell count. This staging system has been used by some countries for managing HIV patients where the CD4 cell count testing is not available [7]. The staging was categorized as 1 to 4 based on clinical severity and progression from primary infection to advanced stage. The adult and adolescents were defined as individuals aged ≥ 15 years. WHO, 2007 [8] classifies the clinical staging of HIV/AIDS based on the clinical conditions or symptoms (Table 3).

Clinical Stages	Clinical Conditions or Symptoms
Primary HIV Infection	· Asymptomatic · Acute retroviral syndrome
Clinical Stage 1	· Asymptomatic · Persistent generalized lymphadenopathy

Clinical Stage 2	· Moderate unexplained weight loss (<10% of presumed or measured body weight)
	· Recurrent respiratory infections (sinusitis, tonsillitis, otitis media, and pharyngitis)
	· Herpes zoster
	· Angular cheilitis
	· Recurrent oral ulceration
	· Papular pruritic eruptions
	· Seborrheic dermatitis
	· Fungal nail infections
Clinical Stage 3	· Unexplained severe weight loss ("/>10% of presumed or measured body weight)
	· Unexplained chronic diarrhea for "/> 1 month
	· Unexplained persistent fever for "/> 1 month ("/>37.6ºC, intermittent or constant)
	· Persistent oral candidiasis
	· Oral hairy leukoplakia
	· Pulmonary tuberculosis
	· Severe presumed bacterial infection (e.g., pneumonia, empyema, pyomyositis, bone or joint infection, meningitis, bacteremia)
	· Acute necrotizing ulcerative stomatitis, gingivitis or periodontitis
	· Unexplained anaemia (haemoglobin<8 g/dl)
	· Neutropenia (neutrophils <500 cells/μL)
	· Chronic thrombocytopenia (platelets < 50, 000 cells/ μL)
Clinical Stage 4	· HIV wasting syndrome, as defined by the CDC (see Table 1, above)
	· *Pneumocystis* pneumonia
	· Recurrent severe bacterial pneumonia
	· Chronic herpes simplex infection (orolabial, genital, or anorectal site for "/>1 month or visceral herpes at any site)
	· Esophageal candidiasis (or candidiasis of trachea, bronchi, or lungs)
	· Extrapulmonary tuberculosis
	· Kaposi sarcoma
	· Cytomegalovirus infection (retinitis or infection of other organs)
	· Central nervous system toxoplasmosis
	· HIV encephalopathy
	· Cryptococcosis, extrapulmonary (including meningitis)
	· Disseminated nontuberculosis mycobacteria infection
	· Progressive multifocal leukoencephalopathy
	· Candida of the trachea, bronchi, or lungs
	· Chronic cryptosporidiosis (with diarrhea)
	· Chronic isosporiasis
	· Disseminated mycosis (e.g., histoplasmosis, coccidioidomycosis, penicilliosis)
	· Recurrent nontyphoidal *Salmonella* bacteremia
	· Lymphoma (cerebral or B-cell non-Hodgkin)
	· Invasive cervical carcinoma
	· Atypical disseminated leishmaniasis
	· Symptomatic HIV-associated nephropathy

http://dx.doi.org/10.5772/61259

· Symptomatic HIV-associated cardiomyopathy

· Reactivation of American trypanosomiasis (meningoencephalitis or myocarditis)

Table 3. WHO Clinical Staging of HIV/AIDS for Adult and Adolescents [8].

3.2.2. CDC classification system for HIV infection

The CDC classification of HIV/AIDS is based on the level of CD4 cell count and on previously diagnosed HIV-related conditions (Table 4) [7]. For example, if a patient had met the criteria for category B but currently is asymptomatic, the patient would remain in category B. The categorization is shown in Table 5. Patients in categories A3, B3 and C1-C3 are considered to have AIDS.

CD4 Cell Count Categories	CLINICAL CATEGORIES		
	A: Asymptomatic, Acute HIV or PGL	*B: Symptomatic Conditions, not A or C	**C: AIDS-Indicator Conditions
1. ≥ 500 cells/μL	A1	B1	C1
2. 200-499 cells/μL	A2	B2	C2
3. < 200 cells/μL	A3	B3	C3

PGL: persistent generalized lymphadenopathy for *B and **C Clinical Categories refer to Table 5

Table 4. CDC Classification System for HIV-Infected Adults and Adolescents [7].

***Category B: Symptomatic Conditions**	Definition: Symptomatic conditions occurring in an HIV-infected adolescent or adult that meet at least one of the following criteria: 1. They are attributed to HIV infection or indicate a defect in cell-mediated immunity 2. They are considered to have a clinical course or management which is complicated by HIV infection 3. Include the following: · Bacillary angiomatosis · Oropharyngeal candidiasis (thrush) · Vulvovaginal candidiasis, persistent or resistant · Pelvic inflammatory disease (PID) · Cervical dysplasia (moderate or severe)/cervical carcinoma in situ · Hairy leukoplakia, oral · Herpes zoster (shingles), involving two or more episodes or at least one dermatome · Idiopathic thrombocytopenic purpura · Constitutional symptoms, such as fever ("/>38.5°C) or diarrhea lasting "/>1 month · Peripheral neuropathy

****Category C: AIDS-Indicator Conditions**	· Bacterial pneumonia, recurrent (two or more episodes in 12 months) · Candidiasis of the bronchi, trachea, or lungs · Candidiasis, esophageal · Cervical carcinoma, invasive, confirmed by biopsy · Coccidioidomycosis, disseminated or extrapulmonary · Cryptococcosis, extrapulmonary · Cryptosporidiosis, chronic intestinal ("/>1 month in duration) · Cytomegalovirus disease (other than liver, spleen, or nodes) · Encephalopathy, HIV-related · Herpes simplex: chronic ulcers ("/>1 month in duration), or bronchitis, pneumonitis, or esophagitis · Histoplasmosis, disseminated or extrapulmonary · Isosporiasis, chronic intestinal ("/>1-month in duration) · Kaposi sarcoma · Lymphoma, Burkitt, immunoblastic, or primary central nervous system · *Mycobacterium avium* complex (MAC) or *Mycobacterium kansasii*, disseminated or extrapulmonary · *Mycobacterium tuberculosis*, pulmonary or extrapulmonary · *Mycobacterium*, other species or unidentified species, disseminated or extrapulmonary · *Pneumocystis jiroveci* (formerly *carinii*) pneumonia (PCP) · Progressive multifocal leukoencephalopathy (PML) · *Salmonella* septicemia, recurrent (nontyphoid) · Toxoplasmosis of brain · Wasting syndrome caused by HIV (involuntary weight loss "/>10% of baseline body weight) associated with either chronic diarrhea (two or more loose stools per day for ≥1 month) or chronic weakness and documented fever for ≥1 month

Table 5. B and **C Clinical Categories of HIV infection [7].

3.3. Immunologic changes in HIV infection

3.3.1. Depletion of CD4+T cells causes immunodeficiency

Untreated HIV-1 infection is associated with a gradual loss of peripheral $CD4^+$ T cells. Loss of $CD4^+$ T cells and systemic immune activation are the major hallmarks of HIV infection [9]. There are two major phases of HIV disease, acute and chronic infection. Acute infection is associated with gradual loss of $CD4^+$ T cells in the mucosal tissue [10] while chronic infection is characterized by immune activation which is associated with massive production of proinflammatory cytokines [11]. This subsequently leads to decrease in peripheral $CD4^+$ T cells and profound immunodeficiency.

The major mechanism of $CD4^+$ T cell depletion in HIV patients is due to apoptosis, in which the number of apoptotic cells exceed the number of HIV-infected cells [12]. Other causes of $CD4^+$ T cell depletion include impairment of *de novo* production of T lymphocytes by the thymus [9], induction of syncytium formation, alteration of membrane permeability, mitochondrial dysfunction as well as killing by HIV-specific $CD8^+$ T cells due to immune activation [9].

3.3.2. Loss of function of CD4+ T cells

Functional defects in the immune system of HIV-infected individuals exacerbate the immune deficiency caused by depletion of CD4+ T cells. These functional defects include a decrease in T cell responses to antigens as well as weak humoral immune responses even though total serum Ig levels may be elevated [13]. The defects might be due to the direct effects of HIV on $CD4^+$ T cells through:

1. Binding of gp120 (viral encoded membrane glycoprotein) to newly synthesized intracellular CD4+ T cells that result in the interference of normal protein processing in the endoplasmic reticulum as well as block the surface expression of $CD4^+$ T cells.This makes the cell incapable of responding to antigenic stimulation and,

2. $CD4^+$ T cells which bound to gp120 may not be available to interact with class II major histocompatibilty complex (Class II MHC) molecules on antigen presenting cells (APCs), thus T cell responses to antigens would be inhibited. Alternatively, gp120 binding to $CD4^+$ may deliver signals that downregulate helper T cell function.

In addition, HIV-infected T cells are unable to form tight synapses with APCs, therefore interferes with T cell activation [13]. Failure of the activation process will lead to incapability of the T cells particularly $CD4^+$ T cells to interact with other immune cells and subsequently lead to failure of elimination of the virus [13].

3.3.3. Cytokine dysregulation and coagulopathy in HIV infection

Cytokines play an important role in controlling the homeostasis of the immune system. Cytokine dysregulation is a major immunopathogenic factor in HIV infection [14]. The rise in serum levels of pro-inflammatory and inflammatory cytokines contribute to viral replication and many manifestations of immunodeficiency [15]. Cytokine production can increase viral replication due to its activation role in HIV infected cells [16]. Such cytokines include IL-2, IL-4 and interferon type II (IFN-γ) which primarily are required for expansion aid of antiviral T cells and antibody responses [16].

3.3.3.1. Cytokine dysregulation

Infection with HIV results in dysregulation of the cytokine profile *in vivo* and *in vitro*. During the course of HIV-1 infection secretion of T-helper 1 (Th1) cytokines, such as interleukin (IL)-2 and antiviral interferon (IFN)-gamma important for intracellular infection is generally decreased, whereas production of T-helper 2 (Th2) cytokines required for extracellular infection such as IL-4, IL-10, proinflammatory cytokines (IL-1, IL-6, IL-8) and tumour necrosis factor (TNF)-alpha, is increased [13, 14, 17]. This altered balance of Th1 and Th2 responses may partially explain the susceptibility of HIV-infected individuals to infection by intracellular microbes. In addition, Th2 cytokines also may inhibit macrophage-mediated killing of microbes [13] and consequently lead to failure of macrophage activation in the killing process of the virus.

Tumour necrosis factor-alfa (TNF)-α, IL-1 and IL-6 which are produced by monocytes and macrophages, play an important role in activation of neutrophils, monocytes and macrophages to initiate bacterial and tumor cell killing, increase adhesion molecule expression on the surface of neutrophils and endothelial cells, stimulate T and B lymphocytes proliferation as well as initiate the production of other proinflammatory cytokines [1, 2]. In addition, these cytokines can cause systemic symptoms such as fever and weight loss as well as influence the production of acute phase protein in the liver [1]. Inflammation is one of the components of innate immune response. Thus, production of appropriate amounts of TNF, IL-1 and IL-6 is important in response to infection [1]. Increased production of these cytokines, particularly TNF-α has been found in acute and inflammatory conditions (e.g., trauma, sepsis, infection, rheumatoid arthritis) [18]. The observed increase in proinflammatory and inflammatory cytokines following cell injury or infection subsequently leads to immune dysfunction.

3.3.3.2. Coagulopathy in HIV patients

Normal levels of protein S, protein C and antithrombin activities are necessary for coagulation process. In HIV patients, protein S, protein C and antithrombin activities decrease with an increase in plasma D-dimer [19, 20]. Binding of viral and bacterial components to Toll-like receptors (TLRs) stimulate the procoagulant tissue factor to initiate the coagulation cascade. This leads to thrombin activation which then cleaves the fibrinogen to fibrin [21]. Plasmin cleaves the fibrin to produce fibrin degradation products. An increase in monocyte tissue factor expression leads to increase in D-dimer in HIV infection [21]. Decrease protein S, protein C and antithrombin activities as well as increase in plasma D-dimer are the predisposing factors which will increase the risk HIV patients to thrombosis.

3.4. Prognostic markers of HIV infection

Prognostic markers are important tools for monitoring the HIV disease progression. Proper monitoring of the disease may reduce the morbidity as well as mortality rate. Some markers have been identified for monitoring the HIV disease progression. The markers is classified as immunologic (CD4+ T cells), virologic (RNA viral load), serologic (serum $\beta_2$microglobulin and neopterin) [22] as well as biomarkers (lipid peroxidation) [23]. Among the markers, CD4+ T cell count and RNA viral load are two most commonly used prognostic markers for clinical progression of HIV infection [24, 25].

3.4.1. Immunologic marker of infection

The CD4+ T cell count is the most important laboratory indicator of immune function in HIV-infected patients. It is also the strongest predictor of subsequent disease progression and survival according to findings from clinical trials and cohort studies [22, 26].

Measurement of CD4+ T cell count is necessary prior to the initiation of HAART. Since the CD4+ T cell count reflects the status of overall immune function of HIV-infected patients, the measurement is important as a guide for initiation of HAART to HIV patients as well as to start or discontinue the prophylaxis for opportunistic infection (OI). Most of OIs occur in patients with CD4+ T cell counts<200 cells/mm^3 [27], however some patients may have OIs at higher CD4+ T cell counts. For patients who are on therapy, adequate response is defined as an increase in CD4+ T cell counts in the range of 50 to 150 cells/mm^3 during the first year of HAART. Patients who has faster response will show the response within the first 3 months of treatment and subsequent increase in the range of 50 to 100 cells/mm^3 per year until it reaches a steady state [27]. Patients who has undergone the therapy at a low CD4+ T cell counts [28] or at an older age [29] may have a minimal increase in CD4+ T cell counts despite virologic suppression.

3.4.2. *Virologic marker of infection*

RNA viral load is the best indicator of progression to AIDS and death followed by $CD4^+$ T cell count, serum neopterin levels and serum $\beta_2$microglobulin. It strongly predicts the rate of decrease in $CD4^+$T cell counts and progression to AIDS and eventual death, but the prognosis of HIV is best predicted by combination of both plasma HIV-1 RNA and $CD4^+$ T cells [21].

In addition, it is also a marker of response to HAART. The main goal of HAART is to achieve and maintain durable viral suppression. A patient's pre-HAART viral load level and the magnitude of viral load decline after initiation of HAART provide prognostic information about the probability of disease progression [30]. Thus, the most important use of the viral load is to monitor the effectiveness of therapy after initiation of HAART. The minimal changes in the viral load is considered to be statistically significant (2 standard deviations) when there is a three-fold change (equivalent to a 0.5 $\log_{10}$ copies/mL change) in the viral load [31]. Optimal viral suppression is defined as presence of persistent viral load below the level of detection (HIV RNA <20 to 75 copies/mL, depending on the assay used) [31].

Data from previous studies and clinical trials reported that reduction in viral load following initiation of HAART are associated with reduced risk of progression to AIDS or death [30]. Therefore, RNA viral load measurement is an established surrogate marker for treatment response.

3.4.3. *Serologic markers*

Beta-2 microglobulin is a low molecular weight protein, which comprises the light chain of class 1 MHC proteins and is noncovalently bound to the heavy chain [2]. It is present on the surface of all nucleated cells. Dissociation during metabolism and degradation leads to its release to all biological fluids. In HIV disease, an increased level of Beta-2 microglobulin in cerebrospinal fluid (CSF) correlates with the disease progression and a decrease level indicates successful therapy [32].

Similarly, neopterin, a marker of immune activation is a low molecular weight compound derived from guanosine triphosphate [5]. It is produced by monocyte/macrophages upon stimulation with IFN-γ. The production is increased in HIV infection and infection by intracellular organisms such as parasite, autoimmune disease, malignant tumours, allograft rejection, neurological as well as cardiovascular disease [33]. However, it has slightly low predictive value compared to beta-2 microglobulin [5]. Neopterin and beta-2 microglobulin levels were proved to be significant predictors of AIDS risk in HIV-1 seropositive patients. The predictive value of both parameters is equal to $CD4^+$ T cell counts. Therefore, neopterin and beta-2 microglobulin are recommended to be used as an additional marker to predict AIDS risk for HIV-1 seropositive patients and is beneficial particularly in the setting where the CD4+ T cell count measurement is not available [34].

3.4.4. Biomarker

Oxidative stress is a condition in which there is increased amounts of reactive oxygen or nitrogen species. This condition is now recognized to be a prominent feature of many acute and chronic disease and even in normal ageing process. Lipid peroxidation was found to be one of the biomarkers to assess oxidative stress status in human disease including HIV [23]. A study done by Friis-Moller *et al.* [35] have shown that HIV-infected patients have oxidative imbalance early in the disease; low serum and tissue antioxidants and elevation of peroxidation products. Besides, high plasma levels of malondialdehyde (MDA), reduced plasma glutathione (GSH) and decreased superoxide dismutase activities were also found [36].

4. Haematologic aspects of HIV infection

4.1. Normal haemopoiesis

Haemopoiesis is the formation of blood or blood cells in the living body. It involves the production of three (3) major cell lines which are red blood cells, white blood cells and platelets [37]. In humans, this process occurs in the bone marrow. In certain diseases, the process can be altered either directly or indirectly. Patients with HIV infection will have altered haemopoiesis [38], affecting both red and white blood cells and platelet formation.

Haemopoietic stem cells (HSCs) are the earliest cells recognized in the bone marrow (Figure 2). HSCs produce all blood cells [37]. About 5% of the HSCs in the bone marrow are functioning at one time, thus maintaining the haemopoietic system for the lifetime in a human body. Growth factors, also play an important role for production and differentiation of blood cells in the bone marrow. Erythropoietin, a type of hormone which is mainly produced by the kidney and thrombopoietin, which is mainly produced by the liver, are the growth factors that are necessary for production and proliferation of red blood cells and platelets respectively.White blood cells have five (5) major components which include neutrophil, monocyte, eosinophil, basophil and lymphocyte. The lymphocytes are further subdivided into B-lymphocytes and T-lymphocytes, which are important for functional activity.

In most circumstances, HIV infection causes reduction in blood cell formation [40]. These include red blood cell (anaemia), platelet (thrombocytopenia) and white blood cell (leucope-

http://dx.doi.org/10.5772/61259

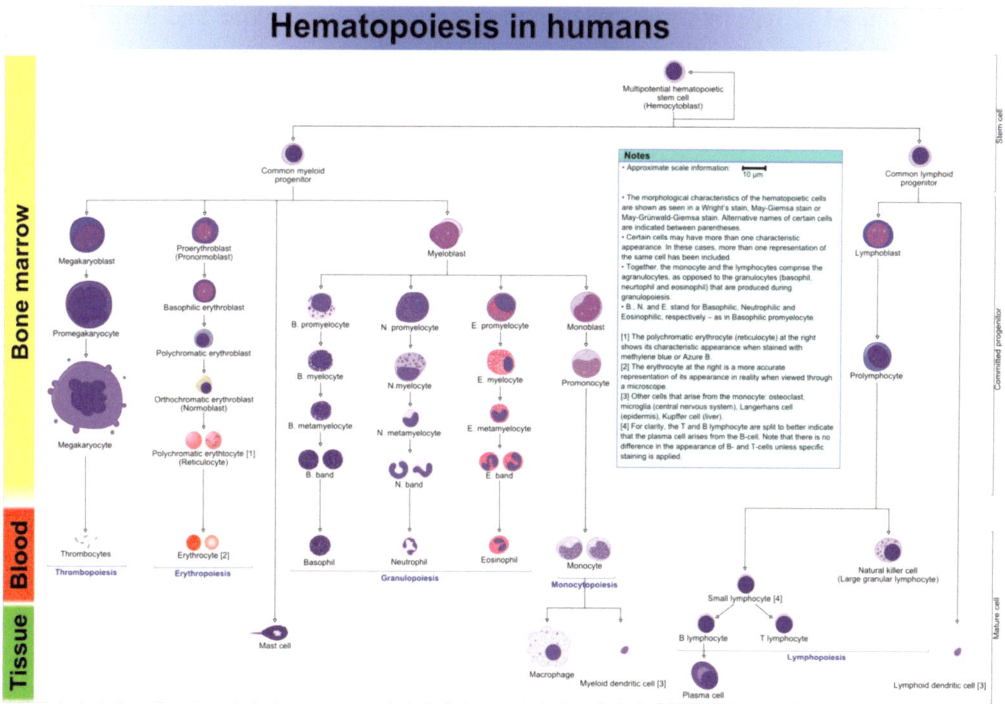

The diagram illustrates the hematopoiesis process that occurs in the bone marrow which gives rise to production of various cell lines from the marrow stem cell.

Figure 2. Production of red and white blood cells and platelets in the bone marrow [39]

nia) or any combination of these lineages (Table 6). The cause of these changes in HIV infection are not fully understood.

White blood cell	Normal Value ($x10^9/l$)	%	Reduce lineage
1. Neutrophil	2.0 – 7.0	40 – 80	Neutropaenia
2. Monocyte	0.2 – 1.0	2 – 10	Monocytopaenia
3. Eosinophil	0.02 – 0.5	1 – 6	
4. Basophil	0.02 – 0.1	<1 – 2	
5. Lymphocyte	1.0 – 3.0	20 - 40	Lymphopaenia

Table 6. Haematological abnormalities in HIV infection and normal adult reference values.

4.2. Haematological changes in HIV infection

Haematological abnormalities are common complications of HIV infection. These abnormalities increase as the disease advances. On both antiretroviral-treated and untreated individuals, different types of haematological abnormalities are common [41, 42, 43, 44] (Table 6).

Since the impact of HIV infection can be found in the peripheral blood and bone marrow, disorders of the haemopoietic system include anaemia, leucopenia, thrombocytopenia and thrombosis. These could be because of direct effects of the virus on the bone marrow, suppression of bone marrow by secondary infections or neoplasms causing ineffective haematopoiesis, nutritional deficiencies or side effects of the drugs used [44]. The disorders commonly occur throughout the course of HIV infection.

4.2.1. Blood abnormalities

The majority of the HIV cases present haematological abnormalities in the middle or advanced stages of the infection. However, some of the changes such as low haemoglobin and platelets have been reported in the early stages of HIV infection [44].

4.2.1.1. Anaemia

Anaemia refers to decrease in the haemoglobin (Hb) concentration with reference to healthy individuals of the same age group, sex, physiological state and environment (altitude).Normal haemoglobin for men is more than 13 g/dL while for women is 12 g/dL [38]. This can be classified based on the etiology or morphology of the red blood cell. The normal red blood cell shows a normochromic normocytic morphology. Anaemia is one of the commonest abnormalities seen in HIV, occurring in more than 50% of patients [40]. In a study done in HIV patients without myelosuppressive therapies, 8% of asymptomatic HIV-seropositive patients, 20% of those with symptomatic middle-stage HIV disease, and 71% of those with Centers for Disease Control (CDC)-defined AIDS were found to be anaemic [40]. Anaemia can be the earliest haematological manifestation, especially in children with HIV infection. Normochromic normocytic anaemia is the usual feature, but sometimes the HIV patients can present with a hypochromic microcytic anemia [45, 46, 47, 48, 49].

The causes of anemia in HIV patients are multifactorial. Inflammatory cytokines released by lymphocytes such as tumour necrosis factor (TNF), Interleukin-1 (IL-1) and interferon gamma play an important role in the pathogenesis of anaemia. These cytokines have been shown to inhibit red cell production (erythropoiesis) *in vitro* [51]. TNF levels were found to be consistently elevated in HIV infection and this condition is correlated with viral load [52]. Presence of dyserythropoiesis and opportunistic infections have also resulted in functional and morphological abnormalities of red blood cells [41]. This can alter the normal function of red blood cell as oxygen carrier or alter its normal biconcave shape. Other factors that contribute to the development of anaemia include underlying chronic disease, mixed nutritional deficiencies, opportunistic infections and side effects from the treatment [53]. As HIV disease progresses, the prevalence and severity of anaemia also increases [48, 54].

Disseminated Mycobacterium avium complex (MAC) disease may be present in HIV patients. It has been reported that about 76% of patients with this infection have severe anemia [52]. Another isolated red cell disorder, chronic pure red cell aplasia has been reported in HIV patients infected with parvovirus B19 [55]. This indicates that the underlying infection due to immunosuppression can give rise to anaemia.

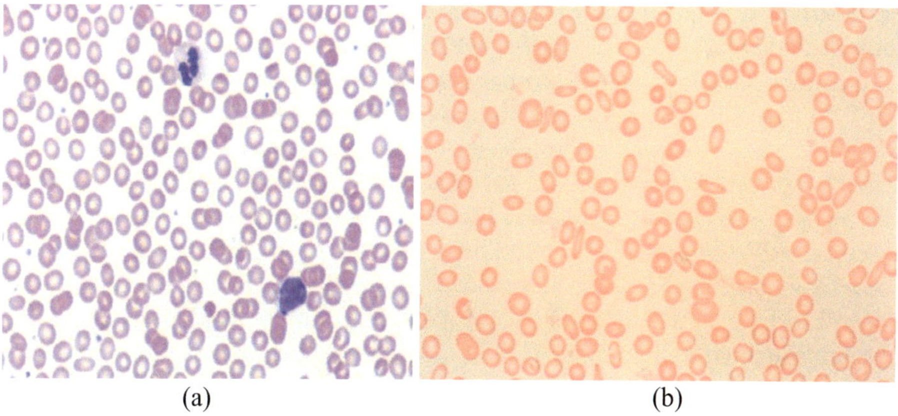

The peripheral blood smear in Figure 3(a) appears normal morphology, this condition is a normochromic, normocytic anemia. The utilization of iron is impaired due to a cytokine-mediated blockage in transfer of iron from the storage pool to the erythroid precursors in the bone marrow. The RBC's in Figure 3(b) appear smaller than the normal morphology and have an increased zone of central pallor. This feature shows a hypochromic (less hemoglobin in each RBC) and microcytic (smaller size of each RBC) anemia.

Figure 3. (a) Normochromic normocytic red cells and (b) Hypochromic microcytic red cells [50]

Nutritional anaemia in HIV patients frequently arises from an inadequate balanced diet intake and malabsorption. Infection and drug toxicity are common causes of gastrointestinal disease. Vitamin B12 deficiency is seen in up to one-third of HIV-positive subjects. Iron and folate deficiency are also common in this type of patients [38]. Bone marrow infiltration by tumour, such as lymphoma, is more common among HIV patients as compared to the normal population.The infiltration can suppress the production of red blood cells which can lead to anaemia. Anaemia is known to occur as an adverse effect of drug therapy for HIV infection or its complications. Myelosuppression can be caused by dose limiting toxicity of zidovudine [56]. Other drugs such as primaquine, dapsone and ganciclovir can lead to anaemia in HIV patients [52]. HIV patients with lymphoma on chemotherapy may present with anaemia due to the myelosuppressive treatment.

4.2.1.2. Thrombocytopaenia

Platelets are produced in the bone marrow. Normal platelet count is between 150 – 400 x 10^9/L. Reduction in the number of platelet count can be due to ineffective and/or reduced production of platelets in the bone marrow or increase destruction/ consumption of platelets in the peripheral blood. In HIV disease, thrombocytopaenia is the second most frequent hematological complication of HIV infection. It is found in 3% to 40% of individuals with HIV infection and could occur at any stage [57]. Presence of thrombocytopaenia is independent of the disease progression.

The mechanism of thrombocytopenia in HIV infection is mainly due to ineffective platelet production and at the same time increased platelet destruction [58]. There is a significant platelet sequestration and destruction in the spleen in HIV-associated thrombocytopenia.

Platelet destruction normally occurs early in the course of the disease. The destruction is often antibody mediated [59]. There are HIV-specific antibodies that have been shown to share a common epitope with antibodies against glycoprotein on the platelet surface (platelet GPIIb/IIIa) [59]. Nonspecific absorption of immune complexes onto platelets also occurs which predisposes the cell to immune thrombocytopaenia. Interestingly, there was a study that correlated the presence of lupus anticoagulant and anticardiolipin antibodies in HIV patients with the presence of thrombocytopaenia [60]. The other common cause of reduced platelet production in HIV patients is direct infection of megakaryocytes by the virus itself [61]. This gives rise to abnormal megakaryocytes morphology in the marrow. Other causes of thrombocytopenia include marrow infiltration by opportunistic infection or lymphoma, presence of complications such as thrombothic thrombocytopaenic purpura, and myelosuppressive effects of drug therapy.

4.2.1.3. Leucopaenia

Leucopaenia is the reduction in total white blood cell (WBC) count. In adults, normal WBC count is between 4.5 to 11.0 x 10^9/L. Leucopaenia is frequently seen in HIV patients and predominantly due to lymphopenia, decrease in the number of lymphocyte count, mainly $CD4^+$ lymphocytes. Leucopaenia generally correlates with the disease progression in HIV patients [62]. Reduction in absolute number of $CD4^+$ T-cells occurs as one of the earliest immunologic abnormalities of HIV infection and is one of the important prognostic indicators of risk of developing opportunistic infections.

Production of granulocytes and monocytes is also reduced, but less well recognized feature as compared to lymphopaenia. Occurance of neutropaenia is hinged on several other factors which are commonly seen in patients with advanced HIV disease. It can also occur due to concurrent infections, immune mediated or therapy related factors. Another cause of neutropaenia might be decreased bone marrow production of granulocytes due to inhibition of granulocyte progenitors. It has been postulated that a glycoprotein present in the marrow of infected patients might have an inhibitory effect [62]. Despite cellularity changes, morphological changes may occur in HIV patients. The changes are mainly due to dysplasia [38]. Peripheral blood smear will show some neutrophil changes such as detached nuclear fragments, abnormal nuclear fragmentation either hypofragmentation or hyperfragmentation, and abnormal nuclear granulation.

4.2.1.4. Haematological changes in HIV infection with correlation to CD4 cell count

In 2012, Parinithia and Kulkarni had done a study among 250 HIV patients to determine the haematological changes that occur in HIV patients as well as to evaluate its correlation with the CD4 cell count. They reported that among the HIV patients studied, anaemia, lymphopenia and thrombocytopenia was found in 210 (84%), 163 (65.2%) and 45 (18%) cases respectively [61]. Majority of the cases (70%) had CD4 cell counts below 200 cells/mm^3, 54 cases (21.6%) had CD4 cell counts between 200 to 499 cells/mm^3 and in 21 cases (8.4%), the CD4 count is more than 500 cells/mm^3. In patients with CD4 cell counts less than 200 cells/mm^3, anaemia, leucopenia, lymphopenia and thrombocytopenia was observed in 91.4% 26.8%, 80% and 21.7%

cases respectively [61]. This study revealed that there was a significant increase in the number of cases of anaemia and lymphopenia with decreasing CD4 cell counts. Thrombocytopenia was also seen but did not show significant increase with disease progression.

5. Bone marrow associated haematological abnormalities

Bone marrow abnormalities are frequently seen in HIV infected patients.However, these changes do not seem to be specific, but maybe typical for HIV patients. The most common findings are dysplasia affecting one or more cell lineages. Bone marrow examination is not routinely done in HIV infected patients. It is usually performed to evaluate peripheral cytopenias or when systemic infections or malignancies are suspected.

5.1. Cellular abnormalities

The cellularity of the bone marrow can be assessed based on trephine biopsy. It can be normal, reduced or increased, depending on the patients' condition. Normally the bone marrow will show normal or increased cellularity. However, the marrow cellularity does not always correlate with the peripheral blood findings. The commonly observed pancytopenia (reduction in the 3 major cell lineages, which are red cells, white cells and platelets) in the peripheral blood is often associated with an active marrow [45], suggesting dysmyelopoiesis or increased peripheral destruction. Other than cellularity, the morphology and function of the cells can be altered. These include presence of severe nutritional deficiencies in advanced stages of HIV infection, bone marrow suppression by opportunistic infections or neoplasm, underlying chronic and toxic side effects of antiretroviral compounds (or other medications used to treat the complications of HIV disease). Megaloblastic changes where the red cell series are macrocytic, are occasionally seen in the bone marrow aspiration of HIV patients and this may reflect myelodysplastic changes or concurrent effect of treatment [45]. There is possibility of HIV directly infecting the haematopoietic precursor cells and inhibiting their differentiation and maturation [45].

The increased number of plasma cells has been observed in some HIV patients. This may be related to repeated infections that always occur in immunocompromised patients. Haemophagocytosis is frequently seen in a bone marrow examination, especially in patients with CMV and herpes simplex infection. Features of increased macrophage activity may also be seen in tuberculosis [63] and histoplasmosis infection associated with HIV disease [64].

5.2. Opportunistic infections

An opportunistic infection is an infection caused by pathogens, particularly opportunistic pathogens, such as bacterial, viral, fungal or protozoal infections that usually do not cause disease in a healthy host with a healthy immune system. All HIV-infected individuals are in the immunosuppressive state. They are susceptible to a wide array of opportunistic infections and are at higher risk to pathogenic organisms that plague the general population [65]. Infectious agents reported to attack the bone marrow in patients with HIV include Mycobacterium avium complex, Mycobacterium tuberculosis, Mycobacterium xenopi and kansasi, Histoplasma, Cryptococcus, Toxoplasma, Cytomegalovirus and Pneumocystis carinii [66]. These infections may cause marrow changes either directly by the the organism itself or indirectly by causing reactive changes.

5.3. HAART and other medication that cause bone marrow changes

Introduction to highly active antiretroviral therapy (HAART) has resulted in a highly significant decline in mortality [67]. However, some of these drugs frequently cause haematologic toxicity. Several studies have shown that zidovudine and dideoxycytidine inhibit erythroid colony forming units (CFU-E) that are needed for erythroid formation and granulocyte macrophage colony forming units that is important for granulocyte formation [68]. Leucopenia can be seen in HIV patients treated with Ganciclovir. Pyrimethamine and sulfadiazine used in the treatment of toxoplasmosis cause leucopenia and thrombocytopenia. Chemotherapeutic agents used in the treatment of malignancies, especially lymphoma result in myelosuppression which is often dose limiting. Alpha interferon used in the treatment of Kaposi sarcoma in HIV patient is frequently associated with haematologic toxicity [69].

5.4. Lymphoma in HIV disease

Lymphoma is a group of diseases caused by malignant lymphocytes that accumulate in lymph nodes [37]. Lymphadenopathy or enlargement of the lymph nodes is the main clinical feature. It can be subdivided into Hodgkin's lymphoma and non-Hodgkin's lymphoma.

Patients with HIV disease have an increased incidence of lymphoma as compared to general population, especially diffuse non-Hodgkin's lymphoma subtype [70]. This is often of high grade lymphoma and mostly of B cell origin [70, 71]. The increased risk of lymphoma appears to be related to many factors, which are mainly related to a variety of genetic lesions, including infection by Epstein-Barr virus (EBV), c-myc gene rearrangement, bcl-6 gene rearrangement, ras gene mutations, and p53 mutations/deletions [72]. The malignant lymphoma, probably arises as a monoclonal outgrowth from a pool of proliferating B lymphocytes, which have been stimulated by the infective agents such as EBV and CMV.These opportunistic infections contribute to the pathogenesis of lymphoma more seen in HIV infection. Lymphoma in HIV patients tends to metastasize to brain or spread extranodal [73]. The relapse rate is high and overall patients will have a poor prognosis. However, with the introduction of HAART treatment, the risk of lymphoma has decreased and the clinical outcome improved [73].

6. Conclusion

The HIV epidemic clearly has broad and significant implications and impact on individuals infected and affected globally. Possibility of HIV patient developing severe HIV-related disease or not, depends on the degree of suppression of the immune system as well as the extensive reduction in the blood count. Therefore, it is important to identify those patients who are at risk of having the disease for proper assessment of infection and/or disease progression and subsequent monitoring. Prompt and consistent treatment should be given to those who are early diagnosed and side effects or drug toxicity assessment clearly made for effective consideration of drug change or drug discontinuation. Recently, with the introduction of HAART most of the immunological and haematological complications has been reduced, though some patients still develop unpredictable complications.

Author details

Wan Majdiah Wan Mohamad[1*], Wan Suriana Wan Ab Rahman[1],
Suhair Abbas Ahmed Al-Salih[2] and Che Maraina Che Hussin[2]

*Address all correspondence to: wmajdiah@usm.my

1 School of Dental Sciences, USM Health Campus, Kubang Kerian, Kelantan, Malaysia

2 School of Medical Sciences, USM Health Campus, Kubang Kerian, Kelantan, Malaysia

References

[1] Calder PC. Immunological Parameters: What do they mean? The Journal of Nutrition 2007;137 773S-780S.

[2] Parslow TG, Stites DP, Terr AI, Imboden JB. Medical Immunology, Lange Medical Books/McGraw-Hill, Medical Publishing Division, 10th edition; 2001. p148.

[3] O'Garra A & Arai N. The molecular basis of T helper 1 and T helper 2 cell differentiation. Trends Cell Biol. 2000; 10(12): 542-550.

[4] Bukowski RM, Olencki T, McLain D, Finke JH. Pleiotropic effects of cytokines: clinical and preclinical studies.Stem Cells 1994;12 Suppl 1: 129-40.

[5] De Wolf F & Lange JMA.Serologic and Immunologic Markers in the Course of HIV-1 Infection. Clinics in Dermatology 1991; 9 1-11.

[6] World Health Organization. WHO case definitions for AIDS surveillance in adults and adolescents.Weekly Epidemiological Record 69. 1994; 273-275.

[7] HIV Classification: CDC and WHO Staging Systems. 2014. http://aidsetc.org/guide/hiv-classification-cdc-and-who-staging-systems. Accessed April 2014.

[8] World Health Organization. WHO Case Definitions of HIV for Surveillance and Revised Clinical Staging and Immunological Classification of HIV-Related Disease in Adults and Children. 2007; http://www.who.int/hiv/pub/guidelines/HIVstaging150307.pdf?ua=1 Accessed 2007.

[9] Fevrier M, Dorgham K, Rebollo A. CD4+ T cell depletion in human immunodeficiency virus (HIV) infection: Role of apoptosis. 2011; 3(5) 586-612.

[10] Mehandru S, Poles MA, Tenner-Racz K, Horowitz A, Hurley A, et al. Primary HIV-1 infection is associated with preferential depletion of CD4+ T lymphocytes from effector sites in the gastrointestinal tract. J Exp Med 2004; 761-770.

[11] Cossarizza A, Ortolani C, Mussini C, Borghi V, Guaraldi G, Mongiardo N, Bellesia E, Franceschini MG, De Rienzo B, Franceschi C. Massive activation of immune cells with an intact T cell repertoire in acute human immunodeficiency virus syndrome. J Infect Dis. 1995;172:105–112.

[12] Holm GH, Zhang C, Gorry PR, Peden K, Schols D, De Clercq E, Gabuzda D. Apoptosis of bystander T cells induced by human immunodeficiency virus type 1 with increased envelope/receptor affinity and coreceptor binding site exposure. J Virol. 2004;78:4541–4551.

[13] Abbas AK, Lichtman AHH, Pillai S. Cellular and Molecular Immunology, Saunders Elsevier, 6th edition;2007. p482-483.

[14] Kedzierska K & Crowe SM. Cytokine and HIV-1: interactions and clinical implications. Antivir Chem Chemother 2001;12(3) 133-150.

[15] Munoz-Fernandez MA, Navarro J, Garcia A, Punzón C, Fernández-Cruz E, Fresno M. Replication of human immunodeficiency virus-1 in primary human T cells is dependent on the autocrine secretion of tumor necrosis factor through the control of nuclear factor-kappa B activation. J Allergy ClinImmunol 1997;100 838-845.

[16] Keating SM, Jacobs ES, Norris PJ. Soluble mediators of inflammation in HIV and their implications for therapeutics and vaccine development. Cytokine Growth F R 2012;23 193-206.

[17] Clerici M & Shearer GM. The Th1-Th2 hypothesis of HIV infection: new insights. Immunol Today1994;15 575–581.

[18] Popa C, Netea MG, van Riel PLCM, van der Meer JWM, Stalenhoef AFH. The role of TNF-α in chronic injury conditions, intermediary metabolism and cardiovascular risk. The Journal of Lipid Research. 2007; 48 751-762.

[19] Jong E, Louw S, Meijers JC, et al. The hemostatic balance in HIV-infected patients with and without anti-retroviral therapy: partial restoration with antiretroviral therapy. AIDS Patient Care STDS. 2009;231001–1007. [PubMed]

[20] Pontrelli G, Martino AM, Tchidjou HK, et al. HIV is associated with thrombophilia and high D-dimer in children and adolescents. AIDS 2010;24 1145–1151.

[21] Funderburg NT, Mayne E, Sieg SF, et al. Increased tissue factor expression on circulating monocytes in chronic HIV infection: relationship to in vivo coagulation and immune activation. Blood 2010;115161–167.

[22] Mellors JW, Munoz A, Giorgi JV, et al. Plasma viral load and CD4+ lymphocytes as prognostic markers of HIV-1 infection. Ann Intern Med1997;126(12) 946-954.

[23] Dalle-Donne I, Rossi R, Colombo R, Giustarini D, Milzani A. Biomarkers of oxidative damage in human disease. Clinical Chemistry 2006;52(4) 601-623.

[24] Hammer SM, Saag MS, Schechter M, et al. Treatment for adult HIV infection: 2006 recommendations of the International AIDS Society-USA panel. Top HIV Med. 2006;14 827-843.

[25] Gilks CF, Crowley S, Ekpini R, et al. The WHO public-health approach to antiretroviral treatment against HIV in resource-limited settings. Lancet 2006;368 505-510.

[26] Egger M, May M, Chene G, et al. Prognosis of HIV-1-infected patients starting highly active antiretroviral therapy: a collaborative analysis of prospective studies. Lancet 2002;360(9327)119-129.

[27] Mocroft A, Furrer HJ, Miro JM, et al. The incidence of AIDS-defining illnesses at a current CD4 count >/= 200 cells/muL in the post-combination antiretroviral therapy era. Clin Infect Dis 2013;57(7)1038-1047.

[28] Kaufmann GR, Perrin L, Pantaleo G, et al. CD4 T-lymphocyte recovery in individuals with advanced HIV-1 infection receiving potent antiretroviral therapy for 4 years: the Swiss HIV Cohort Study. Arch Intern Med 2003;163(18) 2187-2195.

[29] Moore RD & Keruly JC. CD4+ cell count 6 years after commencement of highly active antiretroviral therapy in persons with sustained virologic suppression. Clin Infect Dis 2007;44(3) 441-446.

[30] Murray JS, Elashoff MR, Iacono-Connors LC, Cvetkovich TA, Struble KA. The use of plasma HIV RNA as a study endpoint in efficacy trials of antiretroviral drugs. AIDS 1999;13(7) 797-804.

[31] Havlir DV, Bassett R, Levitan D, et al. Prevalence and predictive value of intermittent viremia with combination hiv therapy. JAMA 2001;286(2) 171-179.

[32] Svatonova J, Borecka K, Adam P, Lanska V. Beta-2 microglobulin as a diagnostic marker in cerebrospinal fluid: A follow-up study. Article ID 495402. Disease Markers 2014; 1-6.

[33] Murr C, Widner B, Wirleitner B, Fuchs D. Neopterin as a marker for immune system activation. Curr Drug Metab 2002; Apr 3(2) 175-187.

[34] Fuchs D, Kramer A, Reibnegger G, Werner ER, Dierich MP, Goedert JJ, Wachter H. Neopterin and beta-2 microglobulin as prognostic indices in human immunodeficiency virus type1 infection. Infection 1991; 19 Suppl 2S98-102.

[35] Friis-Moller N, Reiss P, Sabin CA. Class ofantiretroviral drugs and the risk of myocardial infarction. N Engl J Med 2007;3561723-1735.

[36] Day BJ & Lewis W. Oxidative stress in NRTI induced toxicity: evidence from clinical experience and experiments in vitro and in vivo. CardiovascToxicol 4. 2004; 207-216.

[37] Hoffbrand AV, Moss PAH, Pettit JE. Essential Haematology, Blackwell publishing; 6th edition. 2011.p246.

[38] Hoffbrand AV, et al. Postgraduate Haematology.Blackwell publishing; 6th edition. 2011. p954

[39] Rad A. Hematopoiesis in humans.2006.http://commons.wikipedia.org/wiki/File:Hematopoiesis (human) diagram.png. Assessed August 11 2006.

[40] Zon LI, Groopman JE. Hematologic manifestations of the human immunodeficiency virus (HIV).Semin Hematol 1988;25208-218.

[41] Zon LI, Arkin C, Groopman JE. Haematological manifestations of human immunodeficiency virus (HIV). Br J Haematol 1987;66251-256.

[42] Gange SJ, Lau B, Phair J, Riddler SA, Detels R, Margolick JB. Rapid declines in total lymphocyte count and hemoglobin in HIV infection begin at CD4 lymphocyte counts that justify antiretroviral therapy. AIDS. 2003;14:119–121.

[43] Muluneh A, Fessahaye A. Hematologic abnormalities among children on HAART in Jimma University Specialized Hospital, Southwestern Ethiopia. Ethiop J Health Sci. 2009;14(2) 83–89.

[44] Basu A, Ghosh K, Banerjee K. Bone marrow involvement in HIV infection: light, electron and immuno electron microscopic studies. Indian J Hematol& Blood Transf 1999;17(4) 76-86.

[45] Dikshit B, Wanchu A, Sachdeva KR, Sharma A, Das R. Profile of hematological abnormalities of Indian HIV infected individuals. BMC Blood Disorders. 2009;14:5.

[46] Akinbami A, Oshinaike O, Adeyemo T. Hematologic abnormalities in treatment-naïve HIV patients. Lagos, Nigeria. Infect Dis: Res Treat 2010;14 45–49.

[47] Behler C, Shade S, Gregory K, Abrams D, Volberding P. Anemia and HIV in the antiretroviral era: potential significance of testosterone. AIDS Res Hum Retrovir 2005;14(3) 200–206.

[48] Belperio PS, Rhew DC. Prevalence and outcomes of anemia in individuals with human immunodeficiency virus: a systematic review of the literature. Am J Med 2004;14(7) 27–43.

[49] Patwardhan MS, Golwilkar AS, Abhyankar JR, Atre MC. Hematological profile of HIV positive patients. Indian J PatholMicrobiol. 2002;14(2) 147–150.

[50] http://library.med.utah.edu/WebPath/HEMEHTML/HEME250.html. Assessed Jun 13 2015.

[51] Henry DH, Hoxie JA. Hematological manifestations of AIDS. In: Hoffmann R, Benz EJ, Shattil SJ, Furie B, Cohen HJ, Silberstein LE, and others (eds). Haematology basic

principles and practice, 4th edition. Philadelphia, Churchill Livingstone 2005; 2: 585-612.

[52] Coyle TE. Hematologic complications of human immunodeficiency virus infection and the acquired Immunodeficiency syndrome. Med Clin North Am 1997; 81(2) 449-470.

[53] Enawgaw B, et al. Determination of hematological and immunological parameters among HIV positive patients taking highly active antiretroviral treatment and treatment naïve in the antiretroviral therapy clinic of Gondar University Hospital, Gondar, Northwest Ethiopia: a comparative cross-sectional study. BMC Hematology 2014;14:8.

[54] Volberding P. The impact of anemia on quality of life in human immunodeficiency virus-infected patients. J Infect Dis 2002;14:110–114.

[55] Bain BJ. The haematological features of HIV infection. Br J Haematol 1997;99 1-8.

[56] Mehta S, Jutur S, Gautam D.Hematologic Manifestations of HIV/AIDS.Medicine Update-2011.

[57] Liebman HA. Viral-associated immune thrombocytopenic purpura. Haematology the Education Program of the American Society of Haematology.American Society of Haematology.Education Program. 2008. p212–218.

[58] Kuter DJ, Phil D, Gernsheimer TB. Thrombopoietin and Platelet Production in Chronic Immune Thrombocytopenia.Hematol Oncol Clin North Am. 2009; 23(6) 1193–1211.

[59] Kumar V, et al. Robbins and Cotran Pathologic Basis of Disease. Elsevier Saunders; 9th edition. 2010. p659.

[60] Cohen AJ, Philips TM, Kessler CM. Circulating coagulation inhibitors in acquired immune deficiency syndrome. Ann Intern Med 1986;104 175-180.

[61] Parinitha S & Kulkarni M. Haematological Changes in HIV Infection with Correlation to CD4 cell count. Australas Med J 2012; 5(3) 157-162.

[62] Aboulafia DM, Mitsuyasu RT. Hematologic abnormalities in AIDS. Hematol Oncol Clin North Am 1991;5(2): 195-214.

[63] Chandra P, Chaudhery SA, Rosner P, Kagen M. Transient histiocytosis with striking phagocytosis of platelets. Arch Intern Med 1975;135 989-991.

[64] Cooperberg AA, Schwartz J. The diagnosis of disseminated histoplasmosis from marrow aspiration. Ann Intern Med 1964;61 289-295.

[65] Haburchak DR, Windle ML, Bartlett J. Preventing Opportunistic Infections in Patients With HIV Medscape emedicine. 2014.

[66] Tripathi AK, Misra R, Kalra P, Gupta N, Ahmad R. Bone Marrow Abnormalities in HIV Disease. JAPI 2005;53705-710.

[67] Kanki PJ, Peeters M, Gueye-Ndiaye A. Virology of HIV-1 and HIV-2: implications for Africa. AIDS 1997;11(suppl B) S33-S42.

[68] Balakrishnan A et al. Zidovudine-induced reversible pure red cell aplasia. Indian J Pharmacol. Jun 2010; 42(3) 189–191.

[69] Pluda JM, Mitsuya H, Yarchoan R. (1991). Hematologic effects of AIDS therapies. Hematol Oncol Clin North Am 1991; 5(2) 229-249.

[70] Ziegler JL, Beckstead JA et al. Non-Hodgkin's lymphoma in 90 homosexual men.Relation to generalized lymphadenopathy and the Acquired Immunodeficiency Syndrome. NEngl J Med 1985;311 565-570.

[71] Lochim HL & Cooper MC. Lymphomas of AIDS.Lancet 1986i:96.

[72] Knowles D. Etiology and pathogenesis of AIDS-related non-Hodgkin's lymphoma. Hematol Oncol Clin Am 2003;17 785-820.

[73] Vishnu P, Aboulafia DM. AIDS-Related Non-Hodgkin's Lymphoma in the Era of Highly Active Antiretroviral Therapy. Advances in Hematology 2012;Volume 2012, Article ID 485943, 1-9.

Chapter 6

The Impact of Modern Antiretroviral Therapy on Lipid Metabolism of HIV-1 Infected Patients

Joel da Cunha, Luciana Morganti Ferreira Maselli,
Sérgio Paulo Bydlowski and Celso Spada

Additional information is available at the end of the chapter

http://dx.doi.org/10.5772/61061

1. Introduction

The highly active antiretroviral therapy (HAART) is the most efficient and safe alternative against HIV-1 infection, to allow the restoration of the immune system, with consequent reduction in mortality rate, increased survival and quality of life of infected patients. Apart from the great benefits of the use of different HAART regimens, laboratory and clinical experience has shown that HAART can induce severe and considerable adverse effects on metabolic complications of lipid metabolism, characterized by signs of dyslipidemia, increased risk of cardiovascular disease and even an increased risk of atherosclerosis. In this context, the class of protease inhibitors has been associated with a higher level of changes of lipid metabolism and an increased risk for cardiovascular disease. In turn, the search for different therapeutic strategies to reverse HAART-associated lipid disorders has led to the use of less metabolically active antiretroviral drugs without compromising antiretroviral efficacy. Thus, the different interactions of antiretroviral drugs are recommended based on their degree of impact on lipid metabolism. Recently, fusion inhibitors, integrase strand transfer inhibitors, entry inhibitors, have been included in the therapeutic arsenal against HIV-1 infection, and are not associated with metabolic disorders, since their mechanisms of action are different from other classes of antiretrovirals. Instead, the use of hypolipidemic drug therapy (statins, fibrates, inhibitors of intestinal cholesterol) becomes necessary when HAART-associated dyslipidemia occurs or persists for a long period and when alterations in diet, exercise and other HAART strategies are ineffective. Several alternatives are available, which, when adequately monitored, may be beneficial in reducing HAART-associated dyslipidemia. Changes in diet and lifestyle, and the adequacy of a hypocaloric diet, are recommendations that seek to reduce the concentrations of total cholesterol and its fractions. These changes bring benefits over short periods of time and reduce the risk for cardiovascular and atherosclerotic diseases in HIV-1 patients. In addition to known HAART regimens, new drugs and formulations have been developed to prevent infection by HIV-1. This new approach based on pre-exposure prophylaxis (PrEP) has shown promising results when administering drugs orally and in vaginal and rectal microbicides. PrEP using intravaginal rings with antiretroviral drugs is emerging as a promising strategy for the prevention of sexual HIV-1 transmission. The use of vaginal rings as controlled release strategy of antiretroviral drugs may improve adherence to PrEP, and provide sustained mucosal levels independent of coitus and daily dosing. Finally, the search for new drugs and methods that allow a greater survival, quality of life or prevention of HIV-1 transmission are constant challenges.

2. HAART as a new perspective of life for HIV+ subjects

For HIV-1-infected patients, the 1990s were marked by the introduction of HAART, which represented a new perspective of life for these patients [1]. The use of HAART was shown to effectively suppress the replication of HIV-1 and dramatically reduce mortality and morbidity rates, which has led to a better and longer quality of life for HIV-1 patients [2]. The HAART regimens, composed of at least three different antiretroviral drugs, are effective in reducing viral load (HIV-1-RNA) to undetectable levels when adhered to recommended prescription [3]. HAART regimens, with their different combination of drugs, inhibit viral replication by acting at different stages of infection [4]. This allows them to reach the viral cycle and/or viral enzymes and thus are classified in different therapeutic groups according to their mechanism of action: nucleoside reverse transcriptase inhibitors (NRTIs), non-nucleoside reverse transcriptase inhibitors (NNRTIs), protease inhibitors (PIs), fusion inhibitors, entry inhibitors (CC chemokine receptor-5 [CCR5] antagonists), and integrase strand transfer inhibitors (InSTIs) [5-10] (Table 1). NRTIs are nucleoside and nucleotide analogues which inhibit reverse transcription during HIV-1 infection. HIV-1 is a virus that has RNA as the genetic material, and is unable to integrate its DNA into host cell. For its integration into the chromosomal DNA of the human cell it must be reverse transcribed into DNA by a reverse transcriptase. The conversion of RNA to DNA therefore, is made by the viral protein reverse transcriptase (RT). NRTIs prevent reverse transcriptase's enzymatic activity and block completion of synthesis of the double-stranded viral DNA, this prevents HIV-1 multiplication. They are analogues of naturally occurring deoxynucleotides and competitively incorporates itself into the growing chain of viral DNA. NRTIs lack a 3′-hydroxyl (3 'OH) group on the deoxyribose moiety thus act as a chain terminator which prevents the next deoxynucleotide from forming another 5′–3′ phosphodiester bond needed to extend the DNA chain [5]. NNRTIs inhibit RT by binding to an allosteric site of the enzyme, and act as non-competitive inhibitors of RT. NNRTIs as a class of drug affect the handling of substrate (nucleotides) by RT by binding near the active site [6]. PIs on the other hand block the viral protease enzyme necessary to produce mature virions upon budding from the host membrane; ultimately these drugs prevent the cleavage of gag and gag/pol precursor proteins. In the presence of protease inhibitors, virus particles produced are defective and mostly non-infectious [7]. Fusion inhibitors and entry inhibitors interfere with binding, fusion and entry of HIV-1 to the host cell by blocking one of several targets. The drugs selzentry and enfuvirtide are the two currently available agents in this class. Selzentry works by targeting CCR5, a co-receptor located on human helper T-cells. Enfuvirtide is a peptide drug that must be injected and acts by interacting with the N-terminal heptad repeat of gp41 of HIV-1 to form an inactive hetero six-helix bundle, which prevents infection of host cells [8, 9]. InSTIs, also known as integrase inhibitors, inhibit the viral enzyme integrase, which is responsible for integration of viral DNA into the DNA of the infected cell. There are several integrase inhibitors currently under clinical trial; the drug raltegravir became the first to receive United States (US) Food and Drug Administration (FDA) approval in 2007. Raltegravir has two metal binding groups that compete for substrate with two Mg^{2+} ions at the metal binding site of integrase. Two other clinically approved integrase inhibitors are elvitegravir and dolutegravir [10]. Apart from the great benefits of the use of different HAART regimens, laboratory and clinical experience has shown that HAART can induce severe and considerable adverse effects on metabolic complications of lipid metabolism, characterized by signs of lipodystrophy, insulin resistance, central adiposity, dyslipidemia, increased risk of cardiovascular disease and even an increased risk of atherosclerosis [11-14]. However, other factors, such as virological, genetic, and individual immunological features, may be involved in the metabolic and lipid alterations observed because not all of the patients exposed to the same HAART regimens are affected [15-17].

3. Lipid changes in HIV infection

The observed changes in lipid metabolism during HIV-1 infection, as shown by changes in high-density lipoprotein (HDL) cholesterol, low-density lipoprotein (LDL) cholesterol, very low-density lipoprotein (VLDL), triglycerides (TG), lipid peroxidation, and their relationship with atherosclerosis in HIV-1 patients, results from the critical role of cholesterol in the mechanism of HIV-1 replication [11, 12, 18, 19]. The HDL is widely known as "good cholesterol", in which many studies have demonstrated that increasing serum levels are considered normal and are associated with a lower risk of cardiovascular disease because it can transport fat molecules out of artery walls, reduce macrophage fat accumulation and therefore regress atherosclerosis [18-20]. HDL has several potential for antiatherogenic properties, for instance, cholesterol is transported from peripheral tissues such as the cells in the arterial walls to the liver by HDL components, where it is used for a composition of lipoproteins and in synthesis of bile acids, steroid hormones, or fat-soluble vitamins [20]. Unlike the HDL, LDL is an important risk factor for the development of atherosclerosis and cardiovascular disease, and, this is the main lipoprotein cholesterol transports to peripheral tissues where they are internalized through the LDL receptor, a key mediator of plasma LDL concentrations [21]. Elevated plasma TG is emerging as an independent risk factor for the metabolic syndrome, type 2 diabetes, and cardiovascular disease, particularly if the levels of HDL are low and the levels of LDL increased [20, 21]. HIV-1 decreases plasma HDL by impairing the cholesterol-dependent efflux transporter ATP-binding cassette protein A1 (ABCA1) in human macrophages, which is a condition that has a high atherogenic risk [22, 23]. The use of PI-based HAART currently constitutes a more potent option against HIV-1 infection, preventing the maturation of viral particles and effectively controlling the infection of new cells by HIV-1. However, observed changes in lipid metabolism in HIV-1 patients have been associated with this class of antiretroviral drugs [13, 14, 24, 25].

Drug class	Generic name drug	Trade name/manufacturer/approval (year)
Nucleoside reverse transcriptase inhibitors (NRTIs)	Abacavir (ABC)	Ziagen® ViiV Healthcare (1998)
	Didanozine (ddl)	Videx® Bristol-Myers Squibb Co. (1991)
	Emtricitabine (FTC)	Emtriva® Gilead Sci. (2003)
	Lamivudine (3TC)	Epivir® GlaxoSmithKline (1995)
	Stavudine (d4T)	Zerit® Bristol-Myers Squibb Co. (1994)
	Tenofovir (TDF)	Viread® Gilead Sci. (2001)
	Zidovudine (AZT)	Retrovir® ViiV Healthcare (1987)
	Zalcitabine (ddC)	Hivid® Roche (1992)
Non-nucleoside reverse transcriptase inhibitors (NNRTIs)	Delavirdine (DLV)	Rescriptor® Pfizer (1997)
	Efavirenz (EFV)	Sustiva® Bristol-Myers Squibb Co. (1998)
	Nevirapine (NVP)	Stocrin® Merck Sharp, Dohme (1998)
	Etravirine (ETR)	Viramune® Boehringer Ingelheim (1996)
	Rilpivirine (RPV)	Intelence® Janssen-Cilag (2008)
		Edurant® Janssen-Cilag (2011)
Protease inhibitors (PIs)	Amprenavir	Agenerase® GlaxoSmithKline (1999)
	Atazanavir	Reyataz® Bristol-Myers Squibb Co. (2003)
	Darunavir	Prezista® Janssen-Cilag (2006)
	Fosamprenavir	Lexiva® ViiV Healthcare (2003)
	Indinavir	Crixivan® Merck & Co. (1996)
	Lopinavir	Kaletra® Abbott (2000)
	Nelfinavir	Viracept® ViiV Healthcare (1997)
	Ritonavir	Norvir® AbbVie Inc. (1996)
	Saquinavir	Invirase® Roche (1995)
	Tipranavir	Aptivus® Boehringer Ingelheim (2005)
Fusion inhibitors	Enfuvirtide/T-20	Fuzeon® Hoffmann La Roche (2003)
Integrase strand transfer inhibitors (InSTIs)	Dolutegravir (DTG)	Tivicay® GlaxoSmithKline (2013)
	Elvitegravir (EVG)	Stribild® Gilead Sci. (2012)
	Raltegravir (RAL)	Isentress® Merck & Co. (2007)
Entry inhibitors (CC chemokine receptor 5 [CCR5] antagonists)	Selzentry	Maraviroc® Pfizer (2007)

Table 1. Antiretroviral drugs.

There is significant support in the literature showing that the PIs are associated with increased hepatic TG-synthesis, VLDL, and to a lesser extent, total cholesterol (TC) [11-14]. Moreover, it was observed that these drugs impair the hydrolysis of TG-rich lipoproteins by lipase, which reduces the storage of free fatty acids (FFA) and interferes with the normal postprandial metabolism of FFA [25, 26]. The PIs are analogous substrates of the aspartyl protease enzyme of the HIV-1 that are involved in the cleavage process of viral proteins and form smaller and functional viral particles with infective capacity. After the cleavage process, the newly formed viral and infectious particles are released from infected cells in mature form [7, 27, 28]. Once the PIs bind to the active site of the protease enzyme, they block the cleavage process, which interferes with the normal process of viral maturation and formation of infectious viral particles in HIV-1 infection [27, 28]. The different mechanisms by which PIs promote these changes remain unknown. However, the main effect of PIs seems to be suppressing the breakdown of the nuclear form of sterol-regulatory element binding protein-1 (nSREBP1) in the liver and adipose tissue. This regulator is a key element in the proteolytic pathway responsible for regulating cellular and plasma levels of fat and cholesterol [29]. Some other classes of antiretroviral drugs are available, including those with excellent activity on suppression of viral replication without adverse effects on lipid metabolism [12, 25, 30]. However, it is clear that the use and recommendation of PIs occurs in situations where other drugs and/or regimens have not achieved the desired effect, either by non-adherence to treatment, viral resistance or lack of immune response [31, 32]. Once the therapy with PIs is initiated, a change to a more conservative therapy without their use is not recommended nor used in clinical practice [33, 34]. Thus, a continuous monitoring of the patient's characteristics for each PI available is required, in order to achieve alternative HAART regimens that could maintain a suppressive response of viremia, with minor effects on lipid metabolism of HIV-1 patients [34, 35].

4. Mechanism of HIV-associated lipid disorders

Lipid disorders during the course of HIV-1 infection and acquired immunodeficiency syndrome (AIDS) had been observed long before the advent of antiretroviral regimens [36, 37]. In the early phase of acute HIV-1 infection, the patient has several clinical signs of immunosuppression, variably characterized by fever, intestinal infections, weight loss and depletion of protein reserves [37, 38]. The possibility of the HIV-1 infection causing changes in lipid metabolism was already postulated because it is evident that plasma viremia may promote a decrease in plasma concentrations of TC, HDL and LDL, and, in later stages of infection, an elevation in the concentration of TG [37, 38]. Specifically, the reduction of HDL likely occurs as a result of an activation of the immune system in early HIV-1 infection, which promotes an increase in lipid peroxidation, alterations in the reverse cholesterol transport, and inflammatory cytokine production. Cytokines are small proteins which function to mediate communication between immune and non-immune cells, and they are produced by various cells of the immune system such as lymphocytes, natural killer (NK) cells, macrophages, dendritic cells, as well as endothelial cells, among others. These molecules orchestrate a variety of processes ranging from the regulation of local and systemic inflammation to cellular proliferation, metabolism, chemotaxis, and tissue repair. Different cytokines produced by these cells mediate the transition from innate to adaptive immunity response [39]. This process promotes an imbalance in the antioxidant system, a decrease in the production of anti-inflammatory cytokines and an elevation of pro-inflammatory cytokines, which increases the chances of developing atherosclerotic diseases [33-40]. The inflammatory process initiated by viral infection, a stimulus of endothelial lipase and phospholipase A2 occurs, which in turn can reduce HDL concentration [41-43]. The inflammatory process may also be characterized by an elevation of interferon-γ levels (IFNγ) originating from lymphocytes and macrophages. IFNγ levels are elevated at early stages of infection and are also correlated with the presence of hypertriglyceridemia [44, 45]. Tumor necrosis factor-α (TNFα) is another potent pro-inflammatory mediator whose concentrations increase in HIV-1 infected ART-naïve patients. TNFα promotes lipid peroxidation and disturbances in the metabolism of free fatty acids and also acts on the suppression of lipolysis mediated by hormones [46].

5. Mechanism of HAART-associated lipid disorders

HAART-associated dyslipidemia is complex and involves immunological, hormonal, genetic predisposition aspects and the effects induced by different antiretroviral drugs [13, 47]. The observed dyslipidemia is characterized by hypertriglyceridemia, hypercholesterolemia, and decreased serum levels of HDL, either accompanied or unaccompanied by increased levels of LDL (Table 2) [47, 48]. Other metabolic and/or clinical common disorders include insulin resistance with hyperinsulinemia, increased C-peptide levels, diabetes mellitus and lipodystrophy syndrome [44-48]. Diabetes mellitus is a group of metabolic disorders in which the blood glucose is higher than normal levels due to insufficiency of insulin release or improper response of cells to insulin. The resultant hyperglycemia produces sever complications [49]. The production and secretion of insulin is realized by pancreatic β-cells, and occurs in response to concentrations of amino acids, fatty acid and glucose. However, glucose is considered the first stimulus to the beta cells which secrete insulin. Regulated insulin release requires tight coupling in the β-cell between glucose metabolism and insulin secretory response [50]. HAART also affects the hydrolysis of TG-rich lipoproteins and tissue lipase, disrupts normal postprandial FFA and lipoprotein catabolism and interferes with peripheral fatty acid trapping. These effects could be due to the interaction of fatty acids with the master transcriptional regulator sterol regulatory element binding protein 1 (SREBP1) [51-56]. Nevertheless, the presence of dyslipidemia in individuals who use HAART is not necessarily accompanied by lipodystrophy and/or an evident insulin resistance, which suggests that the mechanism(s) involved in these disorders maybe independent [47, 51, 56, 57]. The NNRTI-based HAART, zidovudine, stavudine or lamivudine, has eventually become associated with the occurrence of dyslipidemia; however, lipid metabolism disorders are mainly evident in individuals who make use of the PI-based therapy [47, 48, 57, 58]. In as much as the mechanisms involved in PI-associated dyslipidemia are not fully understood, the prevailing hypothesis is based on the structural similarity between the catalytic region of the HIV-1 protease and two homologous human proteins involved in the metabolism of lipids, called cytoplasmic retinoic acid-binding protein type 1 (CRABP-1) and low-density lipoprotein-receptor-related protein type 1 (LRP1).

5.1. CRABP-1

CRABP-1 exhibits 58% homology in its amino acid sequence of the C-terminal region in the catalytic area of the HIV-1 protease. CRABP-1 usually binds intracellular retinoic acid and presents it to Cytochrome P450 3A4 (CYP3A4) (EC 1.14.13.97) enzymes, which convert retinoic acid to cis-9-retinoic acid, bind to retinoid X receptor-peroxisome proliferator-activated receptor γ (RXR-PPARγ) heterodimer, stimulating adipocyte differentiation and inhibiting apoptosis [22, 48, 59]. Hepatic CYP enzymes are responsible for the metabolism of xenobiotic and many pharmaceuticals, but they also utilize endogenous compounds as substrates, such as cholesterol and fatty acids [60]. CRABP-1 shows homology with the viral protease, therefore, it is suggested that PIs bind to CRABP-1 and thereby inhibit the formation of 9-cis retinoic acid, leading to a reduction RXR-PPARy activity, increased apoptosis, and decreased proliferation of peripheral of adipocytes. Such events would cause peripheral lipoatrophy syndrome and hyperlipidemia because of adipocyte loss, decreased lipid storage and lipid release into the bloodstream. The inhibition of CYP3A by ritonavir is another possible mechanism involved in lipid abnormalities in HIV-1 patients and associated PI-based therapy and would promote a reduction in the formation of cis-9-retinoic acid and reduced enzymatic activity of RXR-PPARy. The decrease in RXR-PPARγ activity results in apoptosis of peripheral adipose stores, decreased adiponectin, and insulin resistance. However, central and visceral adipose stores are spared and expand with weight gain, contributing to insulin resistance [22, 48, 60].

5.2. LRP

LRP share 63% homology with the catalytic region of HIV-1 protease. LRP binds to LPL on the capillary endothelium, and the formation of this LRP-LPL complex promotes cleavage of fatty acids from TG, thereby promoting FFA accumulation in peripheral adipocytes. A possible hypothesis is that the binding of PIs to LRP may inhibit the complex normal function of LRP-LPL and interfere with fatty acid storage, leading to hyperlipidemia. Hyperlipidemia is characterized by elevations in cholesterol levels, principally in the LDL and VLDL cholesterol fractions, because fatty acids released into the bloodstream subsequently reach the liver and promote a secondary hepatic synthesis of TG and VLDL [48, 59, 61].

5.3. Mitochondrial alterations

Another proposed mechanism for HAART-associated dyslipidemia is the mitochondrial alterations induced by HAART, especially with PI-based therapy. The hypothesis is that the HAART regimens will cause mitochondrial disturbances by inhibiting the mitochondrial DNA (mtDNA)-polymerase γ, leading to mitochondrial DNA depletion, respiratory chain dysfunction and reduced energy production by cells [62, 63]. This disturbance in the mitochondrial respiratory chain may promote metabolic disorders in adipocytes, promote lipodystrophy syndrome and increase plasma lipid levels. Moreover, interference between PIs and cellular protease could also trigger the development of metabolic alterations because some proteases are essential for mitochondrial biogenesis and metabolic function. Furthermore, functional changes of mitochondria in skeletal tissue promote insulin resistance and consequent dyslipidemia [62-64].

5.4. Genetic factors

HAART-associated lipodystrophy and dyslipidemia may be related to genetic predisposition. Studies on HIV-1 patients with hypertriglyceridemia and low HDL were shown to be associated with different polymorphisms in the *APOCIII* gene. Promoter polymorphisms -455T>C and -482C>T in the *APOCIII* gene are both associated with increased levels of TG containing lipoproteins (VLDL) and low HDL values. Carriers of the -455T>C genetic variant had 30% lower levels of HDL compared to those without this polymorphism and plasma lipid concentrations increase according to the number of these variant alleles. Another variant nucleoside, the -1131T>C promoter polymorphism in the *APOA5* gene, was associated with hypertriglyceridemia in PI-based patients [65-68].

5.5. Paraoxonases

Changes in antioxidant enzymes, such as the family of paraoxonases (PONs), may partially explain some of the mechanisms involved in HAART-associated dyslipidemia and consequently characterize a higher risk for cardiovascular diseases and atherosclerosis [63]. The hypothesis that the PIs can promote reductions in the activity of PONs and an increased risk for atherosclerotic disease in HIV-1 patients has been shown through previous evidence. PON1 is an antioxidant enzyme present in serum is strongly associated with apolipoprotein-A1 (apoAl) from HDL and protects LDL against oxidative modifications [69, 70]. The action of serum PON1 most likely occurs through the involvement of the enzyme in reverse cholesterol transport, a well-established anti-atherogenic propriety of HDL [71]. PON1 has the ability to inhibit LDL oxidation (oxLDL) and significantly reduce the lipid peroxidase enzyme, which decreases the accumulation of cholesterol in peripheral tissues [72]. The oxidative modification of LDL in the arterial wall plays a central role in the pathogenesis of atherosclerosis, which is characterized by the deposition of lipids and the formation of atherosclerotic plaques that cause narrowing of the blood vessels [73]. The inhibition of oxLDL by HDL is attributed to the high antioxidant content of the lipoprotein possibly due to the antioxidant properties of apoA1 and by the presence of other different antioxidant enzymes, such as glutathione peroxidase and PON, which prevent the formation of or degrade bioactive products of oxLDL [68]. Some studies have shown that the activity of PON1 may be affected and/or inactivated by oxidative stress, which could explain its reduced activity during HIV-1 infection [69-71]. In HIV-1 patients and those who undergo HAART, there is a significant increase in oxidative stress. In asymptomatic HIV-1 patients, there is an increased oxidative stress characterized by elevated lipid peroxidation products and/or a quantitative decrease in antioxidants compared to seronegative controls that are considered to be in a healthy condition. Therefore, possible reductions in the activity of PON1 and HDL concentrations may characterize an increased cardiovascular risk in individuals infected with HIV-1 [70, 71, 75]. The PON1 activity that was reduced in ART-naïve patients, and restored in patients treated with HAART suggested that the activity of PON1 is associated with the immune status in HIV-1 patients. However, in individuals treated with lopinavir/ritonavir, even with low plasma viremia, PON1 activity was reduced and a higher atherogenic risk was shown by the high TC:HDL ratio, suggesting that a PI-based regimen affects the mechanisms involved in the oxidation of LDL, which promotes greater atherogenic risk [69-74].

5.6. LDL oxidation

Oxidative modifications to LDL, which are considered the initial event in the pathogenesis of atherosclerosis, are attributed to oxidative stress mechanisms initiated by agents such as superoxide, nitric oxide and hydrogen peroxide (H_2O_2) that transform LDL into oxLDL [77, 77]. The deposition of oxLDL in the arterial intimal layer promotes a cytotoxic effect on the vascular endothelium, followed by inflammation and modification of monocytes into macrophages that phagocytose oxLDL particles to form the foam cells which accumulate in the intima and lead to the development of atheromatous plaques [78]. The oxLDL particles are immunogenic, and serum levels of anti-oxLDL antibodies (Abs) can be used as indicators of oxidative stress [76-78]. The immunoglobulin G (IgG) anti-oxLDL Abs are pro-atherogenic and can predict the progression of coronary and carotid atherosclerosis, whereas IgM anti-oxLDL Abs appear to be associated with a possible protective role against the development of atheromatous plaques [79]. During the process of infection by HIV-1, the increase in atherogenic risk results from changes in lipid metabolism associated with the severity, duration and stages of infection. Different degrees of lipodystrophy occur in patients along with a decrease in LDL receptor expression, which could lead to increased oxidation of LDL particles and the consequent development of atherosclerosis [80]. HIV-1 patients treated with lopinavir/ritonavir have shown higher levels of IgG anti-oxLDL Abs compared to patients treated with efavirenz or nevirapine regimens, and these levels were associated with an increase in the atherogenic indices [78-80].

6. HAART-associated lipodystrophy

Lipodystrophy is a syndrome that includes peripheral fat wasting and central obesity and is a well-documented side effect of HAART (Table 3) [16, 53, 81]. In addition to the decrease in the expression of LDL receptors, and a consequent increase in serum concentrations of LDL, the most obvious mechanism of HAART-associated lipodystrophy and dyslipidemia are the mitochondrial changes induced by HAART [13, 62-64]. The inhibition of mtDNA-polymerase γ, which leads to mitochondrial DNA depletion in respiratory chain dysfunction and a reduced energy production in cells, may promote metabolic disorders in adipocytes and promote increased lipodystrophy syndrome and plasma lipid levels [62-64, 82, 83]. Both therapies, PIs- and NRTIs-based, are associated with the inhibition of mtDNA-polymerase γ [82-84]. The abnormalities observed in lipodystrophy syndrome include lipoatrophy, lipohypertrophy, and metabolic disturbances. Lipoatrophy is associated with the loss of subcutaneous fat, usually in the lower limbs, face and buttocks. The observation of lipoatrophy in HIV-1 patients has been demonstrated in therapy with both PIs- and NRTIs-based therapies. Several studies initially suggested that lipoatrophy in HIV-1 patients is primarily associated with the use of PI-based therapies; however, more recent reports show that the incidence of lipoatrophy was significantly higher in the efavirenz plus two NRTIs group than in the lopinavir or efavirenz plus two NRTIs plus lopinavir groups [85-87]. The association of lipoatrophy with efavirenz use was mainly in combination with either stavudine or zidovudine but not with tenofovir/ lamivudine. Lipohypertrophy consists of the accumulation of adipose tissue. The PI-based therapy has been associated with the development of lipohypertrophy, but several longitudinal studies have failed to demonstrate that this therapy is the main cause of lipohypertrophy in HIV-1 patients [86-89].

Drug class	Drug	Effects on lipids	Effects on glucose
NRTIs	Abacavir (ABC)	↑ Dyslipidemia	No effect
	Didanozine (ddl)	↑ ↑ Dyslipidemia	Insulin resistance
	Emtricitabine (FTC)	↑ Dyslipidemia	No effect
	Lamivudine (3TC)	↑ Dyslipidemia	No effect
	Stavudine (d4T)	↑ ↑ Dyslipidemia	Insulin resistance
	Tenofovir (TDF)	↑ Dyslipidemia	No effect
	Zidovudine (AZT)	↑ ↑ Dyslipidemia	Insulin resistance
NNRTIs	Efavirenz (EFV)	↑ ↑ HDL, ↑ Dyslipidemia	No effect
	Etravirine (ETR)	Neutral effects	No effect
	Nevirapine (NVP)	↑ ↑ HDL, ↑ LDL	
	Rilpivirine (RPV)	Neutral effect	
PIs	Amprenavir/ritonavir	↑ ↑ ↑ Dyslipidemia	Insulin resistance
	Atazanavir/ritonavir	↑ Dyslipidemia	Insulin resistance
	Darunavir/ritonavir	↑ Dyslipidemia	Insulin resistance
	Fosamprenavir/ritonavir	↑ ↑ ↑ Dyslipidemia	Insulin resistance
	Indinavir	↑ ↑ Dyslipidemia	Insulin resistance
	Lopinavir/ritonavir	↑ ↑ ↑ Dyslipidemia	Insulin resistance
	Nelfinavir	↑ ↑ Dyslipidemia	Insulin resistance
	Saquinavir	↑ Dyslipidemia	Insulin resistance
	Tipranavir/ritonavir	↑ ↑ ↑ Dyslipidemia	Insulin resistance
Fusion inhibitors	Enfuvirtide, T-20	Neutral effect	No effect
InSTIs	Dolutegravir (DTG)	Neutral effect	No effect
	Elvitegravir (EVG)	Neutral effect	No effect
	Raltegravir (RAL)	Neutral effect	No effect
Entry inhibitors	Selzentry	Neutral effect	No effect

Table 2. Antiretroviral drugs: impact on lipid and glucose metabolism.

Clinical diagnosis	Treatment options
Lipoatrophy	
Sunken eyes, sunken cheeks, prominent zygomatic arch, prominent veins, skinny or muscular appearance, loose skin folds loss of contour	Switching antiviral therapies: Stavudine or zidovudine to abacavir or tenofovir, other switch, and/or reconstructive procedures
Lipohypertrophy	
Increased abdominal girth with visceral fat accumulation, dorsocervical or supraclavicular fat pad	Diet, exercise, liposuction
Related findings	
Hypertriglyceridemia, usually with depressed HDL, hypercholesterolemia, insulin resistance, glucose intolerance	Statins, fibrates, inhibits intestinal cholesterol absorption, fish oils, diet, exercise, drugs (metformin, acarbose, sulfonylureas, glinides or leptin)

Table 3. Clinical diagnosis and treatment of to HIV-associated lipodystrophy syndrome.

7. Switching antiviral therapies

The search for different therapeutic strategies to reverse HAART-associated dyslipidemia has led to the use of less metabolically active antiretroviral drugs without compromising antiretroviral efficacy. Ritonavir is the most representative drug in HAART-associated dyslipidemia and in combination with lopinavir confers higher risks for cardiovascular disease in HIV-1 patients. Amprenavir and nelfinavir promote lower impacts compared to the therapy with lopinavir/ritonavir [31, 70, 80, 90, 91]. Similarly, the use of indinavir and saquinavir shows even less adverse effect on lipid metabolism in HIV-1 patients receiving HAART. Currently, atazanavir has the least impact on lipid metabolism [92, 93]. In contrast, nelfinavir promotes the elevation of TC, TG and LDL levels, and its replacement by atazanavir permits the reduction of the concentrations of these parameters without affecting antiretroviral activity [94]. A more recent alternative is tipranavir, a non-peptide PI prescribed for patients with multidrug resistance (MDR). However, this drug has shown deleterious effects that promote atherogenic risk by increasing the levels of TC and TG [95]. Another strategy to control dyslipidemia has been the discontinuation of the PI-based regimens and a switch to a NRTI- or NNRTI-based protocol. For ART-naïve patients, HAART regimens that include at least one NNRTI, or abacavir and two NRTIs, might be as efficient as PI-based therapy, although they may not be the standard choice. This exchange of HAART in patients with viral suppression did not reduce antiretroviral efficacy during long-term use [95-96]. A strategy that must be better evaluated is the long-term use of the NRTI/NNRTI class of drugs before the use of PI-based therapy. The use of NRTI-associated nevirapine reduces levels of TC and TG, promotes an increase in HDL and a decrease in atherogenic risk. The use of NNRTIs may also alter the lipid profile due mostly to the use of efavirenz. Using this medication, TG levels were higher when compared with nevirapine usage. However, in studies with a large number of HIV-1 patients, accompanied at intervals of ninety days and with undetectable HIV-1-RNA, the levels of TC, LDL and TG were kept within the desirable limit in the groups treated with nevirapine and efavirenz, including HDL levels within the reference values [95-98]. Only the HIV-1 patients treated with a PI-based regimen showed lipid abnormalities and increased risks for cardiovascular disease [13, 24, 96]. In addition, possible alterations in lipid metabolism resulting from the use of NNRTI-based therapy are easier and faster to reverse with the use of statins, fibrates, diet and lifestyle. Although the individual effects of NRTIs remain unclear, stavudine was associated with TC and TG elevations greater than zidovudine and tenofovir. The addition of fusion inhibitors to the existing therapies, such as enfuvirtide/T-20, had little effect on plasma lipids. The possibility of different HAART strategies eliminating or reducing the dyslipidemia in HIV-1 patients must be evaluated, and the risk of development of variants of the virus with MDR must be taken into account [99]. In HIV-1 patients with favorable historical responses to HAART and accompanied by a physician experienced in HIV-1 infection, the transition from a PI-based to a therapy with nevirapine, abacavir, or even atazanavir may be preferable to the use of a hypolipidemic agent. In practice, many patients will show pre-existing resistance to the drugs, limiting options for the exchange of the treatment [83, 92-94]. Experts must assess the risks of toxicity of the new treatment and the possibility of virologic relapse when switching HAART regimens.

8. Other therapies for HAART-associated dyslipidemia

The use of hypolipidemic drug therapy becomes necessary when HAART-associated dyslipidemia occurs or persists for a long period and when alterations in diet, exercise and other HAART strategies are ineffective. Difficulties in the treatment of dyslipidemia in HIV-1 patients involve potential interaction between drugs, toxicity, intolerance, and low patient adherence to multiple drug regimens. Several alternatives are available, which, when adequately monitored, may be beneficial in reducing HAART-associated dyslipidemia.

8.1. Statins

Statins is the name given to the group of drugs that help lower cholesterol. These will normally be prescribed to people who have harmful cholesterol levels present in their blood, especially if other control methods have failed or if the individual is at risk of developing health complications. Statins benefit users to prevent and treat atherosclerosis, which is the hardening of the arteries as a result of accumulation of cholesterol (atherosclerotic plaques) [100, 101]. They are drugs that inhibit the enzyme HMG-CoA reductase (3-hydroxy-3-methylglutaryl coenzyme A reductase) and are considered the primary drugs for the treatment of primary hypercholesterolemia [100]. In clinical practice, the use of statins has achieved excellent results in reducing TC and LDL, leading to a decreased risk of coronary artery events and in the primary and secondary prevention of heart diseases [100-102]. Statins inhibit the key rate-controlling enzyme in the de novo synthesis of cholesterol, which is responsible for production of >50% of total body cholesterol. Inhibition of HMG-CoA reductase also promotes an increase in the synthesis of hepatic LDL receptors and reduced VLDL production [101-103]. The most important drugs of this class are simvastatin, fluvastatin, atorvastatin, lovastatin, pravastatin and rosuvastatin. All of these drugs reduce LDL concentrations, although the use of simvastatin and atorvastatin has shown superior effects in HIV-1 seronegative patients [101-103]. In HIV-1 patients affected with dyslipidemia, the use of simvastatin, pravastatin, fluvastatin and rosuvastatin promotes reduction of dyslipidemia, but not in complete remission once other factors and elements are associated with the dyslipidemia in these patients [101-104]. The different drugs that compose HAART have metabolizing effects similar to statin (Table 4). In general, statins are metabolized by CYP3A4, and may cause clinically relevant interactions with other agents that are changed by this enzymatic complex, such as oral anticoagulants, ketoconazole, cyclosporine, erythromycin, itraconazole, PIs and NNRTIs [104-106]. Additionally, statins serve as substrates for G-glycoprotein, a known carrier of drugs in the small intestine, which may influence their oral bioavailability [105-107]. The presence of elevated statin levels in plasma increases the risk of liver toxicity, promoting elevations of serum transaminases and possible toxic hepatitis as well as skeletal muscle toxicity and myalgia with elevations of serum creatine kinase (CK) levels, especially in the case of simvastatin and atorvastatin [105-109]. Fluvastatin is metabolized by CYP2C9 enzyme; pravastatin and rosuvastatin are not significantly metabolized by the CYP450 system and have a very low risk of drug interactions. Reductions in the levels of TC and TG were observed in patients with dyslipidemia associated HIV-1 infection undergoing treatment with a PI and the use of rosuvastatin therapy. Simvastatin, lovastatin and atorvastatin should be avoided because they present a high risk of pharmacological interactions with PIs. Moreover, in a recent study, pravastatin had the lowest binding to plasma proteins of the statin agents and dietary advice associated with the statin compound significantly reduced TC levels in HIV-1 patients treated with HAART, without significant adverse events [104-108]. It is reasonable to recommend the use of pravastatin and/or rosuvastatin as a first-line treatment for hypercholesterolemia in PI-treated patients and the use of fluvastatin, characterized by a slightly lower efficacy, as a second-line regimen. Additional benefits are obtained in patients treated with indinavir or pravastatin and fluvastatin, which significantly reduces the levels of TC and LDL, while maintaining good tolerability. Different associations between statins and antiretrovirals present considerable tolerability but always require monitoring of serum transaminases and CK. Different clinical studies and the routine use of fluvastatin, pravastatin, or rosuvastatin have shown that they are most suitable and safe to reduce LDL levels in HIV-1 patients [104-110].

8.2. Fibrates

Fibrates or fibric acid derivatives are the drugs of choice for the treatment of hypertriglyceridemia and play an important role in the control of mixed dyslipidemia. Clinical studies have shown that fibrates may reduce the risk of coronary atherosclerosis in patients with hypercholesterolemia and also in individuals in post myocardial infarction with higher LDL, lower HDL, and TG with discrete increases. Fibrates may be used in combination with statins for hyperlipidemia or when HDL levels are decreased, besides acting in the hepatic synthesis of TG, TC, lipoprotein lipase (LPL) and acetyl-CoA carboxylase, it inhibits peripheral lipolysis and controls blood glucose [111-113]. Fibrates are also metabolized by CYP450 system, but they appear to affect only CYP4A enzymes and do not show clinically relevant interactions

Drug	Metabolism and Interactions
Simvastatin	Considerable CYP3A4 metabolism. ↑ simvastatin levels with PIs and ↓ ↓ levels with efavirenz. Not recommended with atazanavir, atazanavir/ritonavir, fosamprenavir/ritonavir, saquinavir/ritonavir, tipranavir/ritonavir, lopinavir/ritonavir, indinavir/ritonavir, darunavir/ritonavir and nelfinavir. Doses of 80 mg/day with NNRTIs, raltegravir and selzentry.
Lovastatin	Not recommended with atazanavir, atazanavir/ritonavir, fosamprenavir/ritonavir, saquinavir/ritonavir, tipranavir/ritonavir, lopinavir/ritonavir, indinavir/ritonavir, darunavir/ritonavir and nelfinavir. Doses of 80 mg/day with NNRTIs, raltegravir and selzentry.
Atorvastatin	Somewhat CYP3A4 metabolism, ↑ levels with PIs darunavir, lopinavir, saquinavir/ritonavir, fosamprenavir. ↓ levels with efavirenz. Doses of 20 mg/day with PIs, 80 mg/day with NNRTIs, raltegravir and selzentry.
Pravastatin	Reduced interaction with CYP450 metabolism, primarily renal excretion but 50% ↓ with lopinavir/ritonavir, 45% ↓ with nelfinavir, 80% ↑ with darunavir/ritonavir, and 40% ↓ with efavirenz. Doses of 80 mg/day with PIs, NNRTIs, raltegravir and selzentry.
Fluvastatin	Metabolized by CYP2C9, and occasional interactions with nelfinavir and efavirenz. Doses of 80 mg/day with PIs, NNRTIs, raltegravir and selzentry.
Rosuvastatin	Not CYP3A4 metabolized but 5x ↑ levels with lopinavir/ritonavir and darunavir/ritonavir (uncertain). Low starting doses (5-10 mg) recommended with PIs. Doses of 20 mg/day with PIs, 40 mg/day with NNRTIs, raltegravir and selzentry.

Table 4. Statins to HAART-associated dyslipidemia.

with PIs. However, concomitant use of both fibrates and statins can increase the risk of skeletal muscle toxicity and should be avoided [112-114]. In HIV-1 seronegative individuals, the use of a fibrate and a statin in a monotherapy regimen exhibits moderate lipid-lowering effects and good tolerability [114-116]. In HIV-1 patients, fibrates do not have the same efficacy of statins in preventing cardiovascular disease. Studies with HIV-1 patients treated with PI-based therapy and fibrates, including gemfibrozil, bezafibrateor fenofibrate, showed a significant reduction in the concentration of TC, TG and hypertriglyceridemia [113, 115, 116]. Fibrates appear as a suitable alternative for the treatment of dyslipidemia associated with HIV-1, especially in the presence of hypertriglyceridemia. Periodic monitoring of serum creatinine, CK, and transaminases should be performed when using fibrates [115-117]. The association between fibrates and statins has been used with relative safety and demonstrated in different studies with large numbers of HIV-1 patients volunteers, except for the use of the combination of statins and gemfibrozil, which is not recommended [116-118]. The use of statins, fibrates, or associated therapeutic agent has shown positive results in HIV-associated dyslipidemia. and the pravastatin/fenofibrate combination has accelerated the an improvement of lipid parameters and is safe and efficacious [119-120].

8.3. Inhibitors of intestinal cholesterol absorption

Inhibitors of intestinal cholesterol absorption are a class of drugs that prevent the absorption of cholesterol from the small intestine into the circulatory system. Ezetimibe is effective at lowering lipid levels because it has the ability to inhibit the intestinal absorption of cholesterol, and it shows good tolerability because it does not interact with the metabolism of CYPA4 enzymes [121, 122]. In HIV-1 seronegative patients who have dyslipidemia, the monotherapy with ezetimibe or when combined with statins or fenofibrate has shown considerable efficacy and safety [123, 124]. In HIV-1 patients with high serum levels of LDL, the use of ezetimibe has also been considered an effective alternative [122]. Monotherapy using 10 mg/day of ezetimibe has accelerated reductions of more than 20% of serum LDL and, in addition, reduces the concentrations of TC and TG while increasing HDL concentrations [121-124]. Studies have shown that in individuals with HIV-1 that are beyond effective treatments, ezetimibe has no interaction with HAART, and those receiving a PI-based association of fenofibrate/ezetimibe showed greater efficacy compared with pravastatin in monotherapy resolution of dyslipidemia [125-127].

8.4. Fish oil

The ability of fish oil, commonly known as omega-3 fatty acids (namely, eicosapentaenoic acid (EPA) and docosahexaenoic acid (DHA), to reduce elevated TG concentrations has been observed in different studies [128, 129]. HIV-1 patients using both HAART and fish oil showed an effective reduction in the concentration of TG [130]. This ability to reduce TG levels promotes a direct benefit in risk reduction of atherogenic cardiovascular disease through a combination of anti-inflammatory and anti-platelet actions [130-132]. For HIV-1 patients, the use of fish oil associated with fenofibrate showed additive effects in reducing TG. Given these considerable results, the American Heart Association's (AHA) dietary guidelines, recommends that healthy adults have a minimum of two portions of fish per week, and those who have elevated TG should consume 2-4 g of EPA and DHA daily as a dietary supplement [130-133].

8.5. Niacin

Niacin (water-soluble vitamin B3), or nicotinic acid, is a powerful reducing agent of serum lipids when administered at pharmacological doses. Its ability to reduce the levels of lipoproteins and apolipoprotein-B-containing lipoproteins and to raise HDL levels has been shown, characterizing it as an atheroprotective drug [134, 135]. Niacin has beneficial effects on cardiovascular risk factors, including lipoprotein (a), C-reactive protein (CRP), platelet-activating factor (PAF) acetylhydrolase, plasminogen activator inhibitor (PAI)- 1 and fibrinogen [136, 137]. The molecular mechanisms involving the action of niacin are not fully understood, but its effect on hypertriglyceridemia in uninfected individuals is recognized [135-137]. In HIV-1 patients, the use of niacin in an extended release formulation significantly reduced the levels of TC, TG and HDL. However, the use of niacin in HIV-1 patients with dyslipidemia need to be carefully monitored because the presence of adverse events have been commonly shown, including headache, flushing, pruritus, rash, hyperuricemia, and exacerbation of insulin resistance [138, 139].

8.6. Other contributory agents to HIV dyslipidemia

Other agents may contribute to HIV-associated dyslipidemia. The use of recombinant methionyl human leptin was associated with reduced insulin resistance and increased HDL levels

[140]. Tetradecylthioacetic acid (TTA), an agent whose mechanism is still unknown, promotes a reduction in levels of plasma lipoproteins [141]. Additionally, Acipimox, a drug with sustained action and a structure similar to niacin, has been associated with decreased insulin resistance and significantly reduced levels of TG in HIV-1 adults [142]. In a double-blind study, the use of cholestin was able to reduce the levels of TC and LDL without modifying HDL and TG, and without showing adverse effects [143]. The use of L-carnitine (3 g/day) resulted in a significant reduction in serum TG in patients with HIV-associated dyslipidemia [144]. These and other drugs studied aimed to revert the HIV-associated dyslipidemia but require more control to be considered appropriate for the treatment of dyslipidemia.

9. Current antiretroviral drugs and dyslipidemia

Since the introduction of zidovudine (1987) for the treatment of HIV-1 infection, followed by the emergence of the fusion inhibitors, such as enfuvirtide/T-20 (2003), and more recently the introduction of raltegravir (2007) and dolutegravir (2013) (Table 1), both InSTIs drugs, treatment for HIV-1 infection has been adapting to new challenges. Once the inability to eradicate viremia by the different HAART regimens was recognized, new drugs, strategies and therapeutic regimens were developed for greater efficiency associated with safety and reduced adverse effects. The common adverse effects observed by the use of the first class of drugs such as zidovudine, and the dyslipidemia caused by the use of PIs, are obstacles that are being minimized in newer drugs that are in the experimental phase. Currently, more than 30 drugs are approved and available in various forms (the different classes of antiretroviral drugs), and many others are in experimental stages.

9.1. NRTIs

9.1.1. Festinavir

Festinavir (BMS986001) is a thymidine analogue drug, derived from stavudine but with less potential toxicity [145]. It has been used in cases where there is resistance of HIV-1 to abacavir and tenofovir and is an oral drug recommended for HIV-1 patients with MDR. The compound has a 50% effective concentration (EC^{50}) in the inhibition of mtDNA-polymerase γ and is 100 times less toxic to the mtDNA-polymeraseγ in renal proximal tubular cells, muscle cells, and adipocytes and on the cellular levels of adenosine triphosphate and/or lactate production (ATP) than stavudine. The mitochondrial toxic effects of stavudine are the main cause of the adverse effects associated with lipodystrophy and peripheral neuropathy, which has led to the decline in its use and indicated that festinavir, has a minor impact on lipid metabolism [145-147].

9.1.2. Apricitabine

Apricitabine (AVX754, formerly SPD754) is a drug for oral administration and is in the experimental phase (Phase IIB clinical trial). It is structurally related to lamivudine and emtricitabine and, as such, is an analog of cytidine [148]. This drug is well tolerated, and its most common side effects include headache, nausea, muscle aches and diarrhea. The use of apricitabine in HIV-1 patients had no effect on bone marrow, liver or kidney toxicity, and lipase. However, its use causes changes in lipid metabolism, most noticeable by elevated serum TG, indicating that its use should be evaluated in patients who initiated therapy with apricitabine or who already have a dyslipidemic profile [148-150].

9.1.3. GS-7340

GS-7340 is a prodrug of tenofovir called tenofovir disoproxil fumarate (TDF). Unlike tenofovir, GS-7340 is stable in plasma and then converted to tenofovir inside the cell by the cellular enzyme cathepsin, which is highly expressed in lymphoid tissue [151]. Within the cell, the drug is transformed into the active metabolite tenofovir diphosphate, an inhibitor of RT. Phase III studies are underway to better define the safety profile and efficacy, and initially, the drug does not show effects on lipid metabolism. However, formulations with 300 mg promoted adverse effects on the kidneys and bone marrow toxicity [151-153].

Other drugs of the NRTIs class are in the experimental phase, such as racivir (an enantiomer of emtricitabine), elvucitabine (Phase II clinical trial), and amdoxovir (AMDX or DAPD). For these drugs, current data about the adverse effects are insufficient to characterize the impact on lipid metabolism [154-156].

9.2. NNRTIs

9.2.1. Etravirine

Etravirine (ETR, Intelence®) is a drug that has shown efficacy, safety and good tolerability in HIV-1 patients [157]. One of the great advantages of etravirine is as a replacement for other NNRTIs to which the HIV-1 virus is resistant, mainly due to the presence of the K103N and Y181C mutation in the case of efavirenz and nevirapine, respectively. The FDA approved the drug in 2008 for use in patients with multiple drug resistance. However, the drug is a substrate and an inhibitor of different CYP3A4 enzymes, which in turn are contraindicated with antimicrobial and anticonvulsant drugs metabolized by the CYP450 system. In patients receiving HAART and who have alterations in lipid metabolism, the switch to a therapy containing etravirine has shown satisfactory results and the reversal of dyslipidemia [157-160].

9.2.2. Rilpivirine

Rilpivirine (RPV, Edurant®) a NNRTIs class drug is more potent than diarylpyrimidine (DAPY), its adverse effects are considerably reduced compared to older NNRTIs such as efavirenz. After clinical trials, rilpivirine was approved by the FDA in 2011, and its use is combined with emtricitabine and tenofovir. Rilpivirine produces few changes in serum TC, LDL, HDL and TG in HIV-1 patients. In comparison to the treatment with efavirenz, this drug promotes an increase in lipids and in the TC:HDL ratio, which is characterized by an increased risk of cardiovascular diseases in these patients [161, 162].

9.2.3. MK-1439

MK-1439 is a new and effective drug against a variety of HIV-1 mutants that are resistant to NNRTIs [157]. Preclinical studies (Phase l clinical trial) that are currently in progress show that this drug has a good pharmacokinetic profile, with the possibility of a daily dose in low concentrations to obtain an optimal effect. Additionally, it has good absorption, low potential for toxicity and the ability to be used with other antiretroviral agents. MK-1439 showed good results in cases where the K103N mutation of HIV-1 leads to resistance to treatment with nevirapine and efavirenz, as well as in the occurrence of the Y1818C mutation, which leads to a lower susceptibility in treatment with nevirapine, rilpivirine and etravirine. *In vitro* data suggest that MK-1439 has beneficial properties for additional development as a new antiviral drug; however, no data are available about its potential impact on lipid metabolism [163-164].

New NNRTIs class drugs are in various experimental stages such as BILR 355 BS (Phase Ila), (+)-Calanolide A (Phase I), GSK 2248761 (Phase Ilb), MK-4965 (Phase I), MK-6186 (Phase I), RDEA806 (Phase Ila), and UK-453061 (Phase Ilb). These new drugs have not been approved by the FDA and still require different clinical trials to be launched as drugs available for the treatment of HIV-1 infection. Currently, no scientific information regarding their possible effects on lipid metabolism is available.

9.3. Fusion/entry inhibitors

The HIV-1 envelope (Env) glycoprotein complex, which is composed of three receptor-binding gp120 subunits and three fusion protein gp41 subunits, mediates virus entry by fusing viral and cellular membranes and offers an attractive target for developing antiviral agents [165, 166]. In succession to enfuvirtide/T-20, a number of design strategies have been applied to develop new peptide-based fusion inhibitors with improved stability, bioavailability and potency [166, 167]. There are several drug classes that are in two experimental phases. Albuvirtide (FB006M), T649, T2634, T2544, T1249, SC34EK, and SC29EK are in the class of fusion inhibitors. BMS 663068, BMS 626529, vicriviroc (SCH 417690), and cenicriviroc (TAK-652, TBR-652) are in the class of entry inhibitors. These and other drugs are in experimental stages and/or have been suspended, and there are no initial and/or conclusive data about their potential toxic effects and the impact on lipid metabolism.

9.4. InSTIs

Cobicistat (GS-9350) is a new InSTIs drug recently approved by the FDA (2012). This drug, like ritonavir, has the ability to inhibit hepatic enzymes that metabolize other drugs used to treat HIV-1 infection, such as raltegravir [168]. Cobicistat has become increasingly important, and its use has been associated with elvitegravir, permitting it to have higher blood concentrations with use of smaller doses, which theoretically allows for greater suppression of viral replication with elvitegravir, having fewer adverse effects. Cobicistat has been employed in combination with elvitegravir/emtricitabine/tenofovir (Stribild®) [168, 169]. Cobicistat is a potent inhibitor of CYP3A enzymes, which will concurrently affect administered medications metabolized by this pathway. It also inhibits intestinal transport proteins, increasing the overall absorption of several drugs including atazanavir, darunavir, and tenofovir alafenamide fumarate (TAF). Phase III trials of the cobicistat-containing combination antiretroviral therapy regimens in ART-naïve patients have shown a small elevation of serum fasting lipid, with a relative increase in the levels of TC and TG, in addition to bilirubin elevations, jaundice, nausea and diarrhea [168-170]. Other drugs of the InSTI class are experimental, such as MK2048. It is a drug that acts by inhibiting integrase enzyme four times longer and shows superior efficacy to raltegravir. Additionally, it is being investigated for use as part of PrEP [171]. In turn, BI224436 is the first non-catalytic site integrase inhibitor (NCINI) with capacity to inhibit HIV-1 replication. This inhibition of HIV-1 replication occurs via its attachment to a conserved allosteric pocket of the HIV integrase enzyme. This makes the drug distinct in its mechanism of action compared to raltegravir and elvitegravir, which bind at the catalytic site [172, 173]. Another experimental drug is GSK744 (S/GSK1265744, Cabotegravir®), which has a structure similar to that of carbamoyl and omizanddolutegravir. In investigational studies, the agent has been packaged into nanoparticles (GSK744LAP), which confer an exceptionally long half-life of 21–50 days following a single dose. In theory, this would make suppression of HIV-1 possible when dosing as infrequently as once every three months. These drugs do not have sufficient data on their toxicity profile and/or on lipid metabolism; however, they have been previously considered to have low metabolic toxicity [174, 175].

10. Pre-Exposure Prophylaxis (PrEP)

In addition to known HAART regimens demonstrated in HIV-1 patients, new drugs and formulations have been developed to prevent infection by HIV-1. This new approach based on PrEP has shown promising results when administered as oral drugs, vaginal microbicides (VM), and rectal microbicides (RM). PrEP is an important tool for the prevention of HIV-1 infection, and can be combined with condom provision, counseling, and the diagnosis and treatment of sexually transmitted infection (STI), thus providing even greater protection than when used alone [176, 177]. Different clinical trials based on PrEP, have shown reductions in HIV-1 infection rates among men who have sex with men (MSM), and heterosexual HIV-serodiscordant couples, who were prescribed daily oral antiretroviral PrEP with a fixed-dose combination of TDF and emtricitabine (FTC) (Truvada®). The isolated use of TDF also demonstrated safety and efficacy in clinical trials among injecting drug users (IDU) and among men and women in heterosexual HIV-discordant couples [177-180] (Table 5).

10.1. Tenofovir Disoproxil Fumarate (TDF)/Emtricitabine (FTC)

The combination TDF/FTC (Truvada®, TVD), both NRTIs, widely used as part of first-line regimens for the treatment of HIV-1 infection, was approved in July 2012 by the FDA for PrEP in combination with safer sex practices to reduce the risk of sexually acquired HIV-1 in high-risk adults [181]. Currently, prescribing daily oral PrEP with TDF 300mg/FTC 200 is recommended as one prevention option for MSM, heterosexual patners, and IDU at substantial risk of HIV acquisition [181-183]. TDF/FTC has had few serious side effects, which facilitates adherence to its use, however, it can't be administered to subjects with renal failure and

Study	Clinical trial*	Sample size	Limitations	Evidence
Among men who have **sex with men**				
iPrEX trial (n=2499)	Phase lll trial	TDF/FTC (n=1251) Placebo (n=1248)	Adherence	High
US MSM Trial(n=400)	Phase ll trial	TDF/FTC (n=201) Placebo (n=199)	Minimal	High
Among heterosexual men **and women**				
Partners PrEP(n=4758)	Phase lll trial	TDF(n=1589) TDF/FTC (n=1583) Placebo (n=1589)	Minimal	High
TDF2(n=1219)	Phase ll trial	TDF/FTC (n=201) Placebo (n=199)	-High loss to follow-up	Moderate
Among heterosexual Women				
FEM-PrEP(n=2120)	Phase lll trial	TDF/FTC (n=1062) Placebo (n=1058)	-Stopped at interim analysis -Limited follow-up -Very low adherence	Low
West African(n=936)	Phase ll trial	TDF (n=469) Placebo (n=467)	-Stopped early for operational concerns -Small sample size -Limited follow-up time on assigned drug	Low
VOICE(n=3019)	Phase llB trial	TDF(n=1007) TDF/FTC (n=1003) Placebo (n=1009)	-TDF arm stopped at interim analysis -Very low adherence to drug regimen in both TDF and TDF/FTC arms	Low
Among injection drug users				
BTS(n=2411)	Phase lll trial	TDF (n=1204) Placebo (n=1207)	Minimal	High

Table 5. Clinical trials with TDF/FTC (Truvada®) for pre-exposure prophylaxis (PrEP)(GRADE Criteria). Note: Grade quality rating: high=further research is very unlikely to change our confidence in the estimate of effect; moderate=further research is likely to have an important impact on our confidence in the estimate of effect and may change the estimate;low= further research is very likely to have an important impact on our confidence in the estimate of effect and is likely to change the estimate; very low=any estimate of effect is very uncertain. *All trials in this table were randomized, double-blind, prospective clinical trials.

Fanconi syndrome [177-179, 184]. Additionally, its use in PrEP is well tolerated, and the occurrence of headache, nausea, vomiting, abdominal pain, and weight loss may occur infrequently [177-179]. Nausea and vomiting affects about one in six patients at the beginning of the treatment, but these effects often reduce in the first month [177]. Although the use of

TDF/FTC may be in a single daily dose, it is important to assess the risk of developing drug resistance. Thus, it is necessary for all patients to be seronegative for HIV-1 before beginning treatment, to perform laboratory tests every two or three months, in order to confirm their seronegative status for HIV-1 [185]. In individuals with signs and/or symptoms of acute HIV-1 infection, or who reported ppotential HIV-1 exposure in the previous month, HIV-1 infection should be excluded by repeated tests before starting PrEP [177, 179, 185]. Further, the starting of PrEP with TDF/FTC requires that individuals carry out medical examinations and screening for diagnosing possible STI in six-month intervals [185-190]. The main clinical studies of TDF/FTC and TDF monotherapy, which allowed the approval of this therapy as choice for PrEP, are shown in Table 5.

11. Microbicides for prevention of HIV transmission

Recently, strategies for prevention of HIV-1 infection with topical formulations for vaginal application and/or rectal have been receiving attention. Whereas most phase I and phase II clinical trials have found microbicide compounds to be safe and well tolerated, phase III trials completed to date have not demonstrated efficacy in preventing HIV transmission [191]. Different topical microbicides under study for prevention of HIV-1 are grouped into classes of agents, based on where they disrupt the pathway of sexual transmission of HIV. These classes include surfactants/membrane disruptors, vaginal milieu protectors, viral entry inhibitors, reverse transcriptase inhibitors, and other groups whose mechanism is unknown. Surfactants and acidifying agents act non-specifically, either by disrupting viral and cellular membranes, or creating a more hostile environment in the genital tract for viral transmission [191-193] (Table 6).

11.1. Specific microbicide agents

11.1.1. Reverse transcriptase inhibitors

Reverse transcriptase inhibitors are antiretroviral with recognized efficacy and safety in the treatment of HIV-1 infection and prevention of mother-to-child HIV-1 transmission. This class of drugs has allowed the formulation of topical microbicide less toxic and more effective [194]. The nucleotide reverse transcriptase inhibitor tenofovir was the first antiretroviral drug to safely demonstrate in animal models both pre-exposure and post-exposure prophylaxis as proof-of-concept against the sexual transmission of HIV-1 [195, 196]. Two other compounds of class NNRTIs being studied as topical microbicides to prevent HIV-1 infection, are the TMC120 and UC781. Preclinical or clinical testing of these compounds as potential topical microbicides have several features in common, and both compounds show minimal systemic absorption, and good safety profiles in animal studies [200, 201]. *In vitro*, TMC120 and UC781 prevent cell-free and cell-associated virus from infecting co-cultures of monocyte-derived dendritic cells and T cells [202-204].

11.1.1.1. Tenofovir

Tenofovir is active as a diphosphate, rather than a triphosphate, which does not act via HIV DNA chain termination, coupled with the limited phosporylation ability of macrophages. This explains why the drug might be effective in macrophages and other non-dividing cells [197, 198]. Based on the animal studies and with an appreciation for tenofovir's relatively high barrier to resistance compared with other reverse transcriptase inhibitors [196], the compound became the first antiretroviral drug to be assessed as a VM in a clinical trial. In a phase I study (HPTN 050), 0 3% and 1% vaginal tenofovir gel, formulated as a diphosphate, was used once or twice daily for 14 days by HIV-1 infected and uninfected women. The gel was found to be safe, well tolerated, and acceptable to participants [199].

	Drug	Clinical trial*
Specific microbicide agents		
Reverse transcriptase inhibitors (NRTIs and NNRTIs)	Tenofovir (NRTI); (PMPA; nucleotide analogue)	Phase I trial, Phase II (NCT00561496, NCT00540605, NCT00594373), Phase II (NCT00111943), Phase IIb (CAPRISA 004; NCT00441298), and Phase II/IIb (NCT00705679)
	TMC120 (NNRTI)	Phase III trial efficacy study and phase I/II safety
	UC781 (NNRTI)	Phase I trial, Phase I(NCT00441909, NCT00132444, NCT00385554), and Phase I (NCT00408538). Male tolerance study ongoing(NCT00385554)
Entry inhibitors: CCR5 blockers	PSC-RANTES	Protected macaques from SHIV (SF162)
	CPMD167	Full protection of macaques from SHIV (162P4) not achieved alone, but only with addition two peptides BMS-378806and C52-L
Non-specific microbicide agents		
Vaginal milieu protectors/ acidifying agents	Carbopol 974P (BufferGel®)	Phase II/IIb trial (HPTN 035) (NCT00074425)
	Acidform (Amphora®)	Phase III trial: preventionof *N. gonorrhoeae* and *C. trachomatis*
Entry inhibitors: anionic polymers	Naphthalene sulfonate (PRO2000®)	Phase II/IIb trial (NCT00074425), Phase III (NCT00262106)
	Carrageenan (Carraguard®)	Phase III trial
	Cellulose sulfate (Ushercell®)	Phase III trial

	Drug	Clinical trial*
	Cellulose acetate phthalate/CAP	Phase I trial
	Dendrimers: SPL7013(Vivagel®)	Protection from HIV in a macaque model and from HSV models Phase I trial,Phase I trial(NCT00331032), Phase I trial (NCT00442910)
Detergents or surfactants	Nonoxinol 9 (nonoxynol-9®)	No current clinical trials for HIV prevention. Phase III
	C31G (Savvy®)	Phase III trial
	Sodium dodecyl sulphate (SDS)(Invisible Condom)	Phase II trial(NCT00136643)and Phase II/III trial

Note: NNRTI=non-nucleoside reverse transcriptase inhibitor; STI=sexually transmitted infection; SHIV=chimeric simian/human immunodeficiency virus;HSV=herpes simplex virus.

*NCT number: Clinical trials.gov website :http://www.clinicaltrials.gov.

Table 6. Specific and non-specific microbicides agents for prevention HIV-infection.

11.1.1.2. TMC120 and UC781

Two other compounds of class NNRTIs being studied as topical microbicides to prevent HIV-1 infection, are the TMC120 and UC781. Preclinical or clinical testing as potential topical microbicides showed that they possess several features in common, and both compounds show minimal systemic absorption, having revealed goodsafety profiles in animal studies [200, 201]. *In vitro*, TMC120 and UC781 prevent cell-free and cell-associated virus from infecting co-cultures of monocyte-derived dendritic cells and T cells [202-204]. TMC120 (4-[{4-[(2,4,6-trimethylphenyl)amino]pyrimidin-2-yl} amino]benzenecarbonitrile), a diarylpyrimidine, was the first topical microbicide the NNRTIs class, in gel form, with activity and effectiveness proven *in vivo* [201, 203]. The thiocarbanilide UC781 (N-[4-chloro-3-(3-methyl-2-butenyloxy) phyenyl]-2-methyl-furan-3-carbothioamide), presents a good capacity to block cell-free and cell-associated HIV-1 transmission in human cervical tissue-based culture organ [205, 206], and have shown effectiveness as a VM safety studies in rabbits [200]. Additional phase I trials are underway [205, 207] (Table 6).

11.1.2. Entry inhibitors: CCR5 blockers

CCR5 blockers, also known as CC chemokine receptor 5 [CCR5] antagonists, entered the market in 2007 as antiretroviral drugs, such as drugs capable of effectively blocking the fusion of HIV-1 to CCR5 receptors (Selzentry, Maraviroc®) of the target cell. Its effectiveness at blocking HIV-1 fusion raised its possible ability to act as topical microbicide for the prevention of HIV-1 infection [208, 209]. CCR5 is the most important co-receptor for macrophage-tropic viral strains, which can predominate in the early stages of viral transmission (126). Two CCR5 receptor antagonist have been studied as topical microbicides, the PSC-RANTES [208] and CMPD167 [209].

11.1.2.1. PSC-RANTES

PSC-RANTES, a potent synthetic inhibitor of the CCR5 co-receptor, had *in vitro*, showed antiviral activity against all HIV-1 subtypes as well as being able to inhibit the infection of Langerhans cells by HIV-1, which are considered crucial cells for HIV-1 transmission across the vaginal epithelium [210-212].

11.1.2.2. CMPD167

CMPD167, a cyclopentane-based compound formulated as a 5 mmol vaginal gel, provided protection from vaginal simian/human immunodeficiency virus (SHIV) challenge in eight out of ten macaques [209], and, has been assessed in combination with two peptides that block the viral–host cell interaction at different loci, BMS-378806 and C52-L. BMS-378806 binds viral gp120 and prevents attachment to the CD4 and CCR5 receptors [213, 214], whereas C52-L, a modified version of enfuvirtide, inhibits gp41-mediated viral–cell fusion [209, 215]. Although these animal studies evaluating combinations of compounds with different mechanisms are promising, it is not yet clear whether they will correlate with protection from HIV-1 in human trials [209]. An important challenge in considering the CCR5 inhibitors for use as topical microbicides is their inability to block the entry of CXCR4-tropic virus. Although this latter pathway is less important in sexual transmission, it might still have a role in the infection process. Another concern is the pressure that CCR5-inhibiting compounds might place on HIV-1 to shift toward the use of non-CCR5 pathways/co-receptors to gain entry into cells. A clinically effective microbicide most likely will need to block all modes of receptor-mediated entry [191].

11.1.2.3. Cyanovirin-N

Additionally, beyond the fusion inhibitor C52-L, which inhibits viral-cell gp41-mediated fusion [209, 215], another fusion inhibitor that is being evaluated in clinical trials as a topical microbicide is cyanovirin-N, the lectin purified compound from cyanobacterium. A cyanovirin-N, prevents viral–host cell fusion by binding high mannose residues in the HIV-1 envelope [216, 217]. However, it is necessary to consider that some lectins have shown unwanted side-effects, such as human red blood cell agglutination, mitogenic stimulation of peripheral blood mononuclear cells (PBMC), inflammatory activity, and cellular toxicity [218]. Various formulations of cyanovirin-N, including those expressed by lactobacilli, are under development [219] (Table 6).

11.2. Non-specific microbicide agents

11.2.1. Vaginal milieu protectors/acidifying agents

Vaginal milieu protectors are topical microbicides that promote the maintenance and restoration of natural protective mechanisms within the vaginal canal - the acidic pH maintained by lactobacilli. A pH between 4 0 and 5 8 has been shown to inactivate HIV-1 [220-222]. Therefore, various factors affecting this acidic pH, such as the presence of sêmen or bacterial vaginosis, neutralise the baseline acidity of the vagina. Use of microbicidal compounds in this class can act as direct acidifying agents, or as enhancers of lactobacilli production [220-224]. Some representatives of this class that have been evaluated in clinical studies are carbopol 974 (BufferGel®) [223, 224] and acidoform (Amphora®) [225, 226] (Table 6).

11.2.1.1. Carbopol 974P

Different studies on the efficacy of carbopol 974P (BufferGel®) as topical microbicide have been conducted. The compound is a polyacrylic acid that buffers twice its volume of semen to a pH of 5 or less, and has shown spermicidal activity [223], virucidal *in vitro* activity to HIV-1 [221] and herpes simplex virus (HSV) [227], and protection in mouse vaginal models against HSV and *C. trachomatis* [224]. In gel form, inhibits human papillomavirus (HPV) in animal models [228]. Their safety, as topical microbicide, has also been demonstrated in clinical trials phase I [229, 230]. BufferGel was safe and acceptable among men in a penile tolerance study in HIV-1 infected and uninfected men [231], and a study of phase II/IIb (HPTN 035), showed safety and efficacy when compared with a placebo gel and with condoms.

11.2.1.2. Acidoform

Acidoform (Amphora®) is a sexual lubricant, however, acid-buffering and its bioadhesive properties make it appealing for development as a microbicide candidate. Acidform has undergone two phase I safety studies, as well as the male penile tolerance study [232-234]. Clinical studies have shown that acidoform is well tolerated when used alone, and in combination with nonoxinol 9 (N-9) compound, promotes vaginal irritation (80). The presence of moderate vulvar irritation, including itching, tingling, burning, dryness, erythema, ulceration, and vesicles, have been presented, but are instances considered mild [232, 233].

11.2.2. Entry inhibitors

Advances in the drug development against HIV-1 have lead to the identification of new compounds which could be used to target cellular entry and nuclear integration of virus in addition to drugs that commonly target RT and protease. Cellular entry of HIV-1 is a multistep procedure involving a range of cellular and molecular interactions between virus envelope protein and receptors expressed on the surface of the target cells, thus providing many opportunities to block infection [235]. Topical microbicide agents of class entry inhibitors act by blocking the binding of HIV-1 to host cells, as well as inhibit fusion of the viral membranes. This class, stand out as anionic polymers microbicide agents, in which they present negative charges in their structure, interact with viral envelope proteins (gp120 and/or gp41) which interfers with attachment of HIV-1 to CD4+ cells [236]. The gp120 protein of CXCR4-tropic viruses are vulnerable to the actions of anionic polymers by changing the melting capacity of these viruses in the host cell membranes. However, there is controversy about the effectiveness of anionic polymers for CCR5-tropic viruses [236,

237]. Naphthalene sulphonate [238], carrageenan [239], cellulose sulphate [240], cellulose acetate phthalate [241], and dendrimers [242], are the main compounds evaluated in clinical trials, phase l, ll and lll (Table 6).

11.2.2.1. Naphthalene sulphonate

Naphthalene sulphonate (PRO2000® gel), is a sulphfonated polymer with *in vitro* activity against HIV-1, *C. trachomatis, N. gonorrhoeae,* and HSV [243, 244]. Phase I clinical trials have shown that naphthalene sulphonate gel was generally well tolerated [238, 245]. Phase ll/llb revealed safety and efficacy, and a phase III efficacy trial, show that the naphthalene sulphonate gel has better efficacy when compared with BufferGel, gel placebo, or the condom [238, 244, 246].

11.2.2.2. Carrageenan

Carrageenan (Carraguard/R515®) is a sulphonated polysaccharide derived from a seaweed extract, and blocking HIV-1 transmission by binding the HIV-1 envelope. Carrageenan has been found to prevent HIV-1-infected mononuclear cells from migrating across vaginal epithelia to pelvic lymph nodes in mouse models [247]. Phase I safety trials of carraguard gel and similar carageenan-based formulations showed safety in HIV-1 negative men and women [248, 249]. Other clinical trials have shown that carraguard gel was safe in preventing infection by HIV-1 [250, 251]. However, a placebo-controlled phase III study in South Africa, with HIV-1 negative and non-pregnant women, found that although carraguard gel was safe when used over a 2-year period, incident HIV-1 infections occurred at a similar rate in the Carrageenan and placebo groups, with incidence of 3:3 infections per 100 woman-years in the Carrageenan group, and incidence of 3:7 per 100 woman-years in the placebo group, raising major questions about whether poor adherence contributed to the lack of efficacy found in the trial [252].

11.2.2.3. Cellulose sulphate and cellulose acetate phthalate

Cellulose sulphate gel (Ushercell®), acts by binding the V3 loop of the gp120 HIV-1 envelope, and it can inhibit both CXCR4 and CCR5-tropic virus types [253]. Phase III efficacy trials of cellulose sulphate versus placebo showed a higher HIV seroincidence in the trial group [240]. Cellulose acetate phthalate (CAP) is another anionic polymer under investigation as a microbicide agent, that blocks gp120 binding sites, and showed *in vitro* activity against HIV-1 and HSV (types 1 and 2) [255]. CAP has been presented in the form of a film and micronized gel, and has shown ability to block gp120 binding site on CXCR4 and CCR5-tropic virus types [256, 257]. Additionally, the micronised form of CAP provides an acidic environment, which was shown in one study to cause disintegration and loss of infectivity of HIV-1 [258].

11.2.2.4. Dendrimers

Dendrimers are anionic polymers containing macromolecules, and contain a central core, interior branches, and terminal surface groups adapted to specific targets. Because of their size and multiple terminal surface groups, they possess the ability to bind to multiple locations on multiple cells. O SPL7013 (Vivagel®) is a first dendrimer to be formulated as a microbicide gel and tested clinically. It showed protection from chimeric SHIV in a macaque model, and from HSV2 in two different animal models [259].

11.2.3. Detergents or surfactants

Detergents or Surfactants were the first compounds evaluated clinically as topical microbicides. These topical agents act in a nonspecific way disrupt membranes, offering contraceptive properties and activity against a wide range of potential STI pathogens [260, 261]. The agents of this class of topical Microbicides are represented by nonoxynol 9 (N-9), C31G, and sodium lauryl sulfate (SLS) (Table 6).

11.2.3.1. Nonoxinol 9 (N-9)

This prototype detergent compound is the non-ionic surfactant nonoxynol 9 (N-9) that forms a chemical barrier between the vaginal mucosa and the ejaculate. The nonoxynol 9 is a spermicide low cost and easy access sulfactant that proved effective against HIV-1 infection, *in vitro* tests [262]. However, since nonoxynol 9 disrupts the phospholipid membrane of cells, it can cause non-specific damage to vaginal epithelium cells, uterine and cervical tissue thus increasing rather than decreasing the likelihood of HIV-1 infection [260, 261]. In a blinded, randomized controlled efficacy trials of nonoxynol 9, in seronegative sex workers for HIV-1 in Cameroon, the data showed no difference in the rate of HIV-1 infection, though a higher incidence of genital ulcers with the use of nonoxynol 9 compared with placebo was observed [263]. In turn, the efficacy trial in female sex workers in four countries showed an association between N-9 and increased HIV-1 seroincidence when nonoxynol 9 has been used more than three times daily [264]. These findings suggest that the toxicity of nonoxynol 9 on tissue of the vaginal mucosa at higher doses would be a possible cause for increased transmission among frequent users, which led researchers to disregard the use of nonoxynol 9 as a HIV-1 preventive microbicide [191].

11.2.3.2. C31G

C31G (Savvy®), or cetyl betaine and myristamine oxide, is a surfactant with the potential to microbicide and contraceptively spermicide, in addition it has *in vitro* activity against C. trachomatis, HSV, and HIV-1 [265-267]. A clinical study has shown that many patients are reluctant to use it because of associated burning sensations [268]. The C31G co-polymer gel (1%, 0.5% and 1.7%) was evaluated, but the results were inconclusive regarding their safety and efficacy for preventing HIV-1 infection, and clinical trials of C31G have recently been discontinued [268, 269].

11.2.3.3. Sodium Dodecyl Sulphate (SDS)

Sodium dodecyl sulphate (SDS), also called sodium lauril sulphate (SLS) [270, 271], are sulphated (negatively charged) surfactants that denature membrane proteins of pathogens and cells. SDS *in vitro* and in animal models have inhibitory activity against HIV-1 and HSV [272], promoting the reduction of adsorption of the HIV viral envelope glycoproteins in the membrane of the target cell [273]. In the form of a thermoreversible gel acts as a physical barrier and as a denaturing agent of the viral envelope glycoproteins [272, 273]. In similarity with nonoxynol 9, its long time application can cause non-specific damage to the vaginal epithelium cells, uterine and cervical tissue.

12. Intravaginal rings

PrEP using intravaginal rings (IVR) with antiretroviral drugs, is emerging as a promising strategy for the prevention of sexual HIV-1 infection [274]. The use of IVR as controlled release strategy of antiretroviral drugs may improve adherence to PrEP, and provide sustained mucosal levels independent of coitus and daily dosing [275]. The delivery of two or more antiretroviral drugs from conventional IVR designs involves significant technological and manufacturing challenges [276]. Recently, an IVR was developed which allows the release of multiple agents over a wide range of target delivery rates and aqueous solubilities [277-279]. Researchers have evaluated the pharmacokinetics of IVR containing five drugs as a proof-of-concept, described as advanced multipurpose prevention technology, which combines three antiretroviral drugs from different mechanistic classes (tenofovir, nevirapine, and saquinavir) with a proven estrogen-progestogen contraceptive for prevention of HIV-1 infection and unintended pregnancy [280, 281]. Studies with IVR delivering TDF and emtricitabine, as well as a triple-combination IVR delivering TDF, emtricitabine, and selzentry are in progress for safety and pharmacokinetics evaluation. Preliminary results show that no adverse events were observed, although certain toxicological findings were observed. Mild-to-moderate increases in inflammatory infiltrates were observed in the vaginal tissues of some animals in both the presence and absence of IVR [277-281]. New perspectives and challenges are open for the development of IVR delivering multiple drugs, to ensure the safety and efficacy for the prevention of HIV-1 infection [279-281].

13. Diet and lifestyle

Changes in diet and lifestyle, and the adequacy of a hypocaloric diet are recommendations that seek to reduce the concentrations of TC and its fractions, especially LDL [282-284]. These changes bring benefits over short periods of time and reduce the risk for cardiovascular and atherosclerotic diseases. The dietary recommendations are addressed to the entire population and specifically to HIV-1 patients which also indicates measures that should be applied to delay the need for lipid-lowering drugs, even before the treatment of dyslipidemia [282-285]. Changes in diet can directly alter the levels of circulating LDL including saturated fats, cholesterol, and trans-unsaturated fats. The highest impact comes from saturated fats, which are in a solid state at room temperature or under refrigeration. The major sources of saturated fats are meat and meat products (poultry, pork, beef, lard, and sausages), dairy (milk and cheeses), and vegetable oils (derived from palm or coconut). For an adequate daily diet, the recommended consumption is equal or <7% of saturated fats, for the total daily caloric intake. Dietary cholesterol is exclusively found in animal products such as meats (particularly organ meats and tissues such as brain, kidney, and liver), egg yolks, and dairy products. It is recommended to keep dietary cholesterol consumption to <200 mg/day. Trans fats and unsaturated fats are found in breads and cookies, doughnuts, stick margarine, and fried foods [286, 287]. The consumption of unsaturated fats preferred sources include fish such as salmon, mackerel, tuna, and vegetables such as avocado, olives and olive oil and vegetable oils [289]. Other foods that are considered for the maintenance and/or lipid-lowering effects are the omega-3 fats, which are polyunsaturated fats that can lower TG levels. Omega-3 fats are considered as fish oils, they are present in fish such as salmon, tuna and mackerel, but these are also found in krill and flax seed oil. Currently, a diet with 25-35% of daily calories derived from fat sources is recommended, including saturated fats, which must be <7% [289]. In addition, physical activity improves cardiorespiratory function, promotes the reduction of LDL and TG, and decreases insulin resistance (in both uninfected and HIV-1 patients) [290, 291]. Physical exercise has shown reduction effects in TC and TG, also reduced total fat mass, and increased muscle mass in HIV-1 patients with hypertriglyceridemia [291-293]. Additionally, physical exercise is associated with greater cardiovascular fitness, improved muscle strength and endurance, and the reduction of depression and anxiety. In addition, it helps with problems resulting from lipodystrophy (dyslipidemia, insulin resistance, and osteoporosis) and cardiovascular disease [291-293]. However, there are several factors that can directly influence the reduction of metabolic disorders observed in seropositive patients. The common observation of gastrointestinal diseases in patients in advanced stages of infection may reduce the positive effects of a balanced dietary regimen [292, 293].

14. Conclusion

After more than three decades of the emergence of HIV/AIDS, it is clear the advances achieved with HAART in patients infected with HIV-1. A better quality of life, reducing morbidity and mortality, and a greater survival rate are evident in patients who use the therapy. The therapeutic arsenal is wide, and many possibilities occurs in those cases where viral resistance, viral genetic mutations, presence of quasispecies and also adhesion problems of treatment and maintenance due to adverse reactions and side effects such as those produced on lipid metabolism. In turn, the advent of PrEP is undoubtedly the most important and innovative approach to prevent infection by HIV-1, and is already showing excellent results in several clinical studies conducted to date. Additionally, maintaining perspective of low viral load levels in patients who use HAART is considered as one of the keys to reducing the transmission of infection, and associated with PrEP, presents us with a positive scenario for the coming years. Beside the excellent results obtained with HAART , a definitive cure for HIV-1 remains a major obstacle. Nevertheless, nowadays patients infected with HIV-1 have a better perspective of life.

Author details

Joel da Cunha[1,2], Luciana Morganti Ferreira Maselli[1,3], Sérgio Paulo Bydlowski[1] and Celso Spada[2*]

*Address all correspondence to: celso.spada@ufsc.br

1 Laboratory of Genetics and Molecular Hematology (LIM31), University of São Paulo School of Medicine (FMUSP), São Paulo, SP, Brazil

2 Clinical Analysis Department, Health Sciences Center, Federal University of Santa Catarina (UFSC), Florianópolis, SC, Brazil

3 Research Division, Pró-Sangue Hemocentro de São Paulo Foundation, São Paulo, SP, Brazil

The authors state that there are no conflicts of interest regarding the publication of this work.
All authors have equally contributed to this work.

References

[1] Deeks SG, Lewin SR, Havlir DV. The end of AIDS: HIV infection as a chronic disease. Lancet. 2013;382(9903):1525–33.

[2] Passaes CP, Sáez-Cirión A. HIV cure research: advances and prospects. Virology. 2014;454-455:340–52.

[3] Calvo KR, Daar ES. Antiretroviral therapy: Treatment-experienced Individuals. Infect Dis Clin North Am. 2014;28(3):439–56.

[4] Sobieszczyk ME, Talley AK, Wilkin T, Hammer SM. Advances in antiretroviral therapy. Top HIV Med. 2005;13(1):24–44.

[5] Rigourd M, Lanchy JM, Le Grice SF, Ehresmann B, Ehresmann C, Marquet R. Inhibition of the initiation of HIV-1 reverse transcription by 3′-azido-3′-deoxythymidine. Comparison with elongation. J Biol Chem. 2000;275(35):26944–51.

[6] Balzarini J. Current status of the non-nucleoside reverse transcriptase inhibitors of human immunodeficiency virus type 1. Curr Top Med Chem. 2004;4(9):921–44.

[7] Randolph JT, DeGoey DA. Peptidomimetic inhibitors of HIV protease. Curr Top Med Chem. 2004;4(10):1079–95.

[8] Miyamoto F, Kodama EN. Development of small molecule HIV-1 fusion inhibitors: linking biology to chemistry. Curr Pharm Des. 2013;19(10):1827–34.

[9] Boesecke C, Pett SL. Clinical studies with chemokine receptor-5 (CCR5)-inhibitors. Curr Opin HIV AIDS. 2012;7(5):456–62.

[10] Métifiot M, Marchand C, Pommier Y. HIV integrase inhibitors: 20-year landmark and challenges. Adv Pharmacol. 2013;67:75–105.

[11] Carr A, Emery S, Law M, Puls R, Lundgren JD, Powderly WG, et al. An objective case definition of lipodystrophy in HIV-infected adults: a case-control study. Lancet. 2003;361(9359):726–35.

[12] Wohl DA, McComsey G, Tebas P, Brown TT, Glesby MJ, Reeds D, et al. Current concepts in the diagnosis and management of metabolic complications of HIV infection and its therapy. Clin Infect Dis. 2006;43(5):645–53.

[13] Carr A, Samaras K, Burton S, Law M, Freund J, Chisholm DJ, Cooper DA. A syndrome of peripheral lipodystrophy, hyperlipidaemia and insulin resistance in patients receiving HIV protease inhibitors. AIDS. 1998;12(7):F51–58.

[14] Sprinz E, Lazzaretti RK, Kuhmmer R, Ribeiro JP. Dyslipidemia in HIV-infected individuals. Braz J Infect Dis. 2010;14(6):575–88.

[15] Grunfeld C. Dyslipidemia and its treatment in HIV Infection. Top HIV Med. 2010;18(3):112–18.

[16] Freitas P, Carvalho D. Lipodystrophy: beyond generalization? Panminerva Med. 2013;55(3):253–68.

[17] Behrens GM, Stoll M, Schmidt RE. Lipodystrophy syndrome in HIV infection: what is it, what causes it and how can it be managed? Drug Saf. 2000;23(1):57–76.

[18] Campbell SM, Crowe SM, Mak J. Virion-associated cholesterol is critical for the maintenance of HIV-1 structure and infectivity. AIDS. 2002;16(17):2253–61.

[19] Chan R, Uchil PD, Jin J, Shui G, Ott DE, Mothes W, Wenk MR. Retroviruses human immunodeficiency virus and murine leukemia virus are enriched in phosphoinositides. J Virol. 2008;82(22):11228–38.

[20] von Eckardstein A, Nofer JR, Assmann G. High density lipoproteins and arteriosclerosis. Role of cholesterol efflux and reverse cholesterol transport. Arterioscler Thromb Vasc Biol. 2001;21(1):13–27.

[21] National Cholesterol Education Program Working Group on Lipoprotein Measurement: Recommendations on Lipoprotein Measurement. NIH Publication No. 95-3044, Bethesda, MD;1995:31–34.

[22] Hanley TM, Blay Puryear W, Gummuluru S, Viglianti GA. PPARgamma and LXR signaling inhibit dendritic cell-mediated HIV-1 capture and trans-infection. PloS Pathog. 2010;6:e1000981.

[23] Hanley TM, Viglianti GA. Nuclear receptor signaling inhibits HIV-1 replication in macrophages through multiple trans-repression mechanisms. J Virol. 2011;85(20): 10834–50.

[24] Wang X, Chai H, Yao Q, Chen C. Molecular mechanisms of HIV protease inhibitor-induced endothelial dysfunction. J Acquir Immune Defic Syndr. 2007;44(5):493–99.

[25] Sankatsing RR, Wit FW, Vogel M, de Groot E, Brinkman K, Rockstroh JK, et al. Increased carotid intima-media thickness in HIV patients treated with protease inhibitors as compared to non-nucleoside reverse transcriptase inhibitors. Atherosclerosis. 2009;202(2):589–95.

[26] Riddler SA, Li X, Otvos J, Post W, Palella F, Kingsley L, et al. Antiretroviral therapy is associated with an atherogenic lipoprotein phenotype among HIV-1-infected men in the Multicenter AIDS Cohort Study. J Acquir Immune Defic Syndr. 2008;48(3):281–88.

[27] Qiu X, Liu ZP. Recent developments of peptidomimetic HIV-protease inhibitors. Curr Med Chem. 2011;18(29):4513–37.

[28] Rawlings ND, Tolle DP, Barrett AJ. Evolutionary families of peptidase inhibitors. Biochem J. 2004;378(Pt 3):705–16.

[29] Hui DY. Effects of HIV protease inhibitor therapy on lipid metabolism. Prog Lipid Res. 2003;42(2):81–92.

[30] Riddler SA, Li X, Chu H, Kingsley LA, Dobs A, Evans R, et al. Longitudinal changes in serum lipids among HIV-infected men on highly active antiretroviral therapy. HIV Med. 2007;8(5)280–87.

[31] Arribas JR, Pulido F, Delgado R, Lorenzo A, Miralles P, Arranz A, et al. Lopinavir/ritonavir as single-drug therapy for maintenance of HIV-1 viral suppression: 48-week results of randomized, controlles, open-label, proof-on-concept pilot clinical trial (OK Study). J Acquir Immune Defic Syndr. 2005;1:40(3):280–7.

[32] Patick AK, Potts KE. Protease inhibitors as antiviral agentes. Clin Microbiol Rev. 1998;11(4):614–27.

[33] Helleberg M, Kronborg G, Larsen CS, Pedersen G, Pedersen C, Nielsen L. et al. Decreasing rate of multiple treatment modifications among individuals who initiated antiretroviral therapy in 1997-2009 in the Danish HIV Cohort Study. Antiviral Therapy. 2013,18(3):345-354

[34] Carr A, Hudson J, Chuah J, Mallal S, Law M, Hoy J, et al. HIV protease inhibitor substitution in patients with lipodystrophy: a randomized, controlled, open-label, multicentre study. AIDS. 2001;15(14):1811–22.

[35] Prosperi MC, Fabbiani M, Fanti I, Zaccarelli M, Colafigli M, Mondi A, et al. Predictors of first-line antiretroviral therapy discontinuation due to drug-related adverse

events in HIV-infected patients: retrospective cohort study.BMC Infect Dis. 2012;12:296.

[36] Grunfeld C, Pang M, Doerrler W, Shigenaga JK, Jensen P, Feingold KR. Lipids, lipoproteins, triglyceride clearance, and cytokines in human immunodeficiency virus infection and the acquired immunodeficiency syndrome. J Clin Endocrinol Metab. 1992;74(5):1045–52.

[37] Sellmeyer DE, Grunfeld C. Endocrine and metabolic disturbances in human immunodeficiency virus infection and the acquired immune deficiency syndrome. Endocr Rev. 1996;17(5):518–32.

[38] Pedersen C, Lindhardt BO, Jensen BL, Lauritzen E, Gerstoft J, Dickmeiss E, et al. Clinical course of primary HIV infection: consequences for subsequent course of infection. BMJ. 1989;299(6692):154–57.

[39] Dinarello CA. Historical insights into cytokines. Eur J Immunol. 2007;37(Suppl 1):S34–45.

[40] Rose H, Woolley I, Hoy J, Dart A, Bryant B, Mijch A, Sviridov D. HIV infection and high-density lipoprotein: the effect of the disease vs the effect of treatment. Metabolism. 2006;55(1):90–95.

[41] Baker J, Ayenew W, Quick H, Hullsiek KH, Tracy R, Henry, et al. High-density lipoprotein particles and markers of inflammation and thrombotic activity in patients with untreated HIV infection. J Infect Dis. 2010;201(2)285–92.

[42] Zangerle R, Sarcletti M, Gallati H, Reibnegger G, Wachter H, Fuchs D. Decreased plasma concentrations of HDL cholesterol in HIV-infected individuals are associated with immune activation. J Acquir Immune Defic Syndr. 1994;7(11):1149–56.

[43] Chi D, Henry J, Kelley J, Thorpe R, Smith JK, Krishnaswamy G. The effects of HIV infection on endothelial function. Endothelium. 2000;7(4):223–42.

[44] Schroecksnadel K, Frick B, Winkler C, Fuchs D: Crucial role of interferon-gamma and stimulated macrophages in cardiovascular disease. Curr Vasc Pharmacol. 2006;4(3): 205–13.

[45] Cobos Jiménez V, Booiman T, de Taeye SW, van Dort KA, Rits MA, Hamann J, et al. Differential expression of HIV-1 interfering factors in monocyte-derived macrophages stimulated with polarizing cytokines or interferons. Sci Rep. 2012;2:763.

[46] Vaidya SA, Korner C. Sirignano MN, Amero M, Bazner S, Rychert J, et al. Tumor necrosis factor α is associated with viral control and early disease progression in patients with HIV type 1 infection. J Infect Dis. 2014;210(7):1042–46.

[47] Fisher SD, Miller TL, Lipshultz SE. Impact of HIV and highly active antiretroviral therapy on leukocyte adhesion molecules, arterial inflammation, dyslipidemia, and atherosclerosis. Atherosclerosis. 2006;185(1):1–11.

[48] Penzak SR, Chuck SK. Hyperlipidemia associated with HIV protease inhibitor use: pathophysiology, prevalence, risk factors and treatment. Scand J Infect Dis. 2000;32(2):111–23.

[49] Nasri H, rafieian-Kopaei M. Metformin: Current Knowledge. J Res Med Sci. 2014;19(7):658–64

[50] Newsholme P, Brennan L, Rubi B, Maechler P. New insights into amino acid metabolism, beta-cell function and diabetes. Clin Sci (Lond). 2005;108(3):185–94.

[51] Behrens G, Dejam A, Schmidt H, Balks HJ, Brabant G, Körner T et al. Impaired glucose tolerance, beta cell function and lipid metabolism in HIV patients under treatment with protease inhibitors. AIDS. 1999;13(10):F63–70.

[52] Mulligan K, Grunfeld C, Tai VW, Algren H, Pang M, Chernoff DN, et al. Hyperlipidemia and insulin resistance are induced by protease inhibitors independent of changes in body composition in patients with HIV infection. J Acquir Immune Defic Syndr. 2000;23(1):35–43.

[53] Savès M, Raffi F, Capeau J, Rozenbaum W, Ragnaud JM, Perronne C, et al. Factors related to lipodystrophy and metabolic alterations in patients with human immunodeficiencyvirus infection receiving highly active antiretroviral therapy. Clin Infect Dis. 2002;34(10):1396–405.

[54] Sekhar RV, Jahoor F, Pownall HJ, Rehman K, Gaubatz J, Iyer D, Balasubramanyam A. Severely dysregulated disposal of postprandial triacylglycerols exacerbates hypertriacylglycerolemia in HIV lipodystrophy syndrome. Am J Clin Nutr. 2005;81(6): 1405–10.

[55] van Wijk JP, Cabezas MC, de Koning EJ, Rabelink TJ, van der Geest R, Hoepelman IM. In vivo evidence of impaired peripheral fatty acid trapping in patients with human immunodeficiency virus-associated lipodystrophy. J Clin Endocrinol Metab. 2005;90(6):3575–82.

[56] Miserez AR, Muller PY, Spaniol V. Indinavir inhibits sterol-regulatory element-binding protein-1c-dependent lipoprotein lipase and fatty acid synthase gene activations. AIDS. 2002;16(12):1587–94.

[57] Abebe M, Kinde S, Belay G, Gebreegziabxier A, Challa F, Gebeyehu T, et al. Antiretroviral treatment associated hyperglycemia and dyslipidemia among HIV infected patients at Burayu Health Center, Addis Ababa, Ethiopia: a cross-sectional comparative study. BMC Res Notes. 2014;21;7:380.

[58] Crane HM, Grunfeld C, Willig JH, Mugavero MJ, Van Rompaey S, Moore R. Impact of NRTIs on lipid levels among a large HIV-infected cohort initiating antiretroviral therapy in clinical care. AIDS. 2011;25(2):185–95.

[59] Carr A, Samaras K, Thorisdottir A, Kaufmann GR, Chisholm DJ, Cooper DA. Diagnosis, prediction, and natural course of HIV-1 protease inhibitor-associated lipodys-

trophy, hyperlipidaemia, and diabetes mellitus: a cohort study. Lancet. 1999;353(9170):2093–99.

[60] Fleming I. Cytochrome P450-dependent eicosanoid production and crosstalk. Curr Opin Lipidol. 2011;22(5):403–09.

[61] Hu C, Oliver JA, Goldberg MR, Al-Awqati Q. LRP: a new adhesion molecule for endothelial and smooth muscle cells. Am J Physiol Renal Physiol. 2001;281:F739–50.

[62] Zaera MG, Miró O, Pedrol E, Soler A, Picón M, Cardellach F, et al. Mitochondrial involvement in antiretroviral therapy-related lipodystrophy. AIDS. 2001;15(13):1643–51.

[63] Chattopadhyay K, Aldous CA. A brief review on human mtDNA mutations and NRTI-associated mtDNA toxicity and mutations. Mithocondrial DNA. 2014;11:1-3.

[64] Apostolova N, Blas-García A, Esplugues JV. Mitochondrial interference by anti-HIV drugs: mechanisms beyond Pol-γ inhibition. Trends Pharmacol Sci. 2011;32(12):715–25.

[65] Arnedo M, Taffé P, Sahli R, Furrer H, Hirschel B, Elzi L, et al. Contribution of 20 single nucleotide polymorphisms of 13 genes to dyslipidemia associated with antiretroviral therapy. Pharmacogenet Genomics. 2007;17(9):755–64.

[66] Egaña-Gorroño L, Martínez E, Cormand B, Escribà T, Gatell J, Arnedo M. Impact of genetic factors on dyslipidemia in HIV-infected patients starting antiretroviral therapy. AIDS;27(4):529–38.

[67] Fauvel J, Bonnet E, Ruidavets JB, Ferrières J, Toffoletti A, Massip P, et al. An interaction between apo C-IIIvariants and protease inhibitors contributes to high triglyceride/low HDL levels in treated HIV patients. AIDS. 2001;15(18):2397–406.

[68] Foulkes AS, Wohl DA, Frank I, Puleo E, Restine S, Wolfe ML, et al. Associations among race/ethnicity, ApoC-III genotypes, and lipids in HIV-1-infected individuals on antiretroviral therapy. PLoS Med. 2006;3(3):e52.

[69] Parra S, Alonso-Villaverde C, Coll B, Ferré N, Marsillach J, Aragonès G. Serum paraoxonase-1 activity and concentration are influenced by human immunodeficiency virus infection. Atherosclerosis. 2007;194(1):175–81.

[70] Maselli LMF, da Cunha J, Gutierrez EB, Maranhão RC, Spada C, Bydlowski SP. Human paraoxonase-1 activity is related to the number of CD4+ T-cells and is restored by antiretroviral therapy in HIV-1-infected individuals. Dis Markers. 2014;2014:480201.

[71] Aviram M, Rosenblat M. Paraoxonases and cardiovascular diseases pharmacological and nutritional influences. Curr Opin Lipidol. 2005;16(4):393–99.

[72] Mackness MI, Arrol S, Abbott C, Durrington PN. Protection of low-density lipoprotein against oxidative modification by high-density lipoprotein associated paraoxonase. Atherosclerosis. 1993;104(1-2):129–35.

[73] Aviram M, Rosenblat M. Paraoxonases 1, 2, and 3, oxidative stress, and macrophage foam cell formation during atherosclerosis development. Free Radic Biol Med. 2004;37(9):1304–16.

[74] Assmann G, Nofer JR. Atheroprotective effects of High-Density Lipoproteins. Annu Rev Med. 2003;54:321–41.

[75] Ngondi JL, Oben J, Forkah DM, Etame LH, Mbanya D. The effect of different combination therapies on oxidative stress markers in HIV infected patients in Cameroon. AIDS Res Ther. 2006;3:19.

[76] Matsuura E, Hughes GR, Khamashta MA. Oxidation of LDL and its clinical implication. Autoimmun Rev. 2008;7(7):558–66.

[77] Kádár A, Glasz T. Development of atherosclerosis and plaque biology. Cardiovasc Surg. 2001;9(2):109–21.

[78] Navab M, Ananthramaiah GM, Reddy ST, Van Lenten BJ, Ansell BJ, Fonarow GC, et al. The oxidation hypothesis of atherogenesis: the role of oxidized phospholipids and HDL. J Lipid Res. 2004;45(6):993–1007.

[79] Faviou E, Vourli G, Nounopoulos C, Zachari A, Dionyssiou-Asteriou A.Circulating oxidized low density lipoprotein, autoantibodies against them and homocysteine serum levels in diagnosis and estimation of severity of coronary artery disease. Free Radic Res.2005;39(4):419–29.

[80] Cunha J, Maselli LMF, Treitinger A, Monteiro A, Gidlund M, Maranhão RC et al. Serum levels of IgG antibodies against oxidized LDL and atherogenic indices in HIV-1-infected patients treated with protease inhibitors. Clin Chem and Lab Med. 2013;51(2):371–78.

[81] Monnerat BZ, Cerutti Junior C, Caniçali SC, Motta TR. Clinical and biochemical evaluation of HIV-related lipodystrophy in an ambulatory population from the Hospital Universitário Cassiano Antonio de Morais, Vitória, ES, Brazil. Braz J Infect Dis. 2008;12(4):364–68.

[82] Cossarizza A, Riva A, Pinti M, Ammannato S, Fedeli P, Mussini C, et al. Increased mitochondrial DNA content in peripheral blood lymphocytes from HIV-infected patients with lipodystrophy. Antivir Ther. 2003;8(4):315–21.

[83] Pinti M, Salomoni P, Cossarizza A. Anti-HIV drugs and the mitochondria. Biochim Biophys Acta. 2006;1757(5-6):700–07.

[84] Joly V, Flandre P, Meiffredy V, Leturque N, Harel M, Aboulker JP, Yeni P.Increased risk of lipoatrophy under stavudine in HIV-1 infected patients: results of a substudy from a comparative trial. AIDS. 2002;16(18):2447–57.

[85] de Waal R, Cohen K, Maartens G. Systematic review of antiretroviral associated lipodystrophy: lipoatrophy, but not central fat gain, is an antiretroviral adverse drug reaction. PLoS One. 2013;8(5):e63623.

[86] Haubrich RH, Riddler SA, DiRienzo AG, Komarow L, Powderly WG, Klingman K,, et al. Metabolic outcomes in a randomized trial of nucleoside, nonnucleoside and protease inhibitor-sparing regimens for initial HIV treatment. AIDS. 2009;23(9):1109–18.

[87] Kotler DP. HIV lipodystrophy etiology and pathogenesis. Body composition and metabolic alterations: etiology and pathogenesis. AIDS Read. 2003;13 (4 Suppl):S5–9.

[88] Mulligan K, Parker RA, Komarow L, Grinspoon SK, Tebas P, Robbins GK, et al. Mixed patterns of changes in central and peripheral fat following initiation of antiretroviral therapy in a randomized trial. J Acquir Immune Defic Syndr. 2006;41(5):590–97.

[89] Alvrs MD, Brites C, Spriz E. HIV-associated lipodystrophy: a review from a Brazilian perspective. Ther Clin Risk Manag. 2014;10:559-66.

[90] Penzak SR, Chuck SK. Hyperlipidemia associated with HIV protease inhibitor use: pathophysiology, prevalence, risk factors and treatment. Scand J Infect Dis. 2000;32:111–23.

[91] DAD Study Group, Friis-Møller N, Reiss P, Sabin CA, Weber R, et al, for the DAD Study Group. Class of antiretroviral drugs and the risk of myocardial infarction. N Engl J Med. 2007;356(7):1723–35.

[92] Young J, Weber R, Rickenbach M, Furrer H, Bernasconi E, Hirschel B, et al. Lipid profiles for antiretroviral-naive patients starting PI- and NNRTI-based therapy in the Swiss HIV cohort study. Antivir Ther. 2005;10(5):585–91.

[93] Cahn PE, Gatell JM, Squires K, Percival LD, Piliero PJ, Sanne IA, et al. Atazanavir-a once-daily HIV protease inhibitor that does not cause dyslipidemia in newly treated patients: results from two randomized clinical trials. J Int Assoc Physicians AIDS Care (Chic). 2004;3(3):92–98.

[94] Grover SA, Coupal L, Gilmore N, Mukherjee J. Impact of dyslipidemia associated with highly active antiretroviral therapy (HAART) on cardiovascular risk and life expectancy. Am J Cardiol. 2005;95(5):586–91.

[95] Hicks CB, Cahn P, Cooper DA, Walmsley SL, Katlama C, Clotet B, et al. Durable efficacy of tipranavir-ritonavir in combination with an optimised background regimen of antiretroviral drugs for treatment-experienced HIV-1-infected patients at 48 weeks in the Randomized Evaluation of Strategic Intervention in multi-drug reSistant pa-

tients with Tipranavir (RESIST) studies: an analysis of combined data from two randomised open-label trials. Lancet. 2006;368(9534):466–75.

[96] Calza L, Manfredi R, Colangeli V, Tampellini L, Sebastiani T, Pocaterra D, Chiodo F.Substitution of nevirapine or efavirenz for protease inhibitor versus lipid-lowering therapy for the management of dyslipidaemia. AIDS. 2005;19(10):1051–58.

[97] Carr A, Hudson J, Chuah J, Mallal S, Law M, Hoy J, et al. HIV protease inhibitor substitution in patients with lipodystrophy: a randomized, controlled, open-label, multicentre study. AIDS. 2001;15(14):1811–22.

[98] Clotet B, van der Valk M, Negredo E, Reiss P. Impact of nevirapine on lipid metabolism. J Acquir Immune Defic Syndr. 2003;34(suppl1): S79–84.

[99] Dubé MP, Stein JH, Aberg JA, Fichtenbaum CJ, Gerber JG, Tashima KT, et al. Guidelines for the evaluation and management of dyslipidemia in human immunodeficiency virus (HIV)-infected adults receiving antiretroviral therapy: recommendations of the HIV Medical Association of the Infectious Disease Society of America and the Adult AIDS Clinical Trials Group. Clin Infect Dis. 2003;37(5):613–27.

[100] Gould AL, Rossouw JE, Santanello NC, Heyse JF, Furberg CD. Cholesterol reduction yields clinical benefits: impact of statin trials. Circulation. 1998;97(10):946–52.

[101] Baigent C, Keech A, Kearney PM, Blackwell L, Buck G, Pollicino C, et al. Efficacy and safety of cholesterol-lowering treatment: prospective meta-analysis of data from 90 056 participants in 14 randomised trials of statins. Lancet. 2005;366(9493):1267–78.

[102] Boccara F, Simonn T, Lacombe K, Cohen A, Laloux B, Bozec E, et al. Influence of pravastatin on carotid artery structure and function in dyslipidemic HIV-infected patients receiving antiretroviral therapy. AIDS. 2006;20(18):2395–98.

[103] Stein JH, Merwood MA, Bellehumeur JL, Aeschlimann SE, Korcarz CE, Underbakke GL, et al. Effects of pravastatin on lipoproteins and endothelial function in patients receiving human immunodeficiency virus protease inhibitors. Am Heart J. 2004;147(4):E18.

[104] Calza L, Colangeli V, Manfredi R, Legnani G, tampellini L, Procaterra D, Chiodo F. Rosuvastatin for ther treatment of hyperlipidemia in HIV-infected patients receiving protease inhibitors: a pilot study. Aids. 2005;19(10):1103–05.

[105] Fichtenbaum CJ, Gerber JG, Rosenkranz SL, Segal Y, Aberg JA, Blaschke T, et al. Pharmacokinetic interactions between protease inhibitors and statins in HIV seronegative volunteers: ACTG Study A5047. AIDS. 2002;16(4):569–77.

[106] Fichtenbaum CJ, Gerber JG. Interactions between antiretroviral drugs and drugs used for the therapy of the metabolic complications encountered during HIV infection. Clin Pharmacokinet. 2002;41(14):1195–211.

[107] Williams D, Feely J. Pharmacokinetic-pharmacodynamic drug interactions with HMG-CoA reductase inhibitors. Clin Pharmacokinet. 2002;41(5):343–70.

[108] Hare CB, Vu MP, Grunfeld C, Lampiris HW. Simvastatin-nelfinavir interaction implicated in rhabdomyolysis and death. Clin Infect Dis. 2002;35(10):e111–12.

[109] Moro H, Tsukada H, Tanuma A, Shirasaki A, Iino N, Nishibori T, et al. Rhabdomyolysis after simvastatin therapy in an HIV-infected patient with chronic renal failure. AIDS Patient Care STD. 2004;18(12):687–90.

[110] Moyle GJ, Lloyd M, Reynolds B, Baldwin C, Mandalia S, Gazzard BG. Dietary advice with or without pravastatin for the management of hypercholesterolemia associated with protease inhibitor therapy. AIDS. 2001;15(12):1503–08.

[111] Calza L, Manfredi R, Chiodo F. Use of fibrates in the management of hyperlipidemia in HIV-infected patients receiving HAART. Infection. 2002;30(1):26–31.

[112] Mastroianni CM, d'Ettorre G, Forcina G, Lichtner M, Corpolongo A, Coletta S, Vullo V. Rhabdomyolisis after cerivastatin/gemfibrozil therapy in an HIV-infected patient with protease inhibitor-related hyperlipidaemia. AIDS. 2001;15(6):820–21.

[113] Thomas JC, Lopes-Virella MF, Del Bene VE, Cerveny JD, Taylor KB, McWhorter LS, Bultemeier NC.. Use of fenofibrate in the management of protease inhibitor-associated lipid abnormalities. Pharmacotherapy. 2000;20(6):727–34.

[114] Rubins HB, Robins SJ, Collins D, Fye CL, Anderson JW, Elam MB, et al. Gemfibrozil for the secondary prevention of coronary heart disease in men with low levels of high-density lipoprotein cholesterol. N Engl J Med. 1999;341(6):410–18.

[115] Calza L, Manfredi R, Chiodo F. Statins and fibrates for the treatment of hyperlipidaemia in HIV-infected patients receiving HAART. AIDS. 2003;17(6):851–59.

[116] Visnegarwala F, Maldonado M, Sajja P, Minihan JL, Rodriguez-Barradas MC, Ong O, et al. Lipid lowering effects of statins and fibrates in the management of HIV dyslipidemias associated with antiretroviral therapy in HIV clinical practice. J Infect. 2004;49(4):283–90.

[117] Miller J, Brown D, Amin J, Kent-Hughes J, Law M, Kaldor J, et al. A randomized, double-blind study of gemfibrozil for the treatment of protease inhibitor-associated hypertriglyceridaemia. AIDS. 2002;16(16):2195–200.

[118] Keech A, Simes RJ, Barter P, Best J, Scott R, Taskinen MR, et al. Effects of long-term fenofibrate therapy on cardiovascular events in 9795 people with type 2 diabetes mellitus (the FIELD study): randomised controlled trial. Lancet. 2005; 366(9500): 1849–61.

[119] Aberg JA, Zackin RA, Brobst SW, Evans SR, Alston BL, Henry WK, et al. A randomized trial of the efficacy and safety of fenofibrate versus pravastatin in HIV-infected

subjects with lipid abnormalities: AIDS Clinical Trials Group Study 5087. AIDS Res Hum Retroviruses. 2005;21(9):757–67.

[120] Nolan DP, O'Connor MB, O'Connor C, Moriarty M, O'Leary A, Bergin C. HIV-associated dyslipidaemia among HIV antibody-positive patients in Ireland: prevalence andmanagement strategies. Int J STD AIDS. 2010;21(1):75–76.

[121] Negredo E, Moltó J, Puig J, Cinquegrana D, Bonjoch A, Pérez-Alvarez N, et al. Ezetimibe, a promising lipid-lowering agent for the treatment of dyslipidaemia in HIV infected patients with poor response to statins. AIDS. 2006;20(17):2159–64.

[122] Coll B, Aragonés G, Parra S, Alonso-Villaverde C, Masana L. Ezetimibe effectively decreases LDL-cholesterol in HIV-infected patients., Alonso-Villaverde C, Masana L. AIDS. 2006;20(12):1675–77.

[123] Patel SB. Ezetimibe: a novel cholesterol-lowering agent that highlights novel physiologic pathways. Curr Cardiol Rep. 2004;6(6):439–42.

[124] Stein E. Results of phase I/II clinical trials with ezetimibe, a novel selective cholesterol absorption inhibitor. Eur Heart J. 2001;3(Suppl E):E11–16.

[125] Wohl DA, Waters D, Simpson RJ, Richard S, Schnell A, Napravnik S, et al. Ezetimibe alone reduces low-density lipoprotein cholesterol in HIV-infected patients receiving combination antiretroviral therapy. Clin Infect Dis. 2008;47(8):1105–08.

[126] Chastain LM, Bain AM, Edwards KL, Bedimo R, Busti AJ. A retrospective study of the lipid-lowering efficacy and safety of ezetimibe added to hydroxy methylglutaryl coenzyme A reductase therapy in HIV-infected patients with hyperlipidemia. J Clin Lipidol. 2007;1(6):634–39.

[127] Grandi AM, Nicolini E, Rizzi L, Caputo S, Annoni F, Cremona AM, et al. Dyslipidemia in HIV-positive patients: a randomized, controlled, prospective study on ezetimibe+fenofibrate versus pravastatin monotherapy. J Int AIDS Soc. 2014;17:19004.

[128] Phillipson BE, Rothrock DW, Connor WE, Harris WS, Illingworth DR. Reduction of plasma lipids, lipoproteins, and apoproteins by dietary fish oils in patients with hypertriglyceridemia. N Engl J Med.1985;312(19):1210–16.

[129] Harris WS. N-3 Fatty acids and serum lipoproteins: human studies. Am J Clin Nutr. 1997;65(5 Suppl):1645S–54S.

[130] Gerber JG, Kitch DW, Fichtenbaum CJ, Zackin RA, Charles S, Hogg E, et al. Fish oil and fenofibrate for the treatment of hypertriglyceridemia in HIV infected subjects on antiretroviral therapy: results of ACTG A5186. JAIDS. 2008;47(4):459–66.

[131] De Truchis P, Kirstetter M, Perier A, Meunier C, Zucman D, Force G, et al. Reduction in triglycerides level with N-3 polyunsaturated fatty acids in HIV-infected patients taking potent antiretroviral therapy: randomized prospective study. J Acquir Immune Defic Syndr. 2007;44(3):278–85.

[132] Schmidt EB. Marine N-3 polyunsaturated fatty acids and coronary heart disease: come a long way but expect more. Cell Mol Biol (Noisy-le-grand). 2010;56(1):1–3.

[133] Bang HO, Dyerberg J. Plasma lipids and lipoproteins in Greenlandic West Coast Eskimos. Acta Med Scand. 1972;192(1–2):85–94.

[134] Farmer JA. Nicotinic acid: a new look at an old drug. Curr Atheroscler Rep. 2009;11(2):87–92.

[135] Brown BG, Zhao XQ, Chait A, Fisher LD, Cheung MC, Morse JS, et al. Simvastatin and niacin, antioxidant vitamins, or the combination for the prevention of coronary disease. N Engl J Med. 2001;345(22):1583–92.

[136] Meyers CD, Carr MC, Park S, Brunzell JD. Varying cost and free nicotinic acid content in over-the-counter niacin preparations for dyslipidemia. Ann Intern Med. 2003;139(12):996–1002.

[137] Digby JE, Lee JM, Choudhury RP. Nicotinic acid and the prevention of coronary artery disease. Curr Opin Lipidol. 2009;20(4):321–26.

[138] Gerber MT, Mondy KE, Yarasheski KE, Drechsler H, Claxton S, Stoneman J, et al. Niacin in HIV-infected individuals with hyperlipidemia receiving potent antiretroviral therapy. Clin Infect Dis. 2004;39(3):419–25.

[139] Rader DJ. Effects of nonstatin lipid drug therapy on high-density lipoprotein metabolism. Am J Cardiol. 2003;91(7A):18E–23E.

[140] Lee JH, Chan JL, Sourlas E, Raptopoulos V, Mantzoros CS. Recombinant methionyl human leptin therapy in replacement doses improves insulin resistance and metabolic profile in patients with lipoatrophy and metabolic syndrome induced by the highly active antiretroviral therapy. J Clin Endocrinol Metab. 2006;91(7):2605–11.

[141] Fredriksen J, Ueland T, Dyrøy E, Halvorsen B, Melby K, Melbye L, et al. Lipid-lowering and anti-inflammatory effects of tetradecylthioacetic acid in HIV-infected patients on highly active antiretroviral therapy. Eur J Clin Invest. 2004;34(10):709–15.

[142] Hadigan C, Liebau J, Torriani M, Andersen R, Grinspoon S. Improved triglycerides and insulin sensitivity with 3 months of acipimox in human immunodeficiency virus-infected patients with hypertriglyceridemia. J Clin Endocrinol Metab. 2006;91(11):4438–44.

[143] Keithley JK, Swanson B, Sha BE, Zeller JM, Kessler HA, Smith KY. A pilot study of the safety and efficacy of cholestin in treating HIV-related dyslipidemia. Nutrition. 2002;18(2):201–04.

[144] Loignon M, Toma E. L-Carnitine for the treatment of highly active antiretroviral therapy-related hypertriglyceridemia in HIV-infected adults. AIDS. 2001;15(9):1194–95.

[145] Haraguchi k, Takeda S, Kubota Y, Kumamoto H, Tanaka H, Hamasaki, et al. From the Chemistry of Epoxy-Sugar Nucleosides to the Discovery of Anti-HIV Agent 4′-ethynylstavudine-Festinavir. Curr Pharm Des. 2013;19(10):1880–97.

[146] Flexner C, Saag M. The antiretroviral drug pipeline: prospects and implications for future treatment research. Curr Opin HIV AIDS. 2013;8(6):572–78.

[147] Vere Hodge RA, Meeting report: 26 th International Conference on Antiviral Research. Antiviral Res. 2013;100(1):276–85.

[148] Cahn P, Altclas J, Martins M, Losso M, Cassetti I, Cooper DA, Cox S. Antiviral activity of apricitabine in treatment-experienced HIV-1-infected patients with M184V who are failing combination therapy.HIV Med. 2011 Jul;12(6):334–42.

[149] Cox S, Moore S, Southby J. Safety profile of apricitabine, a novel NRTI, during 24-week dosing in experienced HIV-1 infected patients". XVII International AIDS Conference (AIDS 2008). Mexico City. Abstract TUAB0106. Retrieved 2008-08-29.

[150] Cahn P, Cassetti I, Wood R, Phanuphak P, Shiveley L, Bethell RC, Sawyer J. Efficacy and tolerability of 10-day monotherapy with apricitabine in antiretroviral-naive, HIV-infected patients. AIDS. 2006;20(9):1261–68.

[151] Markowitz M, Zolopa A, Squires K, Ruane P, Coakley D, Kearney B, et al. Phase I/II study of the pharmacokinetics, safety and antiretroviral activity of tenofovir alafenamide, a new prodrug of the HIV reverse transcriptase inhibitor tenofovir, in HIV-infected adults. J Antimicrob Chemother. 2014;69(5):1362–69.

[152] Zolopa A, Ortiz R, Sax P. Comparative study of tenofovir alafenamide vs tenofovir disoproxil fumarate, each with elvitegravir, cobicistat, and emtricitabine, for HIV treatment. In: Abstracts of the Twentieth Conference on Retroviruses and Opportunistic Infections. Atlanta, GA, 2013. Abstract 99LB. Foundation for Retrovirology and Human Health, Alexandria, VA, USA.

[153] Ruane PJ, DeJesus E, Berger D, Markowitz M, Bredeek UF, Callebaut C, et al. Antiviral activity, safety, and pharmacokinetics/pharmacodynamics of tenofovir alafenamide (TAF) as 10-day monotherapy in HIV-1-positive adults. JAIDS. 2013;63(4):449–55.

[154] Ghosh RK, Ghosh SM, Chawla S. Recent advances in antiretroviral drugs. Expert Opin Pharmacother. 2011;12(1):31–46.

[155] Desai M, Iyer G, Dikshit RK. Antiretroviral drugs: Critical issues and recent advances. Indian J Pharmacol. 2012;44(3):288–98.

[156] Colucci P, Pottage JC, Robison H, Turgeon J, Ducharme MP. Effect of a single dose of ritonavir on the pharmacokinetic behavior of elvucitabine, a nucleoside reverse transcriptase inhibitor, administered in healthy volunteers. Antimicrob Agents Chemother. 2009;53(2):646–50.

[157] Vingerhoests J, Azin H, Fransen E, De Baere I, Smeulders L, Jochmans D, et al. TMC125 displays a high genetic barrier to the development of resistance: evidence from in vitro selection experiments. J Virol. 2005;79(20):12773–82.

[158] Yanakakis LJ, Bumpus NN. Biotransformation of the antiretroviral drug etravirine: metabolite identification, reaction phenotyping, and characterization of autoinduction of cytochrome P450-dependent metabolism.Drug Metab Dispos. 2012;40(4):803–14.

[159] Casado JL, de Los Santos I, Del Palacio M, García-Fraile L, Pérez-Elías MJ, Sanz J, Moreno S. Lipid-lowering effect and efficacy after switching to etravirine in HIV-infected patients with intolerance to suppressive HAART. HIV Clin Trials. 2013;14(1): 1–9.

[160] Poveda E, Garrido C, de Mendoza C, Corral A, Cobo J, González-Lahoz J, Soriano V. Prevalence of etravirine (TMC-125) resistance mutations in HIV-infected patients with prior experience of non-nucleoside reverse transcriptase inhibitors. J Antimicrob Chemother. 2007;60(6):1409–10.

[161] Goebel F, Yakovlev A, Pozniak AL, Vinogradova E, Boogaerts G, Hoetelmans R, et al. Short-term antiviral activity of TMC278 - a novel NNRTI - in treatment-naive HIV-1-infected subjects. AIDS. 2006;20(13):1721–26.

[162] Tebas P, Sension M, Arribas J, Duiculescu D, Florence E, Hung CC, et al. Lipid levels and changes in body fat distribution in treatment-naive, HIV-1-Infected adults treated with rilpivirine or Efavirenz for 96 weeks in the ECHO and THRIVE trials. Clin Infect Dis. 2014;59(3):425–34.

[163] Côté B, Burch JD, AsanteAsante-Appiah E, Bayly C, Bédard L, Blouin M, et al. Discovery of MK-1439, an orally bioavailable non-nucleoside reverse transcriptase inhibitor potent against a wide range of resistant mutant HIV viruses. Bioorg Med Chem Lett. 2014;24(3):917–22.

[164] Saag MS. New and investigational drugs for HIV infection: mechanisms of action and early research findings. Top Antivir Med. 2012;20(5):162–67.

[165] Lai MT, Feng M, Falgueyret JP, Tawa P, Witmer M, Di Stefano D, et al. In vitro characterization of MK-1439, a novel HIV-1 nonnucleoside reverse transcriptase inhibitor. Antimicrob Agents Chemother. 2014;58(3):1652–63.

[166] Chong H, Yao X, Zhang C, Cai L, Cui S, Wang Y, He Y. Biophysical property and broad anti-HIV activity of albuvirtide, a 3-maleimimidopropionic acid-modified peptide fusion inhibitor. PLoS One. 2012;7(3):e32599.

[167] He Y, Cheng J, Lu H, Li J, Hu J, Qi Z, et al. Potent HIV fusion inhibitors against Enfuvirtide-resistant HIV-1 strains. Proc Natl Acad Sci U S A. 2008;105(42):16332–37.

[168] Nathan B, bayley J, Waters L, Post FA. Cobicistat: a novel pharmaco enhancer for co-formulation with protease and integrase inhibitors. Infect Dis ther. 2013;2(2):111–22.

[169] LePIst EI, Phan TK, Roy A, Tong L, MacLennan K, Murray B, Ray AS. Cobicistat Boosts the Intestinal Absorption of Transport Substrates, Including HIV Protease Inhibitors and GS-7340, *in Vitro*. Antimicrobial Agents and Chemotherapy. 2012;56(10): 5409–13.

[170] Sax PE, DeJesus E, Mills A, Zolopa A, Cohen C, Wohl D, et al. Co-formulated elvitegravir, cobicistat, emtricitabine, and tenofovir versus co-formulated efavirenz, emtricitabine, and tenofovir for initial treatment of HIV-1 infection: a randomised, double-blind, phase 3 trial, analysis of results after 48 weeks. Lancet. 2012;379(9835):2439–48.

[171] Bera S, Pandey KK, Vora AC, Grangenett DP. HIV-1 integrase strand transfer inhibitors stabilize an integrase-single blunt-ended DNA complex.J Mol Biol. 2011;410(5): 831–46.

[172] Fader LD. Malenfant E, Parisien M, Carson R, Bilodeau F, Landry S, et al. Discovery of BI 224436, a non catalytic site integrase inhibitor (NCINI) of HIV-1.ACS Med Chem Lett. 2014;22;5(4):422–27.

[173] Fenwick C, Amad M, Nailey MD, Benthell R, Bös M, Bonneau P, et al. Preclinical profile of BI 224436, a novel HIV-1 non-catalytic site integrase inhibitor. Antimicrob Agents Chemother. 2014;58(6):3233–34.

[174] Taha H, Morgan J, Das A, Das S. Parenteral patent drug S/GSK1265744 has the potential to be an effective agent in pre-exposure prophylaxis against HIV infection.Recent Pat Antiinfect Drug Discov. 2013;8(3):213–18.

[175] Ford SL, Gould E, Chen S, Lou Y, Dumont E, Spreen W, PIscitelli S. Effects of etravirine on the pharmacokinetics of the integrase inhibitor S/GSK1265744.Antimicrob Agents Chemother. 2013;57(1):277–80.

[176] Grohskopf LA, Chillag KL, Gvetadze R, Liu AY, Thompson M, Mayer KH, et al. Randomized trial of clinical safety of daily oral tenofovir disoproxil fumarate among HIV-uninfected men who have sex with men in the United States. J Acquired Immune Defic Syndr. 2013;64(1):79–86.

[177] Grant RM, Lama JR, Anderson PL, McMahan V, Liu AY, Vargas L, et al. Preexposure chemoprophylaxis for HIV prevention in men who have sex with men. N Engl J Med. 2010;363(27):2587–99.

[178] Baeten JM, Donnell D, Ndase P, Mugo NR, Campbell JD, Wangisi J, et al. Antiretroviral prophylaxis for HIV prevention in heterosexual men and women. N Engl J Med. 2012;367(5):399–410.

[179] Thigpen MC, Kebaabetswe PM, Paxton LA, Smith DK, Rose CE, Segolodi TM, et al. Antiretroviral preexposure prophylaxis for heterosexual HIV transmission in Botswana. N Engl J Med. 2012;367(5):423–34.

[180] Choopanya K, Martin M, Suntharasamai P, Sangkum U, Mock PA, Leethochawalit M, et al. Antiretroviral prophylaxis for HIV infection among people who inject drugs

in Bangkok, Thailand (the Bangkok Tenofovir Study): a randomised, double-blind, placebo-controlled phase 3 trial. Lancet. 2013;381(9883):2083–90.

[181] Food and Drug Administration. Truvada approved to reduce the risk of sexually transmitted HIV in people who are not infected with the virus. 2012. http://www.fda.gov/ForConsumers/ByAudience/ForPatientAdvocates/HIVandAIDSActivities/uc.m312264.htm. Accessed November 20, 2014.

[182] Gilead Sciences. Truvada Package Insert. 2013; http://www.gilead.com/pdf/truvada_pi.pdf. Accessed November 20, 2014.

[183] Centers for Disease Control and Prevention. Interim guidance: preexposure prophylaxis for the prevention of HIV infection in men who have sex with men. MMWR Morb Mortal Wkly Rep.2011;60(3):65–68.

[184] Highlights of prescribing information. Truvada (emtricitabine/tenofovir disoproxil fumarate) tablets for oral use. Foster City, Calif.: Gilead Sciences, Inc. Revised June 2013. http://www.gilead.com/pdf/truvada_pi.pdf. Accessed November 20, 2014.

[185] Centers for Disease Control and Prevention (CDC). Interim guidance for clinicians considering the use of preexposure prophylaxis for the prevention of HIV infection in heterosexually active adults. MMWR Morb Mortal Wkly Rep. 2012;61(31):586–59.

[186] US Public Health Service.Centers for Disease Control and Prevention (CDC). preexposure prophylaxis for the prevention of HIV Infection in the United States – 2014 Clinical Practice Guideline. http://www.cdc.gov/hiv/pdf/PrEPguidelines2014.pdf. Accessed November 20, 2014

[187] Guyatt G, Oxman AD, Akl EA, Kunz R, Vist G, Brozek J, Norris S, et al. GRADE guidelines: 1. Introduction-GRADE evidence profiles and summary of findings tables. J Clin Epidemiol. 2011;64(4):383–94.

[188] Van Damme L, Corneli A, Ahmed K, Agot K, Lombaard J, Kapiga S, et al. Preexposure prophylaxis for HIV infection among African women. N Engl J Med. 2012;367(5):411–22.

[189] Peterson L, Taylor D, Roddy R, Belai G, Phillips P, Nanda K, et al. Tenofovir disoproxil fumarate for prevention of HIV infection in women: a phase 2, double-blind, randomized, placebo-controlled trial. PLoS Clin Trials. 2007;2(5):e27.

[190] Marrazzo J, Ramjee G, Nair G, Palanee T, Mkhize B, Nakabiito C, et al. CROI. Atlanta, GA: 2013. Pre-exposure prophylaxis for HIV in women: daily oral tenofovir, oral tenofoviremtricitabine, or vaginal tenofovir gel in the VOICE Study (MTN 003), 2013 Mar 3–6.

[191] Cutler B, Justman J. Vaginal microbicides and the prevention of HIV transmission.Lancet Infect Dis. 2008;8(11):685–97.

[192] McGowan I. Microbicides: a new frontier in HIV prevention. Biologicals. 2006;34(4): 241–55.

[193] Dhawan D, Mayer KH. Microbicides to prevent HIV transmission: overcoming obstacles to chemical barrier protection. J Infect Dis. 2006;193(1):36–44.

[194] Wiysonge CS, Shey MS, Shang J, Kongnyuy EJ, Brocklehurst P. Vaginal microbicides for preventing mother-to-child transmission of HIV infection—no evidence of an effect or evidence of no effect? S Afr Med J. 2007;97(7):530–33.

[195] Tsai CC, Follis KE, Sabo A, Beck TW, Grant RF, Bischofberger N, et al. Prevention of SIV infection in macaques by (R)-9-(2-phosphonylmethoxypropyl)adenine. Science. 1995;270(5239):1197–99.

[196] Wainberg M. The prospect for RT inhibitors as topical microbicides. Microbicides 2004 Conference; London, UK; March 28–31, 2004. Abstract MMM-03.

[197] Balzarini J, Zhang H, Herdewijn P, Johns D, De Clercq E. Intracellular metabolism and mechanism of antiretrovirus action of 9-(2-phosphony lmethoxyethyl)adenine, a potent anti-human immunodefi ciency virus compound. Proc Natl Acad Sci USA. 1991;88(4):1499–503.

[198] Aquaro S, Caliò R, Balzarini J, Bellocchi MC, Garaci E, Perno CF. Macrophages and HIV infection: therapeutical approaches toward this strategic virus reservoir. Antiviral Res. 2002;55(2):209–25.

[199] Mayer KH, Maslankowski LA, Gai F, El-Sadr WM, Justman J, Kwiecien A, et al. Safety and tolerability of tenofovir vaginal gel in abstinent and sexually active HIV-infected and uninfected women. AIDS. 2006;20(4):543–51.

[200] Balzarini J, Naesens L, Verbeken E, Laga M, Van Damme L, Parniak M, et al. Preclinical studies on thiocarboxanilide UC-781 as a virucidal agent. AIDS. 1998;12(10):1129–38.

[201] Di Fabio S, Van Roey J, Giannini G, van den Mooter G, Spada M, Binelli A, et al. Inhibition of vaginal transmission of HIV-1 in hu-SCID mice by the non-nucleoside reverse transcriptase inhibitor TMC120 in a gel formulation. AIDS. 2003;17(11):1597–604.

[202] Fletcher P, Kiselyeva Y, Wallace G, Romano J, Griffin G, Margolis L, Shattock R.. The nonnucleoside reverse transcriptase inhibitor UC-781 inhibits human immunodeficiency virus type 1 infection of human cervical tissue and dissemination by migratory cells. J Virol. 2005;79(17):11179–86.

[203] Van Herrewege Y, Michiels J, Van Roey J, Fransen K, Kestens L, Balzarini J, et al. In vitro evaluation of nonnucleoside reverse transcriptase inhibitors UC-781 and TMC120-R147681 as human immunodeficiency virus microbicides. Antimicrob Agents Chemother. 2004;48(1):337–39.

[204] Van Herrewege Y, Vanham G, Michiels J, Fransen K, Kestens L, Andries K, et al. A series of diaryltriazines anddiarylpyrimidines are highly potent nonnucleoside reversetranscriptase inhibitors with possible applications as microbicides.Antimicrob Agents Chemother. 2004;48(10):3684–89.

[205] Schwartz JL, Kovalevsky G, Lai JJ, Ballagh SA, McCormick T, Douville K, et al. A randomized six day safety study of an antiretroviral microbicide candidate UC-781, a nonnucleoside reverse transcriptase inhibitor. Sex Transm Dis. 2008;35(4):414–19.

[206] Zussman A, Lara L, Lara HH, Bentwich Z, Borkow G. Blocking of cell-free and cell-associated HIV-1 transmission through human cervix organ culture with UC781. AIDS. 2003;17(5):653–61.

[207] Hossain MM, Parniak MA. In vitro microbicidal activity of the nonnucleoside reverse transcriptase inhibitor (NNRTI) UC781 against NNRTI-resistant human immunodeficiency virus type 1. J Virol. 2006;80(9):4440–46.

[208] Lederman MM, Veazey RS, Offord R, Mosier DE, Dufour J, Mefford M, et al. Prevention of vaginal SHIV transmission in rhesus macaques through inhibition of CCR5. Science. 2004;306(5695):485–87.

[209] Veazey RS, Klasse PJ, Schader SM, Hu Q, Ketas TJ, Lu M, et al. Protection of macaques from vaginal SHIV challenge by vaginally delivered inhibitors of virus-cell fusion. Nature. 2005;438(7064):99–102.

[210] Torre VS, Marozsan AJ, Albright JL, Collins KR, Hartley O, Offord RE, et al. Variable sensitivity of CCR5-tropic human immunodefi ciency virus type 1 isolates to inhibition by RANTES analogs. J Virol. 2000;74(10):4868–76.

[211] Kawamura T, Bruse SE, Abraha A, Sugaya M, Hartley O, Offord RE, et al. PSC-RANTES blocks R5 human immunodefi ciency virus infection of Langerhans cells isolated from individuals with a variety of CCR5 diplotypes. J Virol. 2004;78(14): 7602–09.

[212] Kawamura T, Gulden FO, Sugaya M, McNamara DT, Borris DL, Lederman MM, et al. R5 HIV productively infects Langerhans cells, and infection levels are regulated by compound CCR5 polymorphisms. Proc Natl Acad Sci USA. 2003;100(14):8401–06.

[213] Lin PF, Blair W, Wang T, Spicer T, Guo Q, Zhou N, et al. A small molecule HIV-1 inhibitor that targets the HIV-1 envelope and inhibits CD4 receptor binding. Proc Natl Acad Sci USA. 2003;100(19):11013–18.

[214] Guo Q, Ho HT, Dicker I, Fan L, Zhou N, Friborg J, et al. Biochemical and genetic characterizations of a novel human immunodeficiency virus type 1 inhibitor that blocks gp120-CD4 interactions. J Virol. 2003;77(19):10528–36.

[215] Lu M. Stabilizing peptides and their use in the preparation of stabilized HIV inhibitors. World Intellectual Property Organization Patent WO-04/106364A1. 2004.

[216] Bewley CA, Otero-Quintero S. The potent anti-HIV protein cyanovirin-N contains two novel carbohydrate binding sites that selectively bind to Man(8) D1D3 and Man(9) with nanomolar affinity: implications for binding to the HIV envelope protein gp120. J Am Chem Soc. 2001;123(17):3892–902.

[217] Bewley CA. Rapid validation of the overall structure of an internal domain-swapped mutant of the anti-HIV protein cyanovirin-N using residual dipolar couplings. J Am Chem Soc. 2001;123(5):1014–15.

[218] Balzarini J, Van Laethem K, Peumans WJ, Van Damme EJ, Bolmstedt A, Gago F, Schols D. Mutational pathways, resistance profile, and side effects of cyanovirin relative to human immunodeficiency virus type 1 strains with n-glycan deletions in their gp120 envelopes. J Virol. 2006;80(17):8411–21.

[219] Xu Q. Development of a live topical microbicide for women. Microbicides 2008 Conference. New Delhi, India; Feb 24–27, 2008. Abstract 221.

[220] Martin LS, McDougal JS, Loskoski SL. Disinfection and inactivation of the human T lymphotropic virus type III/lymphadenopathy associated virus. J Infect Dis. 1985;152(2):400–03.

[221] Ongradi J, Ceccherini-Nelli L, Pistello M, Specter S, Bendinelli M. Acid sensitivity of cell-free and cell-associated HIV-1: clinical implications. AIDS Res Hum Retroviruses. 1990;6(12):1433–36.

[222] O'Connor TJ, Kinchington D, Kangro HO, Jeffries DJ. The activity of candidate virucidal agents, low pH and genital secretions against HIV-1 in vitro. Int J STD AIDS. 1995;6(4):267–72.

[223] Olmsted SS, Dubin NH, Cone RA, Moench TR. The rate at which human sperm are immobilized and killed by mild acidity. Fertil Steril. 2000;73(4):687–93.

[224] Achilles SL, Shete PB, Whaley KJ, Moench TR, Cone RA. Microbicide efficacy and toxicity tests in a mouse model for vaginal transmission of Chlamydia trachomatis. Sex Transm Dis. 2002;29(11):655–64.

[225] Amaral E, Faundes A, Zaneveld L, Waller D, Garg S. Study of the vaginal tolerance to Acidform, an acid-buff ering, bioadhesive gel. Contraception. 1999;60(6):361–66.

[226] Amaral E, Perdigao A, Souza MH, Mauck C, Waller D, Zaneveld L, Faundes A. Vaginal safety after use of a bioadhesive, acid-buff ering, microbicidal contraceptive gel (ACIDFORM) and a 2% nonoxynol-9 product. Contraception. 2006;73(5):542–47.

[227] Croughan WS, Behbehani AM. Comparative study of inactivation of herpes simplex virus types 1 and 2 by commonly used antiseptic agents. J Clin Microbiol. 1988;26(2):213–15.

[228] Zeitlin L, Hoen TE, Achilles SL, Hegarty TA, Jerse AE, Kreider JW, et al. Tests of Buffergel for contraception and prevention of sexually transmitted diseases in animal models. Sex Transm Dis. 2001;28(7):417–23.

[229] van De Wijgert J, Fullem A, Kelly C, Mehendale S, Rugpao S, Kumwenda N, et al. Phase I trial of the topical microbicide Buff erGel: safety results from four international sites. J Acquir Immune Defic Syndr. 2001;26(1):21–27.

[230] Mayer KH, Peipert J, Fleming T, Fullem A, Moench T, Cu-Uvin S, et al. Safety and tolerability of BufferGel, a novel vaginal microbicide, in women in the United States. Clin Infect Dis. 2001;32(3):476–82.

[231] Tabet SR, Callahan MM, Mauck CK, Gai F, Coletti AS, Profy AT, et al. Safety and acceptability of penile application of 2 candidate topical microbicides: BufferGel and PRO 2000 gel: 3 randomized trials in healthy low-risk men and HIV-positive men. J Acquir Immune Defic Syndr. 2003;33(4):476–83.

[232] Amaral E, Faundes A, Zaneveld L, Waller D, Garg S. Study of the vaginal tolerance to Acidform, an acid-buffering, bioadhesive gel. Contraception. 1999;60(6):361–66.

[233] Amaral E, Perdigao A, Souza MH, et al. Vaginal safety after use of a bioadhesive, acid-buffering, microbicidal contraceptive gel (ACIDFORM) and a 2% nonoxynol-9 product. Contraception. 2006;73:542–47.

[234] Schwartz JL, Poindexter A, Schmitz SW, Mauck C, Callahan MM. Male tolerance of ACIDFORM gel. Contraception. 2005;71(6):443–46.

[235] Sharma AK, George V, Valiathan R, Pilakka-Kanthikeel S, Pallikkuth S. Inhibitors of HIV-1 entry and integration: recent developments and impact on treatment. Recent Pat Inflamm Allergy Drug Discov. 2013;7(2):151–61.

[236] Mitsuya H, Looney DJ, Kuno S, Ueno R, Wong-Staal F, Broder S. Dextran sulfate suppression of viruses in the HIV family: inhibition of virion binding to CD4+ cells. Science. 1988;240(4852):646–49.

[237] Moulard M, Lortat-Jacob H, Mondor I, Roca G, Wyatt R, Sodroski J, et al. Selective interactions of polyanions with basic surfaces on human immunodeficiency virus type 1 gp120. J Virol. 2000;74(4):1948–60.

[238] Van Damme L, Wright A, Depraetere K, Rosenstein I, Vandersmissen V, Poulter L, et al. A phase I study of a novel potential intravaginal microbicide, PRO 2000, in healthy sexually inactive women. Sex Transm Infect. 2000;76(2):126–30.

[239] Johansson E. Results of phase III Carraguard trial. Microbicides 2008 Conference; New Delhi, India; Feb 24–27,2008.

[240] Van Damme L, Govinden R, Mirembe FM, Guédou F, Solomon S, Becker ML, et al. Lack of eff ectiveness of cellulose sulfate gel for the prevention of vaginal HIV transmission. N Engl J Med. 2008;359(5):463–72.

[241] Lacey C. Unacceptable side eff ects of a hyperosmolar vaginal microbicide in a Phase I trial. Microbicides 2008 Conference; New Delhi, India; Feb 24–27, 2008. Abstract B08-527.

[242] Paull J, Chen M, Millwood I. SPL7013 gel (VivaGel(TM)), a topical microbicide in development for prevention of HIV and genital herpes, shown to be well tolerated and comparable with placebo after seven days administration in healthy males. 4th IAS Conference; Sydney, Australia; July 22–25, 2007. Abstract TUAC1LB.

[243] Indevus Pharmaceuticals. PRO2000: product description.Lexington, NA, USA: Indevus Pharmaceuticals, 2006.

[244] Keller MJ, Zerhouni-Layachi B, Cheshenko N, John M, Hogarty K, Kasowitz, et al. PRO 2000 gel inhibits HIV and herpes simplex virus infection following vaginal application: a double-blind placebo-controlled trial. J Infect Dis. 2006;193(1):27–35.

[245] Mayer KH, Karim SA, Kelly C, Maslankowski L, Rees H, Profy AT, et al. Safety and tolerability of vaginal PRO 2000 gel in sexually active HIV-uninfected and abstinent HIV-infected women. AIDS. 2003;17(3):321–29.

[246] Joshi S, Dutta S, Bell B, Profy A, Kuruc J, Fang G, et al. Documenting intermenstrual bleeding in a vaginal microbicide study: case reports and lessons learned. AIDS Res Hum Retroviruses. 2006;22(3):294–96.

[247] Perotti ME, Pirovano A, Phillips DM. Carrageenan formulation prevents macrophage trafficking from vagina: implications for microbicide development. Biol Reprod. 2003;69(3):933–39.

[248] Coggins C, Blanchard K, Alvarez F, Brache V, Weisberg E, Kilmarx PH, et al. Preliminary safety and acceptability of a carrageenan gel for possible use as a vaginal microbicide. Sex Transm Infect. 2000;76(6):480–83.

[249] Bollen LJ, Blanchard K, Kilmarx PH, Chaikummao S, Connolly C, Wasinrapee P, et al. No increase in cervicovaginal proinfl ammatory ctokines after Carraguard use in a placebo-controlled randomized clinical trial. J Acquir Immune Defic Syndr. 2008;47(2):253–57.

[250] van de Wijgert JH, Braunstein SL, Morar NS, Jones HE, Madurai L, Strickfaden TT, et al. Carraguard vaginal gel safety in HIV-positive women and men in South Africa. J Acquir Immune Defic Syndr. 2007;46(5):538–46.

[251] Kilmarx PH, van de Wijgert JH, Chaikummao S, Jones HE, Limpakarnjanarat K, Friedland BA, et al. Safety and acceptability of the candidate microbicide Carraguard in Thai women: findings from a phase II clinical trial. J Acquir Immune Defic Syndr. 2006;43(3):327–34.

[252] Pistorius AG, van de Wijgert JH, Sebola M, Friedland B, Nagel E, Bokaba C, Hoosen AA. Microbicide trials for preventing HIV/AIDS in South Africa: phase II trial participants' experiences and psychological needs. SAHARA J. 2004;1(2):78–86.

[253] Scordi-Bello IA, Mosoian A, He C, Chen Y, Cheng Y, Jarvis GA, et al. Candidate sulfonated and sulfated topical microbicides: comparison of anti-human immunodefi ciency virus activities and mechanisms of action. Antimicrob Agents Chemother. 2005;49(9):3607–15.

[254] Neurath AR, Strick N, Li YY. Water dispersible microbicidal cellulose acetate phthalate film. BMC Infect Dis. 2003; 3:27.

[255] Lu H, Zhao Q, Wallace G, Liu S, He Y, Shattock R, et al. Cellulose acetate 1,2-benzenedicarboxylate inhibits infection by cell-free and cellassociated primary HIV-1 isolates. AIDS Res Hum Retroviruses. 2006;22(5):411–18.

[256] Kawamura T, Cohen SS, Borris DL, Aquilino EA, Glushakova S, Margolis LB, et al. Candidate microbicides block HIV-1 infection of human immature Langerhans cells within epithelial tissue explants. J Exp Med. 2000;192(10):1491–500.

[257] Neurath AR, Strick N, Li YY, Lin K, Jiang S. Design of a "microbicide" for prevention of sexually transmitted diseases using "inactive" pharmaceutical excipients. Biologicals.1999;27(1):11–21.

[258] Jiang YH, Emau P, Cairns JS, Flanary L, Morton WR, McCarthy TD, Tsai CC. SPL7013 gel as a topical microbicide for prevention of vaginal transmission of SHIV89.6P in macaques. AIDS Res Hum Retroviruses. 2005;21(3):207–13.

[259] Bernstein DI, Stanberry LR, Sacks S, Ayisi NK, Gong YH, Ireland J, et al. Evaluations of unformulated and formulated dendrimer-based microbicide candidates in mouse and guinea pig models of genital herpes. Antimicrob Agents Chemother. 2003;47(12): 3784–88.

[260] Hillier SL, Moench T, Shattock R, Black R, Reichelderfer P, Veronese F. In vitro and in vivo: the story of nonoxynol 9. J Acquir Immune Defic Syndr. 2005;39(1):1–8.

[261] Fichorova RN, Tucker DL, Anderson DJ. The molecular basis of nonoxynol-9-induced vaginal inflammation and its possible relevance to human immunodeficiency virus type 1 transmission. J Infect Dis. 2001;184(4):418–28.

[262] Bourinbaiar AS, Lee-Huang S. The efficacy of nonoxynol-9 from an in vitro point of view. AIDS. 1996; 10(5):558–59.

[263] Roddy RE, Zekeng L, Ryan KA, Tamoufe U, Weir SS, Wong EL. A controlled trial of nonoxynol-9 fi lm to reduce male-to-female transmission of sexually transmitted diseases. N Engl J Med. 1998;339(8):504–10.

[264] Van Damme L, Ramjee G, Alary M, Vuylsteke B, Chandeying V, Rees H, et al. Effectiveness of COL-1492, a nonoxynol-9 vaginal gel, on HIV-1 transmission in female sex workers: a randomized controlled trial. Lancet. 2002;360(9338):971–77.

[265] Calis S, Yulug N, Sumnu M, Ayhan A, Hincal AA. A non-antibiotic antimicrobial mixture (C31G): evaluation of the antimicrobial efficiency of C31G on vaginal cultures. Boll Chim Farm. 1992;131(9):335–38.

[266] Krebs FC, Miller SR, Malamud D, Howett MK, Wigdahl B. Inactivation of human immunodeficiency virus type 1 by nonoxynol-9, C31G, or an alkyl sulfate, sodium dodecyl sulfate. Antiviral Res. 1999;43(3):157–73.

[267] Wyrick PB, Knight ST, Gerbig DG Jr, Raulston JE, Davis CH, Paul TR, Malamud D.. The microbicidal agent C31G inhibits Chlamydia trachomatisinfectivity in vitro.Antimicrob Agents Chemother. 1997;41(6):1335–44.

[268] Ballagh SA, Baker JM, Henry DM, Archer DF. Safety of single daily use for one week of C31G HEC gel in women. Contraception. 2002;66(5):369–75.

[269] Bax R, Douville K, McCormick D, Rosenberg M, Higgins J, Bowden M. Microbicides —evaluating multiple formulations of C31G. Contraception. 2002;66(5):365–68.

[270] Roy S, Gourde P, Piret J, Désormeaux A, Lamontagne J, Haineault C, et al. Thermoreversible gel formulations containing sodium lauryl sulfate or n-auroylsarcosine as potential topical microbicides against sexually transmitted diseases. Antimicrob Agents Chemother. 2001;45(6):1671–81.

[271] Howett MK, Neely EB, Christensen ND, Wigdahl B, Krebs FC, Malamud D, et al. A broad-spectrum microbicide with virucidal activity against sexually transmitted viruses. Antimicrob Agents Chemother. 1999;43(2):314–21.

[272] Piret J, Lamontagne J, Bestman-Smith J, Roy S, Gourde P, Désormeaux A, et al. In vitro and in vivo evaluations of sodium lauryl sulfate and dextran sulfate as microbicides against herpes simplex and human immunodeficiency virus. J Clin Microbiol. 2000;38(1):110–19.

[273] Bestman-Smith J, Piret J, Desormeaux A, Tremblay M, Omar R, Bergeron M. Sodium lauryl sulfate abrogates HIV infectivity by affecting viral attachment. Antimicrob Agents Chemother. 2001;45(8):2229–37.

[274] D'Cruz OJ, Uckun FM. Clinical development of microbicides for the prevention of HIV infection. Curr Pharm Des.2004;10(3):315–36.

[275] MalcolmRK, Edwards KL, Kiser P, Romano J, Smith TJ. Advances in microbicide vaginal rings. Antiviral Res. 2010;88(Suppl 1):S30–39.

[276] Baum MM, Butkyavichene I, Gilman J, Kennedy S, Kopin E, Malone AM, et al. An intravaginal ring for the simultaneous delivery of multiple drugs. J Pharm Sci. 2012;101(8):2833–43.

[277] Moss JA, Baum MM, Malone AM, Kennedy S, Kopin E, Nguyen C, et al. Tenofovir and tenofovir disoproxil pharmacokinetics from intravaginal rings. AIDS. 2012;26(6): 707–10.

[278] Moss JA, Malone AM, Smith TJ, Butkyavichene I, Cortez C, Gilman J, et al. Safety and pharmacokinetics of intravaginal rings delivering tenofovir in pig-tailed macaques. Antimicrob Agents Chemother. 2012;56(11):5952–60.

[279] MossJA, Malone AM, Smith TJ, Kennedy S, Kopin E, Nguyen C, et al. Simultaneous delivery of tenofovir and acyclovirvia an intravaginal ring. Antimicrob Agents Chemother. 2012;56(2):875–82.

[280] MossJA, Malone AM, Smith TJ, Kennedy S, Nguyen C, Vincent KL, et al. Pharmacokinetics of a multipurposepod-intravaginal ring simultaneously delivering five drugs in the ovinemodel. Antimicrob Agents Chemother. 2013;57(8):3994–97.

[281] Moss JA, Srinivasan P, Smith TJ, Butkyavichene I, Lopez G, Brooks AA, et al. Pharmacokinetics and preliminary safety study of pod-intravaginal rings delivering antiretroviral combinations for HIV prophylaxis in a macaque model. Antimicrob Agents Chemother. 2014;58(9):5125–35.

[282] Loonam CR, Mullen A. Nutrition and the HIV-associated lipodystrophy syndrome. Nutr Res Rev. 2012;25(2):267–87.

[283] Fields-Gardner C, Campa A; American dietetics association. Position of the American Dietetic Association: nutrition intervention and human immunodeficiency virus infection. J Am Diet Assoc. 2010;110(7):1105–19.

[284] Shah M, Tierney K, Adams-Huet B, Boonyavarakul A, Jacob K, Quittner C, et al. The role of diet, exercise and smoking in dyslipidaemia in HIV-infected patients with lipodystrophy. HIV Med. 2005;6(4):291–98.

[285] Hadigan C, Jeste S, Anderson EJ, Tsay R, Cyr H, Grinspoon S, et al. Modifiable dietary habits and their relation to metabolic abnormalities in men and women with human immunodeficiency virus infection and fat redistribution. Clin Infect Dis. 2001;33(5):710–17.

[286] Expert panel on detection, evaluation, and treatment of high blood cholesterol in adults. Executive summary of the third report of the national cholesterol education program (NCEP). JAMA. 2001;285(19):2486–97.

[287] Grundy SM, Cleeman JI, Merz CN, Brewer HB Jr, Clark LT, Hunninghake DB, et al. Implications of recent clinical trials for the National Cholesterol Education Program Adult Treatment Panel III guidelines. Arterioscler Thromb Vasc Biol. 2004;24(8):e149–61.

[288] Lazzaretti R, Nutritional intervention protects against the development of dyslipidemia in patients who start HAART: a randomized trial. XIV International AIDS Conference; Toronto, Canada; Aug 13–18, 2006. Abstract 2192713.

[289] Schwellenbach LJ, Olson KL, McConnell KJ, Stolcpart RS, Nash JD, Merenich JA, et al.The triglyceride-lowering effects of a modest dose of docosahexaenoic acid alone versus in combination with low dose eicosapentaenoic acid in patients with coronary

artery disease and elevated triglycerides. Journal of the American College of Nutrition. 2006; 25(6):480–85.

[290] Elosua R, Molina L, Fito M, Arquer A, Sanchez-Quesada JL, Covas MI, et al. Response of oxidative stress biomarkers to a 16-week aerobic physical activity program, and to acute physical activity, in healthy young men and women. Atherosclerosis. 2003;167(2):327–34.

[291] Wilson IB, Jacobson DL, Roubenoff R, Spiegelman D, Knox TA, Gorbach SL. Changes in lean body mass and total body weight are weakly associated with physical functioning in patients with HIV infection. HIV Med. 2002;3(4):263–70.

[292] Lindegaard B, Hansen T, Hvid T, van Hall G, Plomgaard P, Ditlevsen S, et al. The effect of strength and endurance training on insulin sensitivity and fat distribution in human immunodeficiency virus-infected patients with lipodystrophy. J Clin Endocrinol Metab. 2008;93(10):3860–69.

[293] Roubenoff R, Wilson IB. Effect of resistance training on self-reported physical functioning in HIV infection. Med Sci Sports Exerc. 2001;33(11):1811-17.

Chapter 7

Oxidative Stress, Redox Regulation and Elite Controllers of HIV Infection: Towards a Functional Cure

Ibeh Bartholomew Okechukwu

Additional information is available at the end of the chapter

http://dx.doi.org/10.5772/60806

1. Introduction

HIV infection has been associated with a high oxidative stress profile. Different stages of the infection are marked with distinct characteristics of redox activity culminating to either potentiation of the disease or an ameliorative process. Both host and viral survival rates require varying degrees of antioxidants to counter the devastating effect of oxidative stress (OS) molecules produced during the onset of the infection. Here, the chapter x-rays and brings to concept the oxidative stress condition and its implication on HIV functional cure. It is obvious that 'excess' free radicals could destroy cell membranes and generate apoptosis, the main cause of lymphocyte-CD4+ depletion in HIV infection. The whole scenario demonstrates that measurement of oxidative stress molecule could function as a potentially HIV biomarker and surveillance parameter in addition to CD4 cell count and that its regulation controls the HIV infection processes.

Generally, people with HIV infection have an unbalanced redox system which is related to a depletion of protective system (glutathione peroxidase; superoxide dismutase; vitamins A, C and E; selenium; etc.), activation of immune signalling molecules (cytokines and chemokines) and an increased production of free radicals (superoxide anion, hydrogen peroxide and hydroxyl radicals). Immunological and biological consequences of this condition include activation of lymphocytes and phagocytising cells, chronic inflammation, increased polyunsaturated fatty acid concentration and lipoperoxidation and direct or indirect effect of several pathologic agents. As the search for HIV functional cure intensifies, oxidative stress condition of natural controllers of HIV infection remains an integral success path for a possible disease cure and management.

2. Free radicals in HIV disease progression

2.1. Free radical production and Reactive Oxygen Species (ROS)

Free radicals are chemical species capable of independent existence and which contain one or more unpaired electrons [1]; they are like loose cannons or rather hot pepper ready to cause biological damage. They consistently react with proteins, lipids, polysaccharides and nucleic acids of biological components and thus damage cell membranes, organelles and importantly DNA [2, 3] with the resultant disease condition [4]. It has been estimated that the average person produces about 10,000–20,000 free radicals attacking each body cell daily [5]. In biological systems, oxygen radicals are known collectively as reactive oxygen species (ROS) possessing high chemical reactivity, with original formation in the mitochondria and smooth endoplasmic reticulum as oxygen reduces along the electron transport chain [6,7]. ROS are formed in other processes that include white blood cells such as neutrophils, which specialise in producing oxygen radicals used in host defence against invading pathogens, cellular exposure to abnormal environment such as hypoxias [8], drugs/xenobiotics [9] and ionising radiation [10]. Hypoxic conditions are created when oxygen is limited and mitochondria pump out ROS which alert the cell to the shortage, but how cells sense hypoxia is a subject of much debate; Bell et al. [11] described these extensively. Reactive oxygen species (ROS), namely, hydroxyl radicals (HO'), superoxide anions (0_2^-), nitric oxide (NO) and hydrogen peroxide (H_20_2), are constantly generated in aerobic organisms in response to both external and internal stimuli [12]; therefore, metabolic activity initiated by immune cells against stimuli creates electron-deficient free radicals. As highly reactive molecules, they damage other molecules by abstracting electrons from them. High doses and/or inadequate removal of ROS results in oxidative stress which causes severe metabolic malfunctions and damage to biological macromolecules. ROS therefore are the main cause of oxidative stress.

2.2. ROS in HIV infection: Do they differ in the different stages of HIV?

Oxidative stress (OS) means any perturbation in the pro-oxidant to antioxidant balances in favour of oxidation, thus resulting in damage to cells. OS increases the replication of HIV and the amount of certain cytokines, among them is tumour necrosis factor-alpha (TNF-α) through the activation of nuclear factor-kappa binding (NF-κB) and indirectly by activation of genes that further promote OS [13]. Oxidant production in HIV infection, however, is through the stimulatory effects of gp125 (an HIV glycoprotein) and tat, the viral-transactivating protein [14]. Mycoplasmas as well enhance the replication of HIV by increasing oxidative stress since they are known to produce H_20_2. HIV coinfection with mycoplasma therefore results in the release of H_20_2 from T-cells.

It has been proposed that CD4+ T-cells are depleted by apoptosis and that T-cells are primed to undergo apoptosis upon cross-linking of CD4 by gp120 of the virus [15]. Subsequent activation perhaps by conventional antigens or superantigens induces apoptosis in these T-cells and increases the progression rate. OS have been implicated to play a rather devastating role in the progression of HIV disease. In this case, certain questions are raised, namely, does the OS condition in HIV infection differ in the various stages of the disease? Does the threshold of OS correspond to the worsening clinical manifestation of the disease as the infection progresses? What is the OS threshold that is associated with the stages of infection?

Generally, chronic OS, with constant generation of free radicals, affects the immune system's fight against HIV through the following mechanisms:

1. *Enhanced HIV replication through activation of NF-kB and genes (TNF genes) that further promote oxidative stress*
2. *Apoptosis of CD4 T-cells and immune dysfunction*
3. *Causing cells to make sensitive abnormal chemicals*
4. *Making the body more sensitive to the toxic effects of certain drugs*

Clinical and immunological classification systems of HIV infection use a four-stage system for both adults and children. Higher numbers indicate advanced degrees of deterioration in clinical and/or immunological status. The recent WHO clinical staging or case definition recognises four (1–4) stages (clinical stage 1, asymptomatic; clinical stage 2, mild symptoms; clinical stage 3, advanced symptoms; clinical stage 4, severe symptoms) [16] as well as the US Centers for Disease Control and Prevention (CDC) which provided a revised classification system for paediatric HIV infection; here, the immunological status staging is used for HIV surveillance. The ranking of the CDC HIV symptoms seems different from the WHO listing. The US CDC clinical staging categories are N, not symptomatic; A, mildly symptomatic; B, moderately symptomatic; and C, severely symptomatic [17]. Similarly, the current CDC HIV surveillance and staging recognises five infection stages in which a confirmed case can be classified as 0, 1, 2, 3 or U [18]. Zero (0) indicates a negative HIV test within six months of the first HIV infection diagnosis. Stages 1–3 are determined by the CD4 test immunologic criteria based primarily on the CD4+ T-lymphocyte count as indicated below: stage 1, ≥1,500 in one-year-olds/≥500 in adults; stage 2, 750–1,499/200–499; and stage 3, 750/<200 [18]. If none of the above apply (e.g. because of missing information on CD4 test results), the stage is U (unknown). These four stages may be referred to, respectively, as the seroconversion and primary HIV infection stage, chronic HIV infection, HIV infection with symptoms and AIDS.

An earlier study by Peterhans showed that viruses could generate ROS from phagocytic cells [19]. Currently, it is known that other viruses (DNA, RNA) could cause cell death through generation of ROS in the infected cell [20,21]. There is confirmed increased free radical production in stage 2 of HIV infection than in stage 4 [22]. Invariably, the antioxidant component is decreased in some cells by half of its amount in stage 2 of the infection [22]. Gaman and her colleagues [23] reported similar patterns of OS increase in stage B/C of chronic lymphocytic leukaemia (CLL) patients. Ibeh et al. using serodiscordant HIV patients showed a high OS condition in serodiscordant-seropositive individuals against their seronegative partners [24]. In a further study, he observed an increased oxidative stress condition in different stages of HIV disease in patients undergoing antiretroviral therapy in Nigeria, where over 50% of the nontreatment group was in stage 2 of the infection [25]. These reports indicate differing OS condition in the various stages of HIV infection and possibly in other viral infections and its capability to serve as a potent surveillance tool (Fig. 1). Further studies should focus on threshold of OS generated and/or needed to determine entrance to the various infection stages. A possible explanation to the observed consecutive more intense overproduction of ROS in the various stages especially in stage 2 is associated partly with changes in the expression of the antiapoptotic/antioxidant compounds Bcl-2 and thioredoxin along the course of the disease by hydrogen peroxide H_2O_2 [26]. It is known that the free radical H_2O_2 plays a central role in activating NF-κB (NF-κB activates HIV replication) through the activation of a factor that binds to a DNA-binding protein; NF-κB in turn stimulates HIV gene expression by acting on the promoter region of the viral long terminal repeat (LTR). NF-κB regulates cellular responses as a 'rapid-acting' primary transcription factor. This makes it to be a first responder to harmful cellular stimuli such as H_2O_2. Known inducers of NF-κB activity include reactive oxygen species (ROS), tumour necrosis factor alpha (TNF-α) and interleukin-1-beta (IL-1β) [27]. If there is no adequate levels of antioxidants, the activity of NF-κB increases in excess amounts and accelerates HIV replication. It is estimated that more than one billion T4 cells are killed and over 50 million HIV replenished on a daily basis in AIDS; this characteristic causes an increase in cytokine synthesis and free radical damage of cells [28].

3. Induction of stress responses and stress response genes: A coping strategy

Oxidative stress is a potent biological stress that weakens and damages cellular components. Naturally, cells devise means of coping, avoiding and responding to this call. Perhaps, the coping mechanism may depend on the degree of the stress, allowing the cell not to overstretch its capabilities. Induction of the antioxidant response element or suppression of inflammatory reactions could limit HIV replication in the host. The master transcription factor known as nuclear factor (erythroid-derived 2)-like 2 (Nrf2) is known to regulate the expression of antioxidants through activation of antioxidant response element (ARE). Fan et al. showed that upregulation of Nrf2 increased the ARE-dependent antioxidants and that HIV-1-related proteins downregulated Nrf2 expression in HIV-1 transgenic rats [29]. Increased oxidative stress induces Nrf2 and stimulates key antioxidant defence mechanism [30] in HIV cells. Cells tend to respond differently to different levels of OS. At a medium level of OS, cells are known to undergo a halt on cell growth and differentiation [31]. In this state, the redox-sensitive transcription factors NF-κB and activator protein-1 (AP-I) are both activated and induce stress protein synthesis through ARE on stress protein genes [128]. Other factors associated with apoptotic pathways are also activated which enables the cell to undergo the characteristic changes known to apoptosis [32, 33]. A higher level of OS is characterised by the pathological changes caused by free radical damage; this becomes apparent and the cell undergoes death characterised by necrosis [34, 35].

However, response to ROS at the cellular level occurs through ARE and oxidative stress-responsive genes (Fig. 1). Following oxidative stress, a signal is transduced by interaction of specific DNA repair enzymes, antioxidant enzymes, heat shock proteins, proteases, protease inhibitors, cytokines and proliferation factors [36]. This adaptive response is biphasic: an 'early' response (1–4 h), which imparts relatively minor protection, and a 'late' response (12–16 h)

http://dx.doi.org/10.5772/60806

which imparts major protection and involves the synthesis of proteins such as repair enzymes [37]. The response also varies with the initiating stress in that some responses are global (e.g. induction of SOD), whereas others are specific to the initiating stress and in other cases, tissue specific (e.g. induction of surfactant proteins in the lung).

4. Lipid peroxidation products: A possible biomarker of HIV disease progression

Lipid peroxidation is a free radical reaction. Any species that has sufficient reactivity to abstract a hydrogen atom from a polyunsaturated fatty acid side chain in membrane lipids may initiate this process [38]. This occurs when hydroxyl radicals and possibly oxygen react with the unsaturated lipids of bio-membrane, resulting in the generation of lipid peroxide radical ($R00^0$), lipid hydroperoxide (R00H) and fragmentation products such as hydroxyoctadecadienoic acid from linoleates, F_2-isoprostanes from arachidonates and neuroprostanes from docosahexaenoates [39], 4-hydroxy-hexanal, 4-hydroxy-2-nonenal and malondialdehyde (MDA) [40] that gives the OS condition. MDA seems to be the most potent biomarker of lipid peroxidation although 4-hydroxy-hexanal and 4-hydroxy-2-nonenal are also specific, sensitive and quantifiable markers (noninvasive) measurable in urine for OS overview [41]. Lipid peroxidation in biological membranes generally proceeds through a complex process involving rearrangement and destruction of the double bonds in polyunsaturated fatty acid. This occurs in three steps, viz. initiation, propagation and termination phases. Peroxidation of membrane lipids can have several outcomes, such as increased membrane rigidity, decreased activity of membrane–bound enzymes, altered activity of membrane receptors (e.g. sodium pumps), altered permeability (increased permissibility), formation of hydrophobic centres that approaches the external phase, alteration of protein structure, mutagenicity (resulting from DNA/RNA damage or binding) and inhibition of growth and protein synthesis [24]. This is caused by the high nucleophilic properties of decomposed aldehyde products formed during lipid peroxidation, which enables them to react with electrophilic sites such as amino and thiol groups [42]. Biomarkers are characteristics that are specific, reliable and can be measured objectively upon evaluation as indicators of normal biological processes, pathogenic processes or pharmacologic responses to a therapeutic intervention.

It is now established that HIV infection is associated with formation of lipid peroxidation products. The importance of evaluating these products is to determine or rather to have a fair idea of the degree of damage the infection has caused the cell. Numerous research works have implicated lipid peroxides as a marker of disease prognosis, drug development and evaluation of efficiency of drugs [43, 44]. A number of scientists have suggested the use of OS marker MDA as a potent additional tool for the assessment and surveillance of HIV/AIDS disease [25,39] and a possible predicator of HIV/AIDS disease progression [45].This is not unlikely knowing that different levels of OS measures as MDA is associated with stages of HIV/AIDS infection classification (Fig. 1).

5. Elite controllers

Elite controllers are referred to as individuals having the ability to spontaneously suppress viral load and maintain HIV control mainly achieved soon after seroconversion. These individuals may not be common in the population, about <1 %, and may best be understood using serodiscordant HIV infection. There is evidence of an increasing number of these individuals in some parts of Africa.

5.1. Serodiscordant infection: Definition

HIV natural resistance can best be described using serodiscordant HIV infection in sexual partners. Serodiscordant HIV infection recognises couples/sexual partners in which one may be either HIV seroconcordant-seropositive or seroconcordant-seronegative or the partners are having different serostatuses [46]. Serodiscordant HIV infection refers, therefore, to partners adequately exposed to HIV infection in which one is HIV positive (seropositive) and the other HIV negative (seronegative).

5.2. Global prevalence

The prevalence of HIV serodiscordant infection in seronegative population has not been well documented. About 0.5 % (one in 200) people are reported in America [47]. Scott-Algara et al. [48] in 2003 reported that between 5 and 15 % of individuals of different populations at risk of HIV infection (regular partners of seropositive subjects, prostitutes and intravenous drug addicts) show no signs of apparent infection by HIV in spite of many years of exposure. However, some studies have indicated an estimate of about 5 % in Africa. Fowke et al. [49] in a cohort study showed that 4.3 % of HIV-1-exposed seronegative prostitutes in Kenya were persistently HIV negative after 12 years of follow-up study. Other reports have shown an increasing number of persistent serodiscordant-seronegatives and the risk of HIV transmission within stable serodiscordant partners across 23 countries of sub-Saharan Africa [50].

5.3. Classification of HIV natural resistance

Those individuals who are serodiscordant-seronegative may possess natural resistance to HIV infection. They can be grouped into two: *highly exposed persistently seronegatives (HEPSs) and long-term nonprogressors (LTNPs)*

5.3.1. Highly Exposed Persistently Seronegatives (HEPSs)

They are individuals who are repeatedly exposed to HIV through different routes of exposure but persistently remain seronegative (do not develop antibody to HIV).

5.3.2. Long-Term Nonprogressors (LTNPs)

About 5–10 % of HIV-infected people remain asymptomatic for about 7–20 years after infection despite being on no antiretroviral therapy. Their immune function is well controlled with CD4+

lymphocytes counts above 6000/mm^3 coupled with a low plasma HIV RNA. Initially, these were based primarily on immunologic control, i.e. maintenance of high CD4 count, but currently LTNPs are known as elite controllers based on viral load calculations/standards. Those with undetectable viremia (HIV RNA<50 copies/ml) are elite controllers, while those with low but detectable viral load (HIV RNA <2000 copies/ml) are known as viremic controllers [51, 52]. These individuals are referred to as LTNP or elite controllers (ECs) [47]. Other subgroups include typical progressors (TPs) where about 80 % of HIV-infected individuals develop AIDS within the median time of ten years [53] and rapid progressors (RPs) which develop within 2–3 years of infection and exist in 10 % of the population [54].

5.3.3. *Viral fitness*

The phenomenon of viral 'fitness' relates to the pathogenicity of certain strains of HIV. HIV replicative capacity (RC) is attributed as a component of viral fitness [55]. RC, therefore, is a measure of the ability of the virus to replicate successfully in a given environment [56] which tends to affect controllers of HIV. In LTNP, a number of genetic defects have been associated with the virus. Such documented defects or genetic lesions include the NF-κB or SP1 site and the nef mutant gene within the long terminal repeats of the virus [57]. According to Learmont et al., some LTNPs have shown to possess this mutant gene (nef) [58]. Also faster rates of disease progression have been observed in Ugandan individuals infected with subtype D compared with subtype A isolates. The current concept is based on the viral load dynamic equilibrium set point that is established between the production of virus (VR) (dependent on the number of activated CD4 cells) and the suppression of replication and elimination of virus-producing CD4 cells by adaptive immunity [51, 52]. Here, the elite controllers fall into extreme low viral load carriers that are undetectable, though other researchers still maintain effective immune clearance of EC as the major factor [58]. From studies, vigorous virus-specific humoral and cell-mediated immune responses have been detected. For example, high titres of potent neutralising antibodies have been found in sera of LTNPs with strong CD8+ cytotoxic T-lymphocyte cells [59]. Genetic differences in human leukocyte antigen (HLA) alleles have also been shown to influence HIV disease susceptibility [60] and disease progression [61]. In particular, HLA B*5701 has been found as reported by Migueles et al. to be highly overrepresented in LTNP. Other immunological factors found include natural killer (Nk) cells in resistant Vietnam population [48] and high levels of IL-2 (interleukin-2) found in resistant infants born to HIV-positive mothers.

A mutant allele of CCR5 with a 32-base pair deletion (CCR5-delta-32) discovered in 1996 confers resistance to the highly exposed group of seronegative individuals [62,63]. It is often seen in populations of European origin (in Caucasians, 1 % are homozygous, while 15–20 % are heterozygous), which encodes a nonfunctional truncated protein. Homozygotes for the Δ-32 allele are believed to exhibit a strong and complete resistance to HIV infection, whereas heterozygotes delayed progression to AIDS as observed in LTNP [64]. This mutation is hypothesised to be absent in African origins and certain Asian populations.

6. Protective effects of antioxidants

Antioxidants are groups of substances which when present at low concentrations, in relation to oxidisable substrates, significantly inhibit or delay oxidative processes while often being oxidised themselves [65]. There exists a balance between their formation and removal (redox state). To maintain an oxido/redox balance, cells protect themselves from the toxicity of excess ROS/RNS in different ways, enzymatic and nonenzymatic antioxidants.

6.1. Relevant HIV antioxidants: Does HIV benefit from their activities?

There are many biochemical processes that oxidise reduced antioxidant molecules to neutralise free radicals and then restore the antioxidant molecules to a reduced state. In HIV infection, antioxidants serve to aid the CD4 cells in removing the virions by reducing the oxidative stress that develops during HIV infection [66]. Antioxidants are useful to the host for defence and neutralisation of free radicals.

6.1.1. Superoxide Dismutase (SOD)

Superoxide dismutase (EC 1.15.1.1) destroys the free radical superoxide by converting it to peroxide which is further destroyed by catalase or glutathione peroxidase (GHPX) reaction. It is known that SOD converts the superoxide radical to the less-reactive H_20_2 [67]. In humans, the three forms of SOD are cytosolic Cu, Zn-SOD, mitochondria Mn-SOD and extracellular SOD (ECSOD). Generally, SOD catalyses the dismutation of $0_2^{\bullet}$- by successive oxidation and reduction of the transition metal ion at the active site in a ping-pong-type mechanism with widely acknowledged high reaction rates [68]. Copper-zinc superoxide dismutase (Cu, Zn-SOD) is also known as SOD-I; the active site is constituted by a copper and a zinc atom bridged by a common ligand.

The HIV TAT domain is a regulatory protein of the virus that enhances the efficiency of virus transcription and has been shown to carry exogenous molecules into cells [69], thus can fuse with protein transduction domains (PTDs) for effective cellular cargo delivery [70]. TAT-PTD linked-SOD1 has been shown to be ferried across the cytoplasm and even the mitochondria where superoxide is generated, making TAT-SOD1 a source of intracellular antioxidant [72]. Currently, Qing et al. [73] in 2013 provided evidence that TAT-SOD1 has protective therapeutic activity against ionisation radiation. Conversely, cells actually infected with HIV have been reported to express less Mn-SOD and to lose their ability to induce antioxidant enzyme in response to TNF. Therefore, expression of TAT protein of HIV suppresses cellular Mn-containing superoxide dismutase (Mn-SOD) [74]. Furthermore, the protective nature of Mn-SOD has been demonstrated by several authors; its overexpression provides oxidant protection against AZT or 3TC-induced endothelial dysfunction [75] and against lung cancer radiation therapy [76].

http://dx.doi.org/10.5772/60806

6.1.2. Glutathione system

The glutathione system (glutathione, glutathione peroxidase, glutathione transferase and glutathione reductase) is a key defence against H_20_2 and other peroxides. The term glutathione is typically used as a collective name to refer to the tripeptide L-gamma-glutamyl-L-cysteinyl glycine in both its reduced and dimeric forms. Glutathione is necessary for maintaining immune-mediated T-cell and phagocytosis. It inhibits HIV replication by acting at the late stages of the virus' life cycle through strong suppression of the production of p24 and gag protein as well as the viral infectivity factor (Vif) [77]. This results in a dramatic decrease in both budding and release of virus particles from chronically infected cells (either macrophages or lymphocytes). Also there is a relative decrease in the expression of gp120 (the protein component of the HIV viral coat), the major envelope glycoprotein rich in intrachain disulphide bonds. Experiments with rats showed that gp120 increases the accumulation of H_20_2 and superoxides; thus, Brook et al. [78] demonstrated that the activity of this HIV protein increases that of the key glutathione peroxidase as a defensive mechanism against ROS. Also glutathione inhibits the reverse transcriptase (RT) process of HIV and its expression [79]. GSH further blocks in a concentration-dependent manner the (intracellular) activation of essential protein-splitting enzymes, such as HIV proteases. The glutathione redox cycle is a major source of protection against low levels of oxidant stress, whereas catalase becomes more significant in protecting against severe oxidant stress [80]. Glutathione reductase enzyme (EC 1.8.1.7), which reduces glutathione disulphide (GSSG) to the sulphhydryl form GSH, is an important cellular antioxidant.

6.1.3. Catalase (CAT)

Catalase (EC 1.11.1.6) is a tetrameric haem-enzyme consisting of 4 identical tetrahedrally arranged subunits of 60 kDa. It is highly efficient that it is difficult to be saturated by H_20_2 at any concentration [81]. Catalase reacts with H_20_2 to form water and molecular oxygen, a less/nontoxic product. Catalase protects cells from hydrogen peroxide generated within them. It is actively involved in the HIV disease progression and may serve as one of the marker enzymes where it augments glutathione, SOD and other antioxidants. Serum catalase is known to increase as HIV disease progresses [82, 83].

6.1.4. Vitamins A, C and E

Vitamin A plays a role in the development of both T-helper cells and B-cells. Studies have shown that vitamin A, in the form of retinol or retinoic acid, improves immunity by stimulating immunoglobulin synthesis through its action on T-cells or T-cell products. Retinoic acid inhibits the production of interleukin-6 in a dose-dependent manner by downregulating the expression of interleukin-6 mRNA [84]. Vitamin A acts as an immunostimulant by modulating the growth and function of T-cells, B-lymphocytes and natural killer cells.

Vitamin C (ascorbate, $AscH^-$) can donate a hydrogen atom to a free radical molecule ($R^\cdot$), thereby neutralising it while becoming an ascorbate radical itself (Asc^- or $Asc^{\cdot-}$). But the free radical ($Asc^\cdot$) is very stable because of its resonance structure. Moreover, $AscH^-$ is readily regenerated from the Asc^{-} with NADH or NADPH-dependent reductases [85]. Ascorbate can also neutralise the radical form of other antioxidants such as glutathione ($GS^{\cdot}$) and vitamin E ($^{\cdot}TOC$). Vitamin C also inhibits the replication of human immunodeficiency virus-1 (HIV-1) [86].

Tocopherols (vitamin E) interrupt free radical chain reactions by capturing the free radical; this inherent action displays the antioxidant properties of vitamin E. The free hydroxyl (OH) group on the aromatic ring of tocopherol is responsible for its antioxidant activity. The hydrogen from this group is transferred to the free radical, resulting in a relatively stable free radical form of the vitamin [87]. Vitamin E is an effective antioxidant (peroxyl radical scavenger) for terminating the chain reactions of lipid peroxidation in the cell membrane. The tocopheroxyl radical is the pro-oxidant form of vitamin E and is thought to be regenerated to the antioxidant form by a network of other antioxidants, including vitamin C and glutathione. In the mitochondria membrane, vitamin E that donates a hydrogen to neutralise a free radical can be regenerated (reduced) by coenzyme Q which has two hydrogens to donate and can avoid becoming a free radical by donating both hydrogens; this is an efficient process. Alpha-tocopherol has potent activity against HIV. The anti-HIV-1 activity may be due, in part, to their antioxidant properties. Alpha-tocopherol generally interferes with membrane integrity and fluidity. As HIV-1 is a membrane virus, any alteration of the membrane fluidity of the virus interferes with its ability to bind to cell-receptor sites, thus reducing its infectivity [88]. It stimulates CD4 T-cell and IL-2 proliferation [89]. Vitamin E inhibits CD95 (APO–1/Fas) ligand expression (part of TNF receptor which T-cell uses to undergo apoptosis) and protects T-cell from activation-induced cell death of the CD95/CD95 ligand system of T-cells [90]. Tocopherol completely inhibits and blocks DNA binding NF-κB, resulting to complete inaction [91].

6.1.5. Flavonoids

The flavones and catechins seem to be the most powerful flavonoids for protecting the body against ROS [92]. Flavonoids may have an additive effect to the endogenous scavenging compounds; they increase their function. Flavonoids (quercetin) was reported to exhibit both anti-infective and antireplicative HIV abilities. Quercetin significantly downregulates p24 antigen production, LTR gene expression and viral infectivity in a dose-dependent manner (5–50 mM) and further downregulation of the expression of the pro-inflammatory cytokine TNF-α with concomitant upregulation of anti-inflammatory cytokine IL-13 [93]. A higher level of IL-13 is known to inhibit TNF-α production and also HIV-1 infection. Some flavonoids work on the intracellular replication of viruses, whereas others inhibit the infectious properties of the viruses. Flavonoids have inhibitory activity on reverse RT and RNA-directed DNA polymerase [94, 95]; however, it also has antiintegrase and antiprotease activities [96]. Similarly, myricetin activity was tested against HIV-RT and inhibited the enzyme by 49 % [97]

6.1.6. Metals

Zinc is a metallic divalent cation bound to proteins within cells and cell membranes. Zinc plays catalytic, structural and regulatory roles in more than 200 zinc metalloenzymes that have been identified in biological systems. Zinc fingers are exploited by transcription factors for interacting with DNA and regulating the activity of genes [98]. Another structural role of zinc is in the maintenance of the integrity of biological membranes (membrane stabilisation) by its ability to stabilise thiol groups and phospholipids, resulting in their protection against oxidative injury. These properties affect signalling processes involved in cell-mediated immunity. Zinc also influences gene expression by structural stabilisation of different immunological transcription factors. It induces cytokines, including interleukin (IL)-1, IL-6 and TNF-α [99]. HIV binds to zinc ions in T-cells in order to produce proviral peptides, which form the basis of new infectious viral particles. HIV-1 protease enzyme cuts the viral chains to form new infectious viral particles, as with other proteases (collagenase, angiotensin-converting enzyme (ACE), caboxypeptidase A and neutral endopeptidases); when sufficient zinc ions are bound to the protease, it will remain inactive [100]. Zinc therefore has both an enhancing and inhibiting activity depending on its concentration in the surrounding tissues. In HIV replication, viral RNA is transformed into viral DNA via the enzyme reverse transcriptase; zinc also binds to this enzyme. Zinc influences NK cell-mediated killing and also modulates cytolytic T-cell activity and inhibition of TNF-α [101], in addition to its anti-HIV drug potentiation activity as [102].

Similarly, selenium is found in human and animal tissue as L-selenomethionine or L-selenocysteine. L-selenomethionine is incorporated randomly in proteins known as selenoproteins. The antioxidant activity of selenium is mainly accounted for by virtue of its role in the formation and function of the selenium-dependent glutathione peroxidase (GSHPx) [103]. Selenium effect on boosting cellular immunity is due to the upregulation of the expression of the lymphocyte cells' high affinity to interleukin (IL)-2 receptors, thus providing a vehicle for enhanced lymphocyte cell response as well as preventing oxidative stress to human cells [104,105]. Research has shown that the HIV virus hijacks the host supply of selenium for its own antioxidant protection, thereby inducing or exacerbating a selenium deficiency with increasing disease progression. Thus, HIV may be capable of incorporating host selenium into viral selenoprotein that has glutathione peroxidase activity [106,107].

7. A search for functional cure: Is it functional or sterilising cure?

There is currently no cure for HIV/AIDS, but recent research interest on HIV treatment tends to focus on functional cure which has renewed optimism for HIV cure. The aim of the functional cure is to get rid of all viruses from the system and remove any negative effects of HIV on the body and prevent viral rebound after discontinuation of the antiviral treatment. In other words, people who had been functionally cured would never develop AIDS or other signs of HIV disease as classified by WHO [16] and US CDC [17, 18]. Current HIV themes are now focused on this approach to solve the problem of HIV infection globally.

This type of *HIV cure* does not translate to eradicating all viruses from the body but being able to control viremia without antiviral drugs [108]. The difference between a functional cure or remission and eradication/sterilisation cure is that while the former may de-emphasise the HIV viral reservoir clearance and establish a sufficiently strong immune response with low-level viremia at <50 copies/ml, the latter sees it as a central task to eliminate the virus from all body compartments with a plasma HIV RNA count of <1 copy/ml. In addition, the reservoir is significantly smaller in elite controllers with decreased concentration of HIV DNA. Viral reservoir is simply different areas of the body where viral copies hide quietly and undetected and are unable to be treated until they are stimulated or activated to reproduce. Anatomical reservoirs include the gastrointestinal tract (GIT), lymphoid tissue and the central nervous system (CNS). These compartments may harbour unique long-lived latently infected cells, and penetration of cART may be limited at these sites. What are the phenotypic characteristics of functional cure? First is the undetectable or very low noninfective levels of the virus (<50 copies/ml) though some authors suggested <75 copies/ml for six months [109], and second is a normal range of CD4 cell count when cART is discontinued. Although cART have tremendously improved the lives of individuals with HIV, they come with significant side effects, perhaps not the ideal functional cure which would get HIV-infected patients to the point where cART are no longer needed to keep their infections under control.

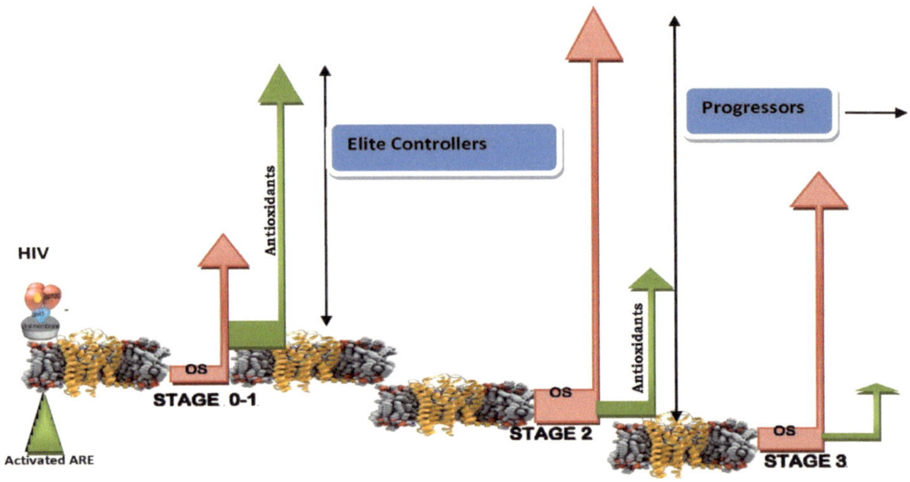

Figure 1. Schematic diagram representing a putative mechanistic model of oxidative stress (OS) activity in elite controllers and in HIV disease progression. (Consequences of oxidant/antioxidant activation in the different stages of HIV infection and interrelationship between OS and HIV control. OS= oxidative stress, ARE= antioxidant responsive element.)

8. Oxidative stress regulation of elite controllers: A reality or a hoax of functional cure

It seems certain that oxidative stress control of HIV elite controllers may contribute to the expected functional cure in HIV patients (Fig. 1). Examination of possible and established cases implicates the action of redox control instead as an approach for the cure. But is this a misconceived theory or a deception?

Epidemiology of elite or aviremic control of HIV infection appears to occur in approximately 1 in 300 HIV-infected persons and represents a distinct phenotype among HIV-infected individuals [110]. Through a recently established international collaboration (HIV Controller Consortium), over 300 elite controllers have been identified and recruited for study [111]. Achieving either a functional cure (long-term control of HIV in the absence of cART) or a sterilising cure (elimination of all HIV-infected cells) still remains a major challenge to scientists. As noted previously, establishment of a latent or 'silent' infection in resting $CD4^+$ T-cells is a major impediment to finding HIV cure. Several randomised clinical trials have shown that treatment intensification even with additional ART has little impact on latent reservoirs. Some potential drugs used to reduce latency, including histone deacetylase inhibitors, currently used and licensed for the treatment of some cancers, methylation inhibitors, cytokines such as IL-7 or activators of NF-κB such as prostratin, show promising activity in reversing latency in vitro when used either alone or in combination [112]. Prodrugs provoked through ferrocene-mediated oxidation currently have been developed to enhance the selectivity and specificity of anticancer drugs. Peng et al. [113] described how the strategies of ROS activation can be employed for further development of new ROS-targeting prodrugs, which must eventually lead to novel approaches and/or combined technology for more efficient and selective treatment of cancers.

The major reason why HIV cannot be cured is the persistence of HIV in a latent form in different cellular reservoirs which may be pre- or post-integration latency. Functional cure strategies tend to reduce effects of this latency. The case report of a German patient with acute myeloid leukaemia, who received a bone marrow transplant from a donor with a 32-base pair deletion in the CCR5 gene, may remain the only current example of a sterilising cure [114]. After transplantation, the patient discontinued cART for 45 months and HIV RNA remained at below 1 copy/ml with no virus found in reservoir compartments. However, a strategy of using bone marrow transplantation with a CCR5 mutant donor is not a realistic cure for HIV, given the toxicity and complexity of the treatment. Similarly, Sangamo Biosciences used zinc finger nucleases, a genome editing technique, to cut off the gene in CD4 cells that controls the expression of CCR5 coreceptor which the virus uses to enter cells, based on the coreceptor theory [115,116]. The data generated from the clinical trials with the drug SB-728-T showed control of viremia, improved CD4 cells and reduced proviral reservoirs with no safety concerns; these were sustained for 56 weeks after disruption of treatment [117,118]. How cost-effective this treatment and its availability to the large population of HIV patients remain to be answered.

There is a possibility that other cases of remission or functional cure exist in patient populations globally who may have started treatment soon after infection. But the figures are not certain on the proportion of these populations that experience functional cure, though some experts have speculated one in seven people. To date, HIV functional cure has not been 100 % successful. In 2010, the Mississippi baby (treatment started early) believed to be functionally cured of HIV after two years of treatment discontinuation now has detectable levels of the virus in her blood [119], though this paved way for rational very early treatment in perinatal HIV infection [120]. Similarly, a German patient who initiated antiretroviral therapy with AZT,

3TC and efavirenz just under three months after exposure to HIV and within one month of confirmed seroconversion, after an acute viral illness had his viral load below limit of detection with stable range of CD4 cell (900–1,000 cells/mm^3). He has shown no HIV RNA or associated proteins in any tissue/organ compartment after treatment interruption for nine years [121]. This case shows evidence of strong and broad CD8 T-cell responses and strong proliferative CD4 T-cell responses. What might be responsible for this? In contrast, analysis of the CCR5 coreceptor showed that the homozygous CCR5 promoter A59029G was present, but no delta 32 deletion was observed [121] and the HLA-I subtype was A 01, 02 B:44, 52. Nevertheless, HIV was recovered later from the patients using a humanised mouse model after transplantation of the patient's purified CD4 T-cells and anti-CD3/anti-CD28 stimulation. This indicated the presence of HIV capable of replication and that other factors other than CCR5 mutation may be responsible for viral control. The French VISCONTI cohort study also reported patients who started treatment early and was able to gain control of the virus replication with undetected viral load after six years of treatment interruption [122]. A period of at least four years of treatment is suggested prior to treatment interruption [123].

In most studies, preferential attention has been given to latent resting CD4+ T-lymphocytes as a source of HIV persistence in the cell and CCR5 coreceptor mutation as responsible for HIV control. While explanations for functional cure have proved inadequate, ROS has been demonstrated to contribute to disease progression and drug design [124]. New strategies for HIV functional cure should incorporate use of ROS-activated prodrugs [113]. Adequate data on OS condition of spontaneous controllers (natural resistance) and the posttreatment controllers (PTC)/functional cure are not available. Luc Montagner, codiscoverer of the HIV, identified oxidative stress as one of the four factors responsible for its variability [125]. Besides, recent report that P13K/Akt inhibitors can drastically sensitise HIV-infected macrophages (reservoir) to oxidative-stress-induced cell death [126] indicates possible ROS therapeutic approach to achieve HIV cure as well as the cytoprotective effect of the virus-activated P13K/AKt in human microglial cell line and macrophages against apoptotic challenge [127]. In addition, HIV infection increases the cellular levels of ROS, especially superoxide anion and peroxynitrite which accelerates HIV replication in macrophages [28]. Recently, Bhaskar et al. demonstrated that a marginal increase of about ~25mV in *E*GSH is sufficient to switch HIV-1 from latency to reaction using Grx1-roGFP2 biosensor [128], suggesting possibility of purging HIV-1 by redox modulators which shows how fluctuations in *E*GSH modulate expression of antioxidant gene in infected HIV patients [129].

9. Conclusion

HIV host reservoir of latently infected cells stands as the barrier to a successful longed-for cure that would free HIV-positive patients from a lifetime of taking antiretroviral drugs. Antiretrovirals known to protect uninfected cells reduce the viral load and stave off full-blown AIDS. However, they do not eliminate the HIV reservoir in the host. Though the virus is not completely eradicated in EC, the reservoir could not replicate, so low viral load is recorded and antiretrovirals are unnecessary. OS however has been implicated in HIV replication and

http://dx.doi.org/10.5772/60806

disease progression; so it can be used as a surveillance tool. The chapter presents oxidative stress and redox regulation of controllers of HIV infection as a means to achieve a functional cure. Therefore, ROS should be seen as a viable strategy to achieving HIV functional cure.

Author details

Ibeh Bartholomew Okechukwu*

Address all correspondence to: barthokeyibeh@yahoo.com

Medical Biotechnology Department,National Biotechnology Development Agency, Abuja, Nigeria

References

[1] Fakoya EAO, Ositesi OO, Fakoya TA, Oduson OL: Antioxidant nutrients and disease interaction. Nig J Nutr Sci 1998,19(1):6-17.

[2] Valko M, Izakovic M, Mazur M, Rhodes CJ, Telser J: Role of oxygen radicals in DNA damage and cancer incidence. Mol Cell Biochem 2004,266:37-56.

[3] Kukreja RC, Hess ML: The oxygen free-radical system-From equations through membrane–protein interactions to cardiovascular injury and protection. Cardiovasc Res 1992,26:641-655.

[4] Karthikeyan R, Manivasagam T, Anantharaman P, Balasubramanian T, Somasundaram ST: Chemopreventive effect of Padina boergesenii extracts on ferric nitrilotriacetate (Fe-NTA)-induced oxidative damage in Wistar rats. *J Appl Phycol* 2011,257(2): 257–263. doi:10.1007/s10811-010-9564-0.

[5] Valko M, Rhodes CJ, Moncol J, Izakovic M, Mazur M: Free radicals, metals and antioxidants in oxidative stress-induced cancer. Chem Biol Interact 2006,160:1-40.

[6] Valko M, Leibfritz D, Moncola J, Cronin M, Mazura M, Telser I: Free radicals and antioxidants in normal physiological functions and human disease. Int J Biochem Cell Biol 2007,39(1):44-84.

[7] Halliwell: Reactive oxygen species in living systems, source, biochemistry and role in human disease. Ameri J Med 1991,91(3)S3:14S–22S.

[8] Thomas L. Clanton: Hypoxia-induced reactive oxygen species formation in skeletal muscle. J Appl Physiol 2007,102(6):2379-2388. DOI: 10.1152/japplphysiol.01298.2006.

[9] Deavall D, Martin E, Horner J, Roberts R: Drug-Induced Oxidative Stress and Toxicity. J Toxicol 2012, 2012, Article ID 645460, 13pages,.doi:10.1155/2012/645460.

[10] Yamamori T, Yasui H, Yamazumi M, Wada Y, Nakamura Y, Nakamura H, Inanami O: Ionizing radiation induces mitochondrial reactive oxygen species production accompanied by upregulation of mitochondrial electron transport chain function and mitochondrial content under control of the cell cycle checkpoint. J Free Rad Biol Med 2012,53(2):260-70. doi: 10.1016.

[11] Bell E, Klimova T, Eisenbart J, Moraes C, Murphy M, Budinger S, Chandel N: The Q site of the mitochondrial complex III is required for the transduction of hypoxic signaling via reactive oxygen species production. J Cell Biol 2007, 177:1029-1036. doi: 10.1083/jcb.200609074.

[12] Elisa Cabiscol, Jordi Tamarit, Joaquim Ros. Oxidative stress in bacteria and protein damage by reactive oxygen species. Internatl Microbiol 2000,3:3–8.

[13] Droge W, Eck HP, Mihm S: Oxidant-antioxidant status in human immuno deficiency virus infection. In: Packer L, (ed.) Oxygen radicals in Biological Systems. Academic Press, San Diego, CA. U.S.A; 1994: 594-601.

[14] Westendorp MO, Li-Weber M, Frank R, Krammer PH: Sensitization of T cells to CD95-mediated apoptosis by HIV-1 Tat and NFκB. J Virol 1994,68:4177-4185.

[15] Gougeon ML, Montagnier L: HIV infection progression. Sci 1993, 260:1269–1272.

[16] WHO 2005. Interim Who Clinical Staging of HIV/AIDS and HIV/Aids Case Definitions for Surveillance http://www.who.int/hiv/pub/guidelines/clinicalstaging.pdf.

[17] Panel on antiretroviral therapy and medical management of HIV-infected children: *Guidelines for the use of antiretroviral agents in pediatric HIV infection.* 2010; pp1-219. Available at http://aidsinfo.nih.gov/ContentFiles/PediatricGuidelines.pdf (accessed November 20, 2014).

[18] CDC: Terms, Definitions, and Calculations Used in CDC HIV Surveillance Publications. 2014; http://www.cdc.gov/hiv/pdf/prevention_ongoing_surveillance_terms.pdf. (accessed November 18, 2014).

[19] Peterhans E: Sendal virus stimulates chemiluminescence in mouse spleen cells. Biochemical and Biophysical Research Communications 91(1): 383–392.

[20] Peterhans E, Grob M, Bürge T, Zanoni R: Virus-induced formation of reactive oxygen intermediates in phagocytic cells. Free Rad Res Comm 1987, 3(1–5):39–46.

[21] Vierucci A, De Martino M, Graziani E: A mechanism for liver cell injury in viral hepatitis: effects of hepatitis B virus on neutrophil function in vitro and in children with chronic active hepatitis. Pediatric Res 1983, 17(10): 814–820.

[22] Favier A, Sappey C, Leclerc P, Faure P, Micoud M: Antioxidant status and lipid peroxidation in patients infected with HIV. Chem Biol Interact 1994, 91(2-3):165-80.

[23] Gaman AM, Buga A, Gaman M, Popa-Wagner A: The Role of Oxidative Stress and the Effects of Antioxidants on the Incidence of Infectious Complications of Chronic

Lymphocytic Leukemia. Ox Med Cellu Long 2014, 2014, Article ID 158135, 6 pages, doi:10.1155/2014/158135.

[24] Ibeh BO, Obidoa O, Nwuke C: Lipid peroxidation correlates with HIV mRNA in serodiscordant heterosexual HIV partners of Nigerian origin. Indian J Clin Biochem 2011,26(3):249–256.

[25] Ibeh BO, Emeka-Nwabunni: Increased oxidative stress condition found in different stages of HIV disease in patients undergoing antiretroviral therapy in Umuahia (Nigeria). Immunopharm Immunot 2012,34(6):1060-1066 (doi: 10.3109/08923973.2012.681327).

[26] Elbim C, Pillet S, Prevost MH, Preira A, Girard PM, Rogine N, Hakim J, Israel N, Gougerot-Pocidalo MA: The role of phagocytes in HIV-related oxidative stress. J Clin Virol. 2001 Feb;20(3):99-109.

[27] Chandel NS, Trzyna WC, McClintock DS, Schumacker PT: Role of oxidants in NF-kappa B activation and TNF-alpha gene transcription induced by hypoxia and endotoxin. J Immunol 2000,165 (2):1013–1021. doi:10.4049/jimmunol.165.2.1013.

[28] Westendrop MO, Shatrov VA, SchulzeOsthof K, Frank R, Kraft M, Los M, Krammer PH, Droge W, Lehmann V: HIV-1 Tat potentiates TNF-induced NF-kappa B activation and cytotoxicity by altering the cellular redox state. EMBO J 1995,14(3):546-554.

[29] Fan X, Staiteih BS, Jesen JS, Mould KJ, Greenberg JA, Joshi PC, Koval M, Guidot DM: Activating the Nrf2-mediated antioxidant response element restores barrir function in the alveolar epithelium of HIV-1 transgenic rats. Am J Physiol Lung Cell Mol.Physiol 2013,305(3):L267-277.

[30] Reddy PV, Gandhi N, Samikkannu T, Saiyed Z, Agudelo M, Yndart A, Khatavkar P, Nair MP: HIV-1 gp 120 induces antioxidant response element-mediated expression in primary astrocytes: role in HIV associated neurocognitive disorder. Neurochem Int. 2012,61(5):807-814.

[31] Clopton EK, Saltman P: Low-level oxidative stress causes cell cycle specific arrest in cultured cells. Biochem. Biophys. Ress. Comm 1995,210:189–196.

[32] Sen CK, Packer L: Antioxidant and redox regulation of gene transcription. FASEB J 1996,6:607-620.

[33] Buttke T, Sandstrom O: Oxidative stress as a mediator or apoptosis (review). Immunol. Today 1994,15:7-10.

[34] Bonfoco E, Krainc D, Ankarcronia M, Nicotera P, Lipton SA: Apoptosis and necrosis: two distinct events induced, respectively, by mild and intense insults with N-methyl-D-aspartate or nitric oxide/superoxide in cortical cell cultures. Proc. Natl. Acad. Sci.U.S.A 1995,92:7162–7166.

[35] Awodele O, Olayemi SO, Nwite JA, Adeyemo TA: Investigation of the levels of oxidative stress parameters in HIV and HIV-TB co-infected patients. J infect Dev Ctries 2012,6(1):79-85.

[36] Janssen YM, van Houten BV, Borm PJ, Mossman BT: Biology of disease: cell and tissue responses to oxidative damage. Lab Invest 1993,69:261-274.

[37] Davies JM: Regulation of gene expression in adaption to oxidative stress. In: Poli G, Albano E, Dianzani MU (eds.) Free Radicals: From Basic Science to Medicine. Birkhauser Verlag, Basel-Boston-Berlin; 2003: 18-30.

[38] Aruoma IO. Experimental tools in free radical Biochemistry. Free Rad Trop.Dis 1993,10:225-242.

[39] Yoshida Y, Umeno A, Shichiri M: Lipid peroxidation biomarkers for evaluating oxidative stress and assessing antioxidant capacity in vivo. J Clin Biochem Nutr 2013,52(1):9–16.

[40] Uchida A: Activation of stress signaling pathways by end product of lipid peroxidation. J Biol chem 2000,274:2234-2242.

[41] Guichardant M, Lagarde M: Analysis of biomarkers from lipid peroxidation: A comparative study. Eur J Lipid Sci Technol 2009,111:75–82. doi: 10.1002/ejlt.200800069.

[42] Aust SD, Svingen BA: Lipid peroxidation in cellular membrane. In: Free radicals in biology. Pryor W.a. (Ed.). Academic press, New York. 1982, pp 91–113.

[43] Niki E: Biomarkers of lipid peroxidation in clinical material. Biochimica et Biophysica Acta (BBA) 2014, 809–817.

[44] Niki E. Lipid peroxidation products as oxidative stress biomarkers. Biofactors 2008,34(2):171-180.

[45] Erin M Siegel, Nitin Patel, Beibei Lu, Ji-Hyun Lee, Alan G. Nyitray, Neal E Craft, Krystyna Frenkel, Luisa L. Villa, Eduardo L. Franco, Anna R. Giuliano. Biomarkers of oxidant load and type-specific clearance of prevalent oncogenic human papillomavirus infection: markers of immune response? Int. J. Cancer 2012,131: 219–228.

[46] Smith RA: Serodiscordant couples.1998. The body:couples. http;//www.the body.com/encyclo/couples.(Accessed September 3rd, 2014)

[47] Dutton G: Infected non progressors are proving clues to the control, and potentially the eradication of HIV. The Scientist 2006,20(11):27-31.

[48] Scott-Algara D, Truong LX, Versmisse P, David A, Luong T, Nguyen NG, Theodoru L, Barre-Sinoussi F, Pancino G: Increased NK cell activity in HIV-1 exposed but uninfected vietnames intravascular drug users. J Immu 2003,22:1-11.

[49] Fowke KR, Nagelkerke NJ, Kimani J, Simonsen JN, Anzala AO, Bwayo JJ, Macdonald KS, Ngugi EN, Plummer FA. Resistance to HIV-1 infection among persistently seronegative prostitute in Nairobi, Kenya. Lancet 1997, 349(9052):649-50.

[50] Chemaitelly H, Awad SF, Abu-Raddad LJ: The risk of HIV transmission within HIV-1 sero-discordant couples appears to vary across sub-Saharan Africa. Epidermics 2014,6:1–9.

[51] Grabar S, Selinger-Leneman H, Abgrall S, Pialoux G, Weiss L, Costagliola D: Prevalence and comparative characteristics of long-term nonprogressors and HIV controller patients in the French Hospital Database on HIV. AIDS 2009;23:1163-1169.

[52] Okulicz JF, Marconi VC, Landrum ML et al. Clinical outcomes of elite controllers, viremic controllers, and long-term nonprogressors in the US Department of Defense HIV natural history study. J Infect Dis 2009,200:1714-1723..

[53] Laeyendecker O, Li X, Arroyo M: The effect of HIV subtype on rapid disease progression in rakai, Uganda. 13th Conference on Retroviruses and Opportunistic Infections 2006 (abstract no. 44LB).

[54] AIDS SA: Natural resistance to HIV/AIDS. AIDS SA Up date 1998,6(3):1-5.

[55] Harrigan PR, Bloor S, Larder BA: Relative replicative fitness of zidovudine-resistant human immunodeficiency virus type-1 isolates *in vitro*. J Virol 1998,72:3773-3778.

[56] Croteau G, Doyon L, Thibeault D, McKercher G, Pilote L, Lamarre D: Impaired fitness of human immunodeficiency virus type 1 variants with high-level resistance to protease inhibitors. J. Virol 1997,71:1089-1096.

[57] Kirchhoff F, Greenough TC, Brettler DB, Sullivan JL, Desrosiers RC: Brief report: absence of intact nef sequences in a long-term survivor with nonprogressive HIV-1 infection. N. Engl J Med 1995,332:228-232.

[58] Learmont JC, Geczy AF, Mills J et al. Immunologic and virologic status after 14 to 18 years of infection with an attenuated strain of HIV-1: a report from the Sydney Blood Bank Cohort. N Engl J Med 1999, 340:1715-1722.

[59] Deek SG, Casper C, Carlenor E. Neutralizing antibody responses against autologous and heterogolous viruses in acute versus chronic human immunodeficiency virus (HIV) infection:evidence for a constraint on the ability of HIV to completely evade neutralizing antibody responses.J Virol 2006,80:6155-6164.

[60] Kaul R, Trabattoni D, Bwayo JJ, Arienti D, Zagliani A, Mwangi FM, Kariuki C, Ngugi EN, MacDonald KS, Ball TB, Clerici M, Plummer FA. HIV-1-specific mucosal IgA in a cohort of HIV-1-resistant Kenyan sex workers. AIDS 1999,13:23-29.

[61] Migueles SA, Laborico AC, Imamichi H, Shupert WL, Royce C, McLaughlin M, Ehler L, Metcalf J, Liu S, Hallahan CW, Connors M: The differential ability of HLA B*5701+ long-term nonprogressors and progressors to restrict human immunodeficiency vi-

rus replication is not caused by loss of recognition of autologous viral gag sequences. J Virol 2003,77:6889-6898.

[62] Haung Y, Paxton W, Wolinsky S, Neuman A: The role of a mutantCCR5 allele in HIV-1 transmission and disease progression. Nat Med 1996,2(11):1240-1243.

[63] Theodorou I, Meyer L, Magierowska M, Katlama C, Rouzious C: HIV-1 infection in an individual homozygous for CCR5 delta 32. Seroco study group. Lancet 1997, 349(9060):1219-1220.

[64] Liu R, Paxton WA, Choe S, Ceradini D, Martin SR, Horuk R, MacDonald ME, Stuhlmann H, Koup RA, Landau NR: Homozygous defect in HIV-1 coreceptor accounts for resistance of some multiply-exposed individuals to HIV-1 infection. Cell 1996,86:367-377.

[65] Vaya J, Aviram M: Nutritional antioxidants: Mechanisms of action, Analyses of Activities and Medical Applications. Curr Med Chem Imm 2001,1:99-117.

[66] Pagamara AT, Perno CF, Aquaro S, Bue MC, Dini L, Geraci E: Glutathione inhibits HIV replication by acting at later stages of the virus life cycle. AIDS Res Hum Retroviruses 1996,2(10):1537-1541.

[67] Whittaker M, Whittaker JW: A glutamate bridge is essential for dimer stability and metal selectivity in manganese superoxide dismutase. J Biol Chem 1998,273:22188-22193.

[68] Hsieh YY, Guan C, Tu PJ, Bratt A, Angerhofer R, Lepock MJ, Hickey JA, Tainer HS, Silverman DN: Probing the active site of human manganese superoxide dismutase: the role of glutamine 143. Biochem 1998,37:4731-4739.

[69] Fawell S, Seery J, Daikh Y, Moore C, Chen LL, Pepinsky B, Baroum J: Tat-mediated delivery of heterologous proteins into cells. Proc Natl Acad Sci US 1994,91(2);664-668.

[70] Wadia JS, Dowdy SF: Protein transduction technology. Curr Opin Biotechnol 2002, 13(1):52-56.

[71] Flores SC, Marecki K, Harper SW, Bose SK, Nelson SK, McCord JC: Tat protein of human immunodeficiency virus type1 represses expression of manganese superoxide dismutase in Hela cells. Proc Natl Acad Sci USA 1993, 90: 7620–7636.

[72] Ye N, Liu S, Lin Y, Rao P: Protective effects of intraperitoneal injection of TAT-SOD against focal cerebral ischemia/reperfusion injury in rats. Life Sci 2011,89(23-24)868-874.

[73] Gu Q, Feng T, Cao H, Tang Y, Ge X, Luo J, Xue J, Wu J, Y H, Zhang S, Cao J: HIV-TaT mediated protein transduction of Cu/Zn-superoxide dismutase-1 (SOD1) protects skin cells from ionizing radiation. Radia Oncol 2013,8:253

[74] Flores SC, Marecki K, Harper SW, Bose SK, Nelson SK, McCord JC: Tat protein of human immunodeficiency virus type1 represses expression of manganese Superoxide dismutase in Hela cells. Proc Natl Acad Sci USA 1993,90: 7620–7636.

[75] Glover M, Hebert V, Nicholas K, Xue S, Thibeaux T, Zavecz J, Dugas T: Overexpression of mitochondrial antioxidant manganese superoxide dismutase(MnSOD) provides protection against AZT or 3TC-induced endothelial dysfunction. Antiviral Res 2014,111:136-142.

[76] Tarhini AA, Belani CP, Luketich JD, Argiris A, Ramalingam SS, Gooding W, Pennathur A, Petro D, Kane K, Liggitt D, Smith TC, Zhang X, Epperly MW, Greenberger JS: A phase I study of concurrent chemotherapy (Paclitaxel and Carboplatin) and thoracic radiotherapy with swallowed manganese superoxide dismutase plasmid liposome protection in patients with locally advanced stage III non-small-cell lung cancer. Human Gene Therapy 2011,22(3):336. Doi: 10.1089/hum.2010.078

[77] Palamara AT, Perno CF, Aquaro S, Bue MC, Dini L, Geraci E: Glutathione inhibits HIV replication by acting at later stages of the virus life cycle. AIDS Res. Hum Retroviruses 1996,2(10):1537-1541.

[78] Brooke SM, McLaughlin JR, Cortopassi KM, Sapolsky RM: Effect of GP 120 on glutathione peroxidase activity in cortical cultures and the interaction with steroid hormones. J Neurochem 2002,81(2):277-284

[79] Ho WZ, Douglas SD: Glutathione and N-acetyl cysteine suppression of human immunodeficiency virus replication in human monocyte/macrophages in-vitro. AIDS Res Hum Retroviruses 1992,12(17):1035-1038.

[80] Yan H, Harding JJ: Glycation-induced inactivation and loss of antigenicity of catalase and superoxide dismutase. Biochem J 1997,328:599-605

[81] Lledías FP, Hansberg W: Oxidation of catalase by singlet oxygen. J Biol Chem 1998, 273:10630-10637.

[82] Leff J, Oppegard M, Curiel T, Brown K, Schooley R, Repine J: Progressive increases in serum catalase activity in advancing human immunodeficiency virus infection. Free Rad Biol Med 1992,13(2):143-149.

[83] Ibeh BO, Habu JB, Eze SC: Discordant levels of superoxide dismutase and catalase observed in ART naïve and experienced HIV patients in Southeastern Nigeria. J Infect Dis Therapeu 2013,1:8-16.

[84] Coutsoudis A, Kubendran P, Spooner C: Randomized trial testing the effect of Vitamin A supplementation on pregnancy outcomes and early mother-to-child HIV-1 transmission in Durban, South Africa. AIDS 199,13:1517-1524.

[85] Hossain MA: Ascorbate free radical. J biol Chem 1985,260(24):12920-12926.

[86] Harakeh S, Jariwalla RJ, Pauling L: Suppression of human immunodeficiency virus replication by ascorbate in chronically and acutely infected cells. Proc Natl Acad Sci USA 1990,87:7245-7249.

[87] Packer L, Suzuki Y: Vitamin E and alpha-lipoate: role in antioxidant recycling and activation of the NF-kB transcription factor. Mol Aspects Med 1993,14:229-239.

[88] Harada S, Yusa K, Monde K, Akaike T, Maeda Y: Influence of membrane fluidity on human immunodeficiency virus type 1 entry. Biochem Biophys Res Commun. 2005, 329(2):480-486.

[89] Rufegeri MJ: The occurrences of sexually transmitted infection related to sero converson among HIV discordant couples. Sixteen Interventional AIDS Conference, Toronto 2006, pp 326-343.

[90] Li-Weber M, Weigand MA, Giaisi M, Süss D, Treiber MK, Baumann S, Ritsou E, Breitkreutz R, Krammer PH: Vitamin E inhibits CD95 ligand expression and protects T cells from activation-induced cell death. J Clin Invest 2002,110(5):681–690. doi: 10.1172/JCI200215073

[91] Packer L: Inactivation of NF-kB activation by vitamin E derivatives. Biochem Biophys Res Commun 1993,193:277-283.

[92] De Groot H, Rauen U: Tissue injury by reactive oxygen species and the protective effects of flavonoids. Fundam Clin Pharmacol 1998,12:249–255.

[93] Nair MPN, Saiyed ZM, Gandhi NH, Ramchand CN: The Flavonoid, Quercetin, Inhibits HIV-1 Infection in Normal Peripheral Blood Mononuclear Cells. Amer J infect dis 2009,142:148.

[94] Ng TB, Huang B, Fong WP, Yeung HW: Anti-human immunodeficiency virus (anti-HIV) natural products with special emphasis on HIV reverse transcriptase inhibitors. Life Sci 1997,61:933–949.

[95] Wang H, Xia Y, Yang ZY, Natschke SL, Lee KH. Recent advances in the discovery and development of flavonoids and their analogues as antitumor and anti-HIV agents. Adv Exp Med Biol 1998,439:191–225.

[96] Middleton EJ: Effect of plant flavonoids on immune and inflammatory cell function. Adv. Exp. Med Biol 1998,439:175–182. 9(12):e115323.

[97] South TL, Kim B, Hare DR: Zinc fingers and molecular recognition: structure and nucleic acid bindings studies of an HIV zinc finger-like domain. Biochem. Pharmacol 1990,40:123-129.

[98] Sergio W: Zinc salts that may be effective against the AIDS virus HIV. Med Hyp 1988,26:251-53.

[99] Tamamura H, Otaka A: Interactioin of an anti-HIV peptide, T22, with GP120 and CD4. Biochem. Biophys Res Common 1996,219:555-559.

[100] Fleiger D, Reithmuller G, Ziegler-Heitbrock HWL. Zn2 + inhibits both tumor necrosis factor-mediated NF-KB inductuion. Sci 1995, 270:1194-1197.

[101] Wang Q, Wang Y, Pu S, Zhen YT: Zinc coupling potentiates anti-HIV-1 activity of baicalin. Biochem Biophy Res Comm 2004,324(2):605-610.

[102] Beck MA, Esworth R, HO YS, Chu FF: Glutathione peroxidase in viral induced Myocarditis FASEB J 1998,12:1143–1149.

[103] Baum MK, Campa A: Role of selenium in HIV/AIDS. In: Hatfield DL, Berry MJ, Gladyshev VN, (eds.) Selenium: Its Molecular Biology and Role in Human Health. 2nd ed. New York: Springer; 2006:299-310;

[104] Roy M, Kiremidjian-Schumacher L, Wishe HI, Cohen MW, Stotzky G: Supplementation with selenium and human immune cell functions. I. Effect on lymphocyte proliferation and interleukin 2 receptor expression. Biol Trace Elem Res 1994,41(1-2): 103-114.

[105] Zhao L, Cox AG, Ruzicka JA, Bhat AA, Zhang W, Taylor EW: Molecular modeling and in vitro activity of an HIV-1-encoded glutathione peroxidase. Proc Natl Acad Sci USA. 2000;97(12):6356-6361.

[106] Zhang W, Ramanathan CS, Nadimpalli RG, Bhat AA, Cox AG, Taylor EW: Selenium-dependent glutathione peroxidase modules encoded by RNA viruses. Biol Trace Elem Res 1999,70(2):97-116.

[107] International AIDS Society: New HIV Cure Research Released Today at the XIX International AIDS Conference AIDS 2012. http://www.avert.org/cure-aids.htm#footnote3_itpbkok.Accessed on December 18, 2014.

[108] Olson AD, Meyer L, Prins M, Thiebaut R, Gurdasani D, Guiguet M, Chaix M, Amornkulb P, Babiker A, Sandhu M, Porter K: An evaluation of HIV elite controller definitions within a large seroconverter cohort collaboration. PLoS ONE 2014,9(1):e86719. doi:10.1371.

[109] Lambotte O, Boufassa F, Madec Y, Nguyen A, Goujard C, Meyer L, Rouzioux C: HIV controllers: A homogeneous group of HIV-1—infected patients with spontaneous control of viral replication. Clin Infect Dis 2005,41(7):1053-1056.

[110] Miura T, Ngumbela K, Ramduth D, Pereyra F, Walker B: Perspective: HIV Controllers: Can the Human Genome Project Advance AIDS Vaccine Development? IAVIreport 2007,11(3). http://www.iavireport.org/Back-Issues/Pages/IAVI-Report-11%283%29-PerspectiveHIVControllersCantheHumanGenomeProjectAdvanceAIDSVaccineDevelopment.aspx (Accessed January,2015).

[111] Lewin SR, Rouzioux C: HIV cure and eradication: how will we get from the laboratory to effective clinical trials? AID 2011,25(7):885–897.

[112] Peng X, Gandhi V: ROS-activated anticancer prodrugs: a new strategy for tumor-specific damage. Ther Deliv 2012,3(7):823-833.

[113] Allers K, Hütter G, Hofmann J, Loddenkemper C, Rieger K, Thiel E, Schneider T: Evidence for the cure of HIV infection by CCR5Δ32/Δ32 stem cell transplantation. Blood 2011,117(10):2791-2799.

[114] Didigu CA, Wilen CB, Wang J, Duong J, Secreto AJ, Danet-Desnoyers GA, Riley JL, Gregory PD, June CH, Holmes MC, Doms RW: Simultaneous zinc-finger nuclease editing of the HIV coreceptors ccr5 and cxcr4 protects CD4+ T cells from HIV-1 infection. Blood 2014,123(1):61-69. Epub 2013

[115] Li L, Krymskaya L, Wang J, Henley J, Rao A, Cao LF, Tran CA, Torres-Coronado M, Gardner A, Gonzalez N, Kim K, Liu PQ, Hofer U, Lopez E, Gregory PD, Liu Q, Holmes MC, Cannon PM, Zaia JA, DiGiusto DL: Genomic editing of the HIV-1 coreceptor CCR5 in adult hematopoietic stem and progenitor cells using zinc finger nucleases. Mol Ther 2013,21(6):1259-69.

[116] Ando D, Lalezari J, Blick G, Tang W, Lee G, Nichol G, Zeidan J, Sekaly RP, Deeks S, Mitsuyasu R, Richmond CA: HIV Protected Autologous Zinc Finger Nuclease CCR5 Modified CD4 cells (SB-728-T) Reduce Viral Load (VL) in HIV Subjects During Treatment Interruption (TI): Correlates of Effect, and Effect of Cytoxan Conditioning. 54th Interscience Conference on Antimicrobial Agents and Chemotherapy (ICAAC 2014). Washington, DC, September 5-9, 2014. Abstract H-643.

[117] Zeidan J, Lee G, Fromentin R, Sékaly RP et al: Adoptive Transfer of ZFN CCR5 Modified CD4 T-cells (SB-728-T) in HIV Subjects Leads to Generation of T Memory Stem Cells and a Decrease in the Size of the Latent Reservoir. 54th Interscience Conference on Antimicrobial Agents and Chemotherapy (ICAAC 2014). Washington, DC, September 5-9, 2014. Abstract H-994.

[118] NIH: Mississippi Baby, Now Has Detectable HIV, Researchers.2014 http://www.niaid.nih.gov/news/newsreleases/2014/pages/mississippibabyhiv.aspx. (Accessed February, 2015)

[119] Rainwater-Lovett K, Luzuriaga K, Persaud D : Very early combination antiretroviral therapy in infants: prospects for cure. [Journal Article, Research Support, N.I.H., Extramural] Curr Opin HIV AIDS 2015 Jan,10(1):4-11.

[120] Van Lunzen J, Schulze zur Wiesch J, Schuhmacher U, Hauber I, Hauber J: Functional cure after long term HAART initiated during early HIV infection: a comprehensive case study. Seventh International AIDS Society Conference on HIV Pathogenesis, Treatment and Prevention, abstract TUPE246, Kuala Lumpur, 2013.

[121] Sáez-Cirión A, Bacchus C, Hocqueloux L, Avettand-Fenoel V, Girault I, Lecuroux C, Potard V, Versmisse P, Melard A, Prazuck T: Post-Treatment HIV-1 Controllers with a Long-Term Virological Remission after the Interruption of Early Initiated Antire-

troviral Therapy ANRS VISCONTI Study. PLoS Pathog 2013 9(3): e1003211. doi: 10.1371/journal.ppat.1003211.

[122] Rouzioux C, Hocqueloux L, Sáez-Cirión A: Posttreatment controllers: what do they tell us? Curr Opin HIV AIDS 2015,10(1):29-34.

[123] Salmen S, Berrueta L: Immune modulators of HIV infection: The role of reactive oxygen species. J Clin Cell Immunol 2012,3:121.

[124] Luc montagner: 25 years after HIV discovery: prospects for cure and vaccine. Virol 2010, 397(2):248–254.

[125] Chugh P, Bradel-Tretheway B, Monteiro-Filh CMR, Planelles V, Maggirwar SB, Dewhurst S, Kim B: Akt inhibitors as an HIV-1 infected macrophage-specific anti-viral therapy. Retrovirol 2008,5(1):11.

[126] Chugh P, Fan S, Planelles V, Maggirwar SB, Dewhurst S, Kim B: Infection of human immunodeficiency virus and intracellular viral Tat protein exert a pro-survival effect in a human microglial cell line. J Mol Biol 2007,366(1):67-81.

[127] Ibeh BO, Obidoa O, Uzoegwu PN. High plasma activity of endogenous antioxidants protects CD4+ T-cells in HIV-serodiscordant heterosexual partners in a Nigerian population. Int STD AIDS 2008,19(8):536-540.

[128] Bhaskar A, Munshi MH, Khan SZ, Fatima S, Arya R, Jamee S, Singh A: Measuring Glutathione Redox Potential of HIV-1-infected macrophages. J Biolog Chem 2015,290,1020-1038.

Chapter 8

Novel Prospective Treatment Options

Jeremiah Stanley and Naoki Yamamoto

Additional information is available at the end of the chapter

http://dx.doi.org/10.5772/60961

1. Introduction

The acquired immunodeficiency syndrome (AIDS) caused by the Human immunodeficiency virus (HIV) is by far the most feared disease by any person on the planet. The root cause of this fear stems from its relentless worldwide spread and the absence of an effective therapeutic / preventive modality. Since its discovery in the early 1980s, it has been over three decades of war between mankind and HIV. All attempts to overcome the virus have so far been unsuccessful due to the unique features of HIV such as, the abilty to undergo rapid genetic evolution and to establish latent reservoirs. The higly active anti-retroviral therapy (HAART) is currently the only available strategy to limit the disease progression. However, the principal flaw in HAART is that it fails to eliminate the infection and warrants life long therapy. Long term treatment with anti-retroviral drugs has the disadvantage of poor compliance due to adverse effects and also possesses the risk of selecting resistant mutants. These reasons justify the need to search for novel therapeutic options superior to conventional anti-viral therapy.

Success stories of the Mississippi baby and the Berlin patient have revolutionized the concepts of HIV treatment and offered hope that HIV is not invincible. The strategies that have been developed / being developed against HIV, either affect the virus directly at different phases of its natural course or enhance the immunity to clear the infection from the body. Novel natural and synthetic compounds, peptides, DNA and RNA manipulatory techniques are being explored for their ability to impede the virus. Immune based therapies to accentuate specific anti-HIV immunity have stemmed from the failures encountered with vaccines. Apart from this, various alternative therapies are also being sought by patients. This chapter elaborates the various novel options that are currently being developed for HIV treatment and discusses their potential uses and impediments.

2. Why should we look beyond the HAART?

The major problem faced with HAART is that it only controls the infection and never eliminates it. When used continually on a lifelong basis, the HAART provides an infected individual with a significant improvement of clinical condition, enhancement of the quality of life and drastic reduction of circulating viral load. Nevertheless, treatment cessation at any point results in a rebound viremia, stripping off all the benefits that the patient had enjoyed during therapy. This could be stated as the inherent flaw in HAART, which exerts its inhibitory effect only against the actively replicating viruses in circulation and has little or no effect in destroying the quiescent viruses hidden in the latent cellular and anatomical reservoirs. Due to several reasons, this proviral reservoir gets activated at a later date proceeding to active viral replication and viremia, which can occur unchecked upon discontinuation of HAART [1-4].

Another worrisome aspect of HIV is its ability to undergo rapid genetic evolution as a consequence of its voracious mutating capacity. For a virus with such a feature, lifelong therapy with anti-retroviral drugs can be deleterious by itself, as the constant drug pressure eventually selects the resistant mutant viral populations. Such mutant viruses, resistant to the currently used anti-retroviral drugs have already emerged and are being disseminated in various countries across the globe. There is a possibility that these strains may replace the drug susceptible ones and render the HAART inactive.

Lifelong HAART also faces the practical constraint of continuous patient adherence to the prescribed regimen and also its discontinuation due to adverse drug effects. Optimistic predictions of worldwide HIV control using HAART would be just a mirage if the impending failure of the HAART in the future is not foreseen from the present. In the light of these issues, any attempt to curtail the HIV pandemic warrants the need for novel anti-retroviral agents and/or strategies to supplement, if not to supplant the HAART [5].

3. Novel agents and strategies currently being tried against HIV

All of the therapeutic strategies which are either currently available or under experimental research, involve attacking HIV at any one of the different phases in its infection course. (Figure-1) All these strategies use one or more of the following principles including administration of active chemical compounds, nanotechnology, DNA manipulation, RNA based techniques and cellular transplants.

Apart from these therapeutic strategies which directly impede the viral activity, several immune based therapies are also being developed which intend to enhance the ability of the immune system to overcome HIV on its own. These strategies also act at one or more points in the natural course of HIV infection allowing the immune system to suppress and possibly eliminate HIV [6].

http://dx.doi.org/10.5772/60961

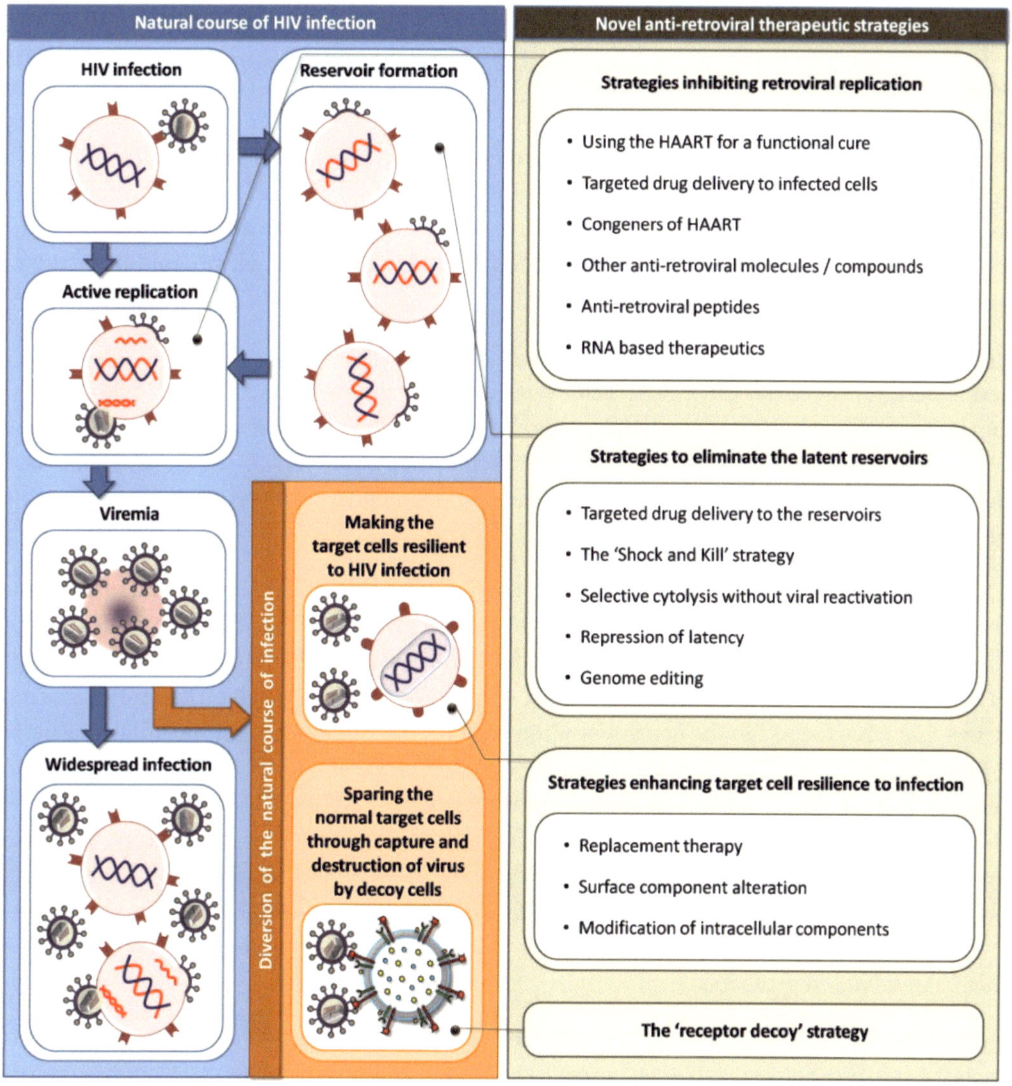

Figure 1. Natural course of HIV infection and the targeting points of therapeutic strategies

4. Agents and strategies inhibiting retroviral replication

4.1. Using the HAART for a functional cure

The HAART and the other anti-retroviral agents halt the natural course of HIV infection at the phase of active viral replication. This section elucidates the newer concepts that propose to maximize the utility of the existing anti-retroviral agents and also sheds light on novel compounds and targets which could be exploited for use against HIV.

The scope of the HAART to achieve a 'functional cure' is being studied extensively. Functional cure is said to be achieved when the infected individual treated aggressively with HAART early in the course of infection, does not develop rebound viremia on cessation of therapy for several months [7]. This concept had stemmed from the story of the Mississippi baby, where a mother seropositive for HIV-1 gave birth to an infant who was also found to be infected. Anti-retroviral therapy was initiated to the baby at 30 hours of birth and was continued till 18 months of age after which the therapy was discontinued. Surprisingly at 30 months of age, the child was tested negative for plasma HIV-1 RNA, proviral DNA in peripheral-blood mononuclear cells and serum HIV-1 antibodies [8].

In an attempt to replicate the observations of the Mississippi baby, the VISCONTI study conducted in France has effectively achieved a functional cure in a cohort of 14 adults who currently are free of viremia even after several years of interruption of anti-retroviral therapy [9]. Likewise, functional cure has been reported in an elderly German patient who had deliberately interrupted treatment after five years and has controlled rebound viremia for nine years after the cessation of treatment [10].

The reason hypothesized behind functional cure is that, early aggressive treatment prevents the build-up of large latent reservoirs and also reduces the viral load low enough that the immune system clears off the residual infection without continued use of antiretroviral drugs [11]. The drawback of this concept is that it necessitates the stoppage of the anti-retroviral drugs that have helped in the control of viremia. It is not known whether this might result in a functional cure or cause a rebound viremia. As it would be unethical to stop treatment in an individual with good viremic control without knowing the correlates of protection, well designed clinical trials must be conducted prior to implementation of this concept, to obtain answers to questions of uncertainty such as; what is the time period within which the treatment should be initiated following infection to favour functional cure? How long should the treatment be given? When is the ideal time for the interruption of treatment? What are the host factors involved in protection?

By the time the functional cure concept offered some hope, the occurrence of rebound viremia in the Mississippi baby smashed all the excitement [12]. It might only be a matter of time before we know whether the other patients claimed to be functionally cured, progress to viremia or remain "cured". Nevertheless, the Mississippi baby and the other studies have hinted that control of viremia is possible on treatment cessation. Further studies are required to find how to prolong this drug-free control of viremia.

4.2. Targeted drug delivery to infected cells

To achieve viremic control by anti-retroviral drugs, the patient should also face a plethora of untoward effects. Drug interactions, synergistic toxicity of combination, frequent dosing and pill burden are the various adverse effects of the HAART causing a poor compliance. Novel techniques based on nanotechnology are being developed to overcome the shortcomings of conventional anti-retroviral drug therapy.

Targeted drug delivery is the technique that is extensively being applied to accentuate the beneficial effects and to simultaneously reduce the adverse effects of anti-retroviral drugs. In the course of infection, HIV gains entry into its target cells by membrane fusion, leaving behind its envelope and surface glycoproteins on the surface of the infected cells. During active replication of HIV within the target cells, the infected cells also express these viral glycoproteins synthesized de novo. Active targeting exploits these viral components on the cell surface to selectively identify the infected cells from the uninfected ones [13]. Active replication of HIV *in vivo*, from the point of infection of a CD4 T-cell to release of viral progeny takes an average of 52 hours for completion [14]. This long generation time of HIV could be effectively utilized to specifically deliver the anti-retroviral drugs to the infected cells by nanotechnology methods. This would prevent the dissemination of the viral progeny and reduce the viral load more effectively than systemically administered anti-retroviral drugs.

The nanoparticles used for targeted drug delivery contain a carrier vessel straddled with a targeting moiety. The carrier nanoparticles are tiny containers which could be loaded with the drug of interest and are capable of delivering their cargo into cells upon fusion. Various types of nanocarriers such as; liposomes, micelles, dendrimers, nanocapsules, nanoemulsions, solid lipid nanoparticles, polymeric nanoparticles, gold nanoparticles and nanocrystals have been successfully loaded with one or more known anti-retroviral agents. The active targeting moiety tagged to the surface of these carriers guides them specifically to the target cells. Recombinant CD4 molecules or Fab fragments of monoclonal anti-gp120 antibodies which possess high affinity to HIV envelope glycoproteins are used to actively target the envelope glycoproteins of HIV present on the surface of the infected CD4 cells [15].

Targeted drug delivery possesses significant advantages over conventional chemotherapy of which, the most important is the reduction of the adverse effect profile of the anti-retroviral agents. This is because, the technique concentrates the drug only to the necessary sites and hence not only it reduces the administered dose, but also avoids the accumulation of drug at unwanted sites. Besides this, some of the nanoparticles have inherent antiretroviral property and function synergistically when loaded. This promising technique however, is not devoid of pitfalls. Nanoparticles face the major problem of opsonization and phagocytic clearance which occurs almost rapidly following their administration. The process of pegylation which involves in coating of the nanoparticles with polyethylene glycol overcomes this disadvantage by making the nanoparticles invisible to immune clearance. However, the fusion kinetics of these 'stealth' nanoparticles is diminished when compared to the non-pegylated ones [16]. Nanocarriers packed with a single drug are more stable and addition of more drugs within the same nanocarrier makes it more unstable. As monotherapy can accelerate viral resistance, stable models of multidrug nanocarriers are now being developed [17]. Poor oral bioavailability, causation of target cell membrane instability and cytotoxicity, complications in renal clearance and high production cost are some of the problems that have to be solved before nanotherapeutics come into effective use [13].

4.3. Congeners of HAART

The currently available anti-retroviral drugs specifically inhibit a select few steps of HIV replication such as HIV entry and fusion, reverse transcription, protease action and integration. Apart from their beneficiary action, the anti-retroviral drugs possess significant adverse reactions which form the principal reason behind poor compliance and drug withdrawal. With the advent of pharamacological techniques, congeners of anti-retroviral drugs are being developed with the aim of minimizing the side effects.

The congeners are molecules of any particular drug class which are engineered to overcome the pitfalls faced by the existing members of the same drug class. They possess minor structural modifications that confer one or more favourable properties such as increased biovailability, increased target site binding affinity or longer half life. By virtue of these properties, the congeners can be effectively administered at reduced dose and interval and hence possess a low adverse effect profile. The congeners are subject to clinical trials and would probably fail or get pass the trial stages to get approved by the United Staes Food and Drug Administration (FDA) and relevant international bodies. Table-1 summarizes the FDA approved anti-retroviral dugs for use in the USA and their congeners in the pipeline (updated to October 2014) [18-21].

Stage of HIV replication inhibited	Anti-retroviral drug class	FDA approved agents	Congeners
Attachment to CCR5 co-receptor	Entry inhibitors	Maraviroc	Cenicriviroc Vicriviroc Adaptavir INCB-9471 PRO-140
Fusion of envelope with cell membrane	Fusion inhibitors	Enfuvirtide	Albuvirtide
Reverse transcription	Nucleoside / Nucleotide Reverse Transcriptase Inhibitors (NRTIs)	Zidovudine Lamivudine Stavudine Didanosine Emtricitabine Abacavir Tenofovir disoproxil fumarate	Tenofovir alafenamide Hexadecycloxy propyl tenofovir Amdoxovir Racivir Festinavir Elvucitabine Dexelvucitabine
	Non-Nucleoside Reverse Transcriptase Inhibitors (NNRTIs)	Nevirapine Efavirenz Delaviridine Etravirine Rilpivirine	Doravirine

Stage of HIV replication inhibited	Anti-retroviral drug class	FDA approved agents	Congeners
Proteolytic cleavage of precursor polyprotein into functional proteins	Protease inhibitors	Ritonavir Nelfinavir Indinavir Saquinavir Atazanavir Foamprinavir Tipranavir Darunavir	-
Integration of viral DNA to the host cell genome	Integrase inhibitors	Raltegravir Dolutegravir	Elvitegravir Cabotegravir

Table 1. Anti-retroviral drugs approved by the FDA and their congeners under consideration

4.4. Reducing the pill burden

One of the practical difficulties faced by the multi-drug HAART regimen is the pill burden. It is glaringly obvious and even scientifically proven that, therapeutic regimens with lesser number of pills have a better patient adherence [22]. In this context, pills with a fixed dose combination of more than one anti-retroviral agent are being developed and few have also been approved by the FDA. Table-2 summarizes the list of combinations approved by the FDA as of October 2014 [18].

Name of the pill	Drugs contained
Epzicom	Abacavir and lamivudine
Combivir	Zidovudine and lamivudine
Truvada	Emtricitabine and tenofovir disoproxil fumarate
Triumec	Abacavir, dolutegravir and lamivudine
Trizivir	Abacavir, zidovudine and lamivudine
Atripla	Efavirenz, emtricitabine and tenofovir disoproxil fumarate
Complera	Emtricitabine, rilpivirine and tenofovir disoproxil fumarate
Striblid	Elvitegravir, cobicistat, emtricitabine and tenofovir disoproxil fumarate

Table 2. Fixed dose combinations of anti-retroviral drugs approved by the FDA

Designing a single drug molecule containing the active moieties of two different anti-retroviral compounds is yet another strategy to reduce the pill burden. These molecules termed 'portmanteau inhibitors' can exert their anti-retroviral action at two different steps of HIV replication and could thereby reduce an extra pill. Caffeoyl-anilide compounds are evaluated for their dual action in inhibiting HIV integrase and blocking the CCR5 receptor mediated entry [23].

4.5. Synergistic enhancers of anti-retroviral drug action

Certain compounds such as pharmacokinetic boosters and virostatics, are being evaluated for their role in potentiating the action of anti-retroviral drugs. The property of pharmacokinetic boosting is exclusively exploited for protease inhibitors which are metabolized and cleared from the body by the cytochrome P-450 CYP3A4 enzyme. The effect of protease inhibitors can be boosted if they are co-administered with compounds that inhibit this enzyme. The protease inhibitor ritonavir with the propensity to inhibit the cytochrome P-450 CYP3A4 enzyme, when co-administered with another protease inhibitor not only enhances its bioavailability, but also acts synergistically to minimize the dosage of both agents [24]. The combination of lopinavir boosted by ritonavir has been identified to provide maximum benefits with minimal adverse effects and hence is approved by the FDA and marketed as a fixed dose combination pill under the name, kaletra. Cobicistat is another unrelated compound which is a potent inhibitor of the cytochrome P-450 CYP3A4 enzyme without having any inherent anti-retroviral activity. As it is also capable of boosting the beneficial effects of integrase inhibitors, it is approved for use along with the fixed combination of elvitegravir, emtricitabine and tenofovir under the trade name, striblid [18, 25].

Virostatics is an abbreviation for the combination of antiviral (viro) and cytostatic drugs (static). This combination intends to reduce viremia by inhibiting HIV replication with anti-retroviral drug and simultaneously reducing the number of the viral target cells (normal CD4 T-cells), using the cytostatic drug. It has been observed that the antiviral drug didanosine functions synergistically with hydroxyurea, an inhibitor of cellular proliferation to achieve viral load reduction. As this strategy depends on hydroxyurea induced immunosuppression for reduction of viremia, more knowledge has to be gained on its practicality, with respect to didanosine resistant HIV mutants and flare-up of opportunistic infections [26, 27]. The anti-parasitic / anti-inflammatory drug leflunomide is also found to have similar synergistic effect to inhibit HIV replication when used along with nucleoside reverse transcriptase inhibitors [28, 29].

4.6. Novel targets and synthetic molecules to inhibit active retroviral replication

From binding to release, the replication of HIV involves several steps of which, only a few steps are targeted by the currently available anti-retroviral drugs and their congeners. As the various sub-cellular and molecular mechanisms of HIV replication are gradually being unraveled, novel compounds are also being identified to target and inhibit one or more steps of HIV replication. Most of these are small synthetic molecules identified based on computational analysis of their structure and ability to dock at the required site and further screened for functionality by *in vitro* bioassays. As the discovery of newer anti-retroviral compounds is an ongoing process, table-3 summarizes a non-exhaustive list of novel synthetic anti-retroviral compounds and the phase of HIV replication they inhibit.

http://dx.doi.org/10.5772/60961

Phase of HIV replication inhibited	Novel mechanism of action	Compound	Reference
Entry and fusion	Binding to HIV gp 120 and prevention of its attachment to CD4 receptor	Temsavir and fostemsavir	[30]
		BMS-488043	[31]
		NBD-556	[32]
		DCM-205	[33]
		Curdlan sulfate	[34]
	Attachment to the CXCR4 co-receptor and prevention of HIV envelope fusion to cell membrane	AMD-11070	[35]
		T-22	[36]
		KRH-1636	[37]
Uncoating	Binding to HIV capsid / cyclophilin-A and prevention of uncoating by stabilizing the capsid	Pyrrolopyrazolone derivatives	[38]
		Quinoxaline derivatives	[39]
	Destabilisation and dissolution of the HIV capsid after entry	PF-3450074 (PF74)	[40, 41]
		I-XW-053	[42]
Reverse transcription and DNA synthesis	Inhibition of reverse transcription by novel nucleoside analogues	Adenosine analogs	[43]
	Inhibition of HIV DNA synthesis and introduction of lethal mutations	Ribonucleoside analogs	[44]
		KP-1461	[45]
	Reversal of susceptibility in NRTI resistant mutants	Foscarnet	[46]
Transcription	Inhibition of viral protein (tat) or inhibition of the leader sequence of HIV mRNA (TAR) or inhibition of tat-TAR interaction to prevent the initiation of transcription	Quinolone derivatives (HM13N, NM13)	[47]
		Acetylpromazine derivatives	[48]
		N1-aryl-propane-1,3-diamine	[49]
	Inhibition of cellular factors responsible for the elongation of HIV mRNA	Flavopiridol derivatives	[50]
		Seliciclib	[51]
		Roscovitine	[52]
		Iron chelators	[53]
		Garcinol derivatives (LTK-14)	[54]
		Ribofuranoside and carbonitrile derivatives	[55]
		Miltefosine	[56]
	Inhibition of post transcriptional processing of HIV mRNA	Mycophenolic acid	[57]

Phase of HIV replication inhibited	Novel mechanism of action	Compound	Reference
Cytoplasmic export of HIV mRNA	Inhibition of host proteins involved in nuclear export of HIV mRNA	PKF050-638	[58]
Translation	Inhibition of cellular ATPases involved in the initiation of HIV mRNA translation	Rhodanine and triazine compounds	[59, 60]
Assembly and release	Binding to capsid protein and Inhibition of assembly	benzodiazepines and benzimidazoles	[61]
	Blocking the ion channel function of the HIV protein vpu	BIT225	[62]
Maturation of progeny after release	Preventing the release of capsid protein from its precursor protein in the progeny virions and thereby rendering them non-infectious	Bevirimat	[63]
Viral DNA integration	Inhibition of lens epithelium derived growth factor protein p75 (LEDGF/p75) which helps in viral DNA integration	2-(quinolin-3-yl) acetic acid derivatives	[21]
		Chicoric acid derivatives	[64]
Enhancing the anti-viral restriction factors of the host cell	Inhibition of HIV virion infectivity factor (vif) to indirectly improve the viral restriction by APOBEC proteins	RN-18	[65, 66]
		VEC-5	[67]
	Direct enhancement of APOBEC proteins	SN-2	[68]
Multiple steps	Inhibition of uncoating and assembly	Thiourea compounds	[69]
		Acylhydrazone derivatives	[70]
	Inhibition of viral entry and transcription	Aminoglcosides (Neomycin, netilmicin)	[47]
Direct destruction of free HIV virions	Cation mediated destruction of HIV envelope	Ceragenins (CSA-54)	[71]
Selective cytolysis of HIV infected cells	Inhibition of acute viral infection and activation of apoptotic pathways specifically in cells infected with HIV	Ciclopirox and deferiprone	[72]

Table 3. Novel synthetic anti-retroviral compounds and their mechanism of action

Although most of these compounds have shown potent *in vitro* anti-retroviral activity, their *in vivo* efficacy needs to be evaluated. A few of the listed drug candidates are undergoing clinical trials and are expected to be available for use in the near future. The concept of using antiviral compounds for treatment of HIV poses a significant drawback. Unlike other viruses,

HIV possesses an immense potential to undergo genetic variation and the anti-retroviral agents rapidly select out resistant mutants. This could be well explained with the experiences faced with the experimental uncoating inhibitor PF74 and the maturation inhibitor bevirimat. The action of both these drugs can be nullified by HIV with simple mutations causing amino acid substitutions and these resistant mutants are expected to emerge rapidly if these drugs get approved for widespread use [41, 73]. While comparing the length of time and amount of work required to approve new anti-retroviral molecules acting on viral components, it is almost an instantaneous process for HIV to develop resistance against the drugs. In this context, compounds that inhibit the genetically more stable host components to produce anti-retroviral effects such as the CCR5 / CXCR4 inhibitors hold promise, until the virus finds an alternative to evade their action.

4.7. Natural derivatives with anti-retroviral property

Apart from the multitude of synthetic anti-retroviral compounds that are being generated every day, many naturally occurring compounds have also been identified to inhibit HIV [74, 75]. Plants, marine organisms, arthropod venoms and bacteria form the principal sources of these compounds. Extracts from natural sources are tested *in vitro* for anti-retroviral activity and the most active component identified, purified and studied for possible mechanism of action. Interestingly, some of the natural compounds have been found to perform better than their synthetic counterparts [73]. Recently, virtual methods are being developed for screening natural compounds for their anti-retroviral property [76]. If the *in vitro* effects could be effectively achieved *in vivo*, it would not be surprising when some of these compounds soon make their way across clinical trials and be available for use in the near future. Table-4 summarizes some recent compounds of renewed interest among various naturally occurring anti-retroviral compounds already identified.

Source	Source organism	Compound	Mechanism of anti-retroviral action	Reference
Plants	*Camellia sinensis* (Green tea)	Epigallocatechin-3-gallate	Inhibits HIV transcription. Also degrades the semen-derived enhancer of virus infection and prevents mucosal transmission	[77, 78]
	Eucalyptus globoidea (Australian Eucalyptus tree)	Globoidnan A	Inhibits HIV integrase	[79]
	Betula pubescens (and several other plants)	Betulinic acid	Prevents the release of capsid protein from its precursor protein in the progeny virions and thereby renders them non-infectious	[73]
	Isatis indigotica (Chinese medicinal plant)	Indirubin-3'-monoxime	Inhibits host cellular machinery responsible for HIV transcription	[80]

Source	Source organism	Compound	Mechanism of anti-retroviral action	Reference
	Salvia miltiorrhiza (Chinese medicinal plant)	Tanshinone II A	Inhibits host cellular machinery responsible for HIV transcription	[81]
	Pelargonium sidoides (German medicinal plant)	Unidentified compounds	Inhibits HIV entry	[82]
	Grapes and berries	Resveratrol	Inhibits tat-induced HIV transactivation. Also possess cystostatic effects on CD4 T-cells similar to hydroxyl urea	[83]
	Grapefruit juice	Unidentified compounds	Neutralizes the CYP3A4 in the GI tract and increases the bioavailabity of anti-retrovirals	[84]
Marine species	*Griffithsia* species (Red algae)	Griffithsin / Grifonin-1	Binds to various HIV surface components including gp41 and gp120 and inhibits entry	[85, 86]
	Corticium simplex (Sponge)	didehydro-cortistatin A	Most potent inhibitor of tat-dependent HIV transcription identified till date	[47, 87]
	Fascaplysinopsis reticulata (Sponge)	Fascaplysin	Inhibits host cellular machinery responsible for HIV transcription. Also inhibits HIV reverse transcriptase	[88]
	Cassiopia *Andromeda* (Jelly fish)	Cnidarian proteins	Various anti-HIV activities including inhibition of HIV protease, inhibition of HIV entry and cytotoxicity of infected cells	[89, 90]
	Galaxura filamentosa (Red algae)			
	Litophyton arboreum (Soft coral)			
Bacteria	*Nostoc ellipsosporum* (Cyanobacterium)	Cyanovirin-N	Binds to various HIV surface components including gp41 and gp120 and inhibits entry	[91]
	Scytonema varium (Cyanobacterium)	Scytovirin		[92]
	Sorangium cellulosum (Myxobacterium)	Ratjadone-A	Inhibits host proteins involved in nuclear export of HIV mRNA	[93]
	Streptomyces species (Actinomycete)	Leptomycin-B	Inhibits the viral protein rev which helps in nuclear export of HIV mRNA	[94]
Arthropods	Bee venom	Melittin	Binds to various HIV surface components and disintegrates the envelope	[95]
	Scorpion venom	Kn2-7	Interacts with HIV envelope and inhibits entry	[96]

Table 4. Anti-retroviral compounds isolated from natural sources

4.8. Anti-retroviral peptides

Eukaryotic organisms are known to secrete antimicrobial peptides as a part of their innate immunity, which have a broad spectrum of activity against various pathogenic microbes [97]. These peptides are usually short sequences of 12 - 20 amino acids, but some of them may also be around 40 amino acids long. Apart from the inherent anti-retroviral peptides produced by the human body, numerous studies have identified several peptides from natural and synthetic sources that are capable of inhibiting HIV replication [98]. With the FDA approval of the fusion inhibitor peptide enfuvirtide, coupled with the growing problem of resistance to anti-retroviral drugs, much interest is being shown in the development of novel anti-retroviral peptides. Currently, there are nearly a thousand HIV inhibiting peptides identified and new members are being added on a daily basis [99].

The anti-retroviral peptides identified till date are predominantly from natural sources ranging from bacteria to plants to primates. Also a significant number of these peptides are derivatives of HIV itself, which structurally mimic the viral substrates and competitively inhibit the various replicatory processes. On the other hand, synthetic production using techniques such as phage display, offer the scope of combination of related or unrelated peptides to achieve maximal anti-retroviral effect. Most of the anti-retroviral peptides inhibit one or more of the phases of HIV replication. Majority of the peptides act extracellularly to inhibit HIV attachment or its fusion while others inhibit the intracellular phases of replication such as reverse transcription, transcription and integration. Apart from the direct administration of peptides for therapy, these agents could also be administered in their complementary DNA form which on recombination with the host cell genome and subsequent expression, makes the target cell resilient to HIV infection (subsequently discussed). Certain peptides possess the unique property of cell penetration and hence being evaluated for their possible role in targeted nanotechnological and cellular delivery techniques [99, 100].

The advantages of therapeutic peptides include their high specificity for the site of action, rapid break down into harmless amino acids which are eliminated easily and hence possess less toxicity and adverse effect profile [98]. However, this rapid breakdown of peptides by the peptidases could also be a drawback since they could be cleared off before they exert their action. Currently, synthetic peptides incorporated with D-isomers of amino acids (instead of the naturally occurring L-isomers) or with added non-peptide moieties, overcome this drawback and possess extended half life [101]. Peptides are highly antigenic and elicit the production of antibodies. Hence the extracellular acting peptides face the problem of antibody mediated clearance. Although the intracellular acting peptides are devoid of the antibody problem, availability of efficient delivery systems into the cell and degradation by the intracellular peptidases are the challenges they face. Poor oral bioavailability, inability to cross biological barriers and high production cost are further problems to be addressed prior to approval for therapeutic use [100, 102]. The FDA however, has approved enfuvirtide, this approval has offered hope for the success of other anti-retroviral peptides currently undergoing clinical trials [103]. With advancements in nanotechnology and cellular delivery systems, peptide therapy might become a reality for HIV infection in due course of time.

4.9. RNA based therapeutics

RNA based therapeutic strategies exert their action between the phases of transcription and translation. Numerous RNA based techniques have been developed which are classified by their mechanism of action. They include; inhibitors of messenger RNA (mRNA) translation (antisense oligonucleotides), the agents of RNA interference (RNAi), catalytically active RNA molecules (ribozymes) and RNAs that bind proteins and other molecular ligands (aptamers) [104, 105] (Table-5). These techniques can be utilized for the treatment of any viral disease by engineering specific, complementary inhibitory RNA particles to the viral transcription components. Among these techniques, RNAi and to a lesser extent antisense oligonucleotides, have been tried out to inhibit retroviral replication. As these techniques can also target the host cellular processes, they are being exploited in strategies to increase the resilience of target cells to HIV infection, which is discussed later [106].

RNAi is an endogenous mechanism which involves the down regulation of mRNA activity during transcription and post transcription phases using short double stranded RNA (dsRNA) called micro RNA (miRNA), which are about 20-30bp long. The identification of this regulatory process has provoked the interest of controlling unwanted viral replication using exogenously administered specific sequences of short dsRNA. The exogenously administered agents of RNAi therapy include small interfering RNA (siRNA) and short hairpin RNA (shRNA). These agents act on the post transcript mRNA and either cause direct sequence specific cleavage when there is a perfect sequence complementarity match, or lead to translational repression and degradation of mRNA when the interfering RNA sequence is of limited complimentarity to the targeted mRNA. As the siRNA get cleared off after their action, their effects are only transient and need repeated administration similar to agents of chemotherapy. On the other hand the action of shRNA is similar to gene therapy, as they get expressed on promoters and cause long term effects. Various viral and non-viral delivery mechanisms and active targeting strategies have been developed to deliver these active agents into the target cells [107, 108].

Systems employing siRNA and shRNA to target the gene products of tat, rev, nef, env, vif and pol have been designed and evaluated for efficacy [47, 106]. However, the use of this technology against viral replicatory processess is threatened by the genetic variation exhibited by HIV. Very simple mutations allow HIV to escape from the action of both siRNA and shRNA [109, 110]. Four possible solutions are being tried to tackle the problem of these escape mutants. The first attempt is to expand the RNAi technique to simulataneously inhibit multiple HIV mRNA targets similar to the concept of multidrug use. Recent studies have demonstrated that concurrent inhibition of HIV mRNA with three different shRNAs can prevent viral escape *in vitro* [111, 112]. In the second possible solution, inhibitory RNAs with a complete match to the most commonly encountered viral escape sequences are being designed. When used along with the inhibitory RNA of the wild type virus, these could prevent a majority of the mutants from escape [113]. The third solution involves identifying novel, genetically conserved sequences of HIV which do not usually undergo mutation. Targeting these stable sites would favour the success of RNAi [114]. Finally, RNAi techniques are also being designed to restrict the 'genetically more stable' host factors that help in HIV replication (discussed later under strategies to enhance target cell resilience to HIV infection).

Apart from the disadvantages posed by the virus per se, RNAi technology has numerous setbacks. The short lived action of siRNA warrants its repetitive administration thereby compounding the treatment cost. The overexpression of shRNA can result in cell death and hence needs strict dose titration. RNA is immunogenic and is rapidly neutralized by antibodies in circulation, hence effective vectors are needed for the *in vivo* administration of RNA. Even after successful intracellular delivery, the administered RNA moieties are easy targets for degradation by cytoplasmic ribonucleases. Engineered RNA with modifications in sugar moieties, nucleotides or their backbone are found to possess improved cytoplasmic stability and are being evaluated for their superiority and efficacy [115].

Due to the numerous setbacks, almost all RNAi techniques that exclusively inhibit the viral targets have stagnated at the level of pre-clinical testing and none have entered into clinical trials. A recent technique which involves the simultaneous use of three shRNAs to specifically inhibit three corresponding targets of HIV, has been found to be safe and effective and is hopeful to enter phase I trials in the near future [111].

5. Strategies to eliminate latent reservoirs

The ability to integrate its nucleic acids with host cell genome and co-exist in a genetically quiescent proviral state is one of the distinct features of HIV, which makes eradication of infection next to impossible. The latent reservoirs of HIV are categorized into two broad groups namely the cellular and the anatomical reservoir. The cellular reservoir comprises the long lived resting CD4 T-cells. With an extended lifespan averaging 400 days, these cells bear the provirus and release the progeny upon activation at a later time [116]. Infection of the cells of the monocyte-macrophage lineage and subsequent compartmentalization of these infected cells into various organs / tissues such as the reticulo-endothelial system, lymph nodes, gastro-intestinal tract, brain and lungs, lead to the formation of anatomical reservoirs. Within the macrophages of these anatomical reservoirs, the HIV either remains quiescent inside the chronically infected cells or maintains a continuous low level replication [117]. Thus, the reservoirs act as Trojan horses spilling the progeny virions into circulation at periodic intervals. Although the mechanisms involved in proviral repression are gradually being unraveled, specific factors / agents reactivating the viral replication are yet to be clearly identified. Although early aggressive treatment helps in achieving a functional cure by limiting the reservoir formation, it does not offer a solution to the already established reservoirs. The new strategies and techniques that are being developed for eradicating the established viral reservoirs are subsequently discussed.

5.1. Targeted drug delivery to the reservoirs

Apart from attempts to limit viral replication in actively infected CD4 T-cells, nanotechnology methods are widely studied for the elimination of the latent viral reservoirs. Strategies include passive and active targeting and the use of surface moieties which enhance the penetration of biological barriers by the nanoparticles.

Upon systemic administration, most of the nanoparticles are instantaneously opsonized with plasma proteins and rapidly cleared off from circulation by the phagocytosis. The macrophages of the reticulo-endothelial system are the principal cells which are involved in the degradation and clearance of the nanoparticles [118]. This forms the basis of passive targeting which aims at achieving high concentrations of anti-retroviral agents in the reticulo-endothelial reservoir as a consequence of phagocytosis of the drug loaded nanoparticles. Studies have demonstrated the achievement of higher drug concentrations in the reticulo-endothelial cells following the administration of liposomes, nanocapsules or polymeric nanoparticles loaded with anti-retroviral drugs [119]. Likewise, passive targeting of the lymphatic reservoir can be achieved by incorporation of the nanoparticles with lipids such as phosphatidylcholine and cholesterol or by surface coating of the nanocarriers with polyethylene glycol [120, 121].

Apart from passive targeting, specific drug delivery to the anatomical reservoirs can be accomplished by active targeting strategies. Nanocarriers tagged on their surface with galactose or mannose residues or anti-HLA-DR monoclonal antibodies, effectively localize in the reticulo-endothelial system which have abundant receptors for these ligands such as the galactose and lectin receptors and the HLA-DR determinant of MHC-II respectively. Active targeting of the cellular reservoirs is based on the aforementioned principle of employing nanocarriers with homing ligands to viral components on infected cell surface. The infected resting CD4 T-cells containing HIV envelope glycoproteins on their surface attract the drug loaded nanoparticles coated with recombinant CD4 molecules or Fab fragments of monoclonal anti-gp120 antibodies [13].

Nanotechnology also offers a solution for the problem of poor drug penetration in certain anatomical sites. One such anatomical reservoir is the brain, where the infected microglial cells rest safely with the protection conferred by the blood brain barrier against the systemically administered anti-retroviral agents. The blood brain barrier functions not only by preventing the permeation of the circulating anti-retroviral compounds into the brain tissue, but also by efflux of a considerable portion of the compounds that have managed to cross through. With the ability to increase the crossing and reduce the efflux of drugs, nanotechnology methods help in reservoir elimination by overcoming the privilege offered by the blood brain barrier [122].

Nanotechnology methods that increase the drug transport across the blood brain barrier function by mimicry of natural substrates, utilization of cell penetrating peptides or by active targeting of molecules of abundance in neuronal vasculature with suitable surface ligands. The non-ionic surfactant 'polysorbate-80' has found to be an effective enhancer of drug delivery to the brain using the principle of substrate mimicry. Upon systemic administration, the drug loaded nanoparticles coated with polysorbate-80 adsorb various apolipoproteins in circulation to form a complex that mimics lipoproteins. Presuming them as natural substrates, the blood brain barrier permits the entry of these complexes by receptor mediated transcytosis resulting in delivery of the drug to the brain tissue [123]. Nanoparticles coated with cell penetrating peptides such as the HIV-1 tat peptide has shown enhanced efficacy in crossing the blood brain barrier. As the microvasculature of the brain is rich in receptors such as transferring receptor, low-density lipoprotein receptor and β2 receptors, their respective ligands such as transferrin, apolipoprotein-E and β2 agonists are considered possible candidates for active targeting.

The use of nanotechnology for reservoir elimination poses some peculiar problems in addition to other drawbacks mentioned earlier. The effectiveness of nanotechniques that rely on anti-retroviral drugs to eliminate the reservoir is questionable as these agents are lethal to the virus only during active replication and do not affect the inactive provirus. The final clearance of the nanoparticles from the anatomical sites, especially from the brain is not clearly known and accumulation overtime with repeated doses can possibly lead to neurotoxicity. Acquisition of more knowledge through carefully designed clinical trials is needed so that the potential of this technology could be put into adequate use [122].

5.2. The 'shock and kill' strategy

Considered as the 'holy grail' of HIV eradication research, this strategy aims at depletion of the latent reservoirs by widespread activation of the provirus using 'shocking agents' and subsequent killing of the actively replicating virions. Reactivation of the quiescent viral genes can be achieved either by inactivating the repressing factors and/or by activating the transcription factors [13].

Deacetylation and methylation of histones and DNA methylation are the few processes that have been identified to favour the proviral repression and hence the inhibitors of these processes are considered as attractive candidates for shocking agents. Inhibitors of the histone deacetylase group of enzymes; valproate and vorinostat have been tried out for viral reactivation with limited success [124]. Congeners of vorinostat such as givinostat, belinostat, panobinostat and droxinostat and other novel histone deacetylase inhibiting compounds such as oxamflatin, romidepsin are being evaluated for their efficacy in reactivating viral replication. Histone methyltransferase inhibitor chaetocin and DNA methyltransferase inhibitors azacytidine and decitabine are also being assessed for their efficacy as shocking agents [125].

Provirus could also be drawn into active replication by making the intracellular milleu conducive for transcription [126, 127]. This could be achieved by activating the transcription factors such as the NF-κB and transcription elongation factor- b. Initial studies that employed NF-κB activators such as interleukin-2 and monoclonal anti-CD3 antibodies failed to relieve the provirus from repression. This led to the identification of a gatekeeper kinase which has to be concurrently activated along with NF-κB to facilitate viral replication. Other compounds such as prostratin and bryostatin-1 are also being evaluated for efficacy in the activation of NF-κB pathways [128]. Activators of elongation factor-b such as hexamethylene bisacetamide, disulfiram and certain quinolones are being evaluated as shocking agents. Apart from these, interleukin-7, agonists of Toll like receptor-9 and novel syenthetic molecules have been identified to activate viral replication in the latent reservoirs [125, 129]. All of these transcription activators are being assessed for stand-alone use or for use in combination with inhibitors of proviral repression.

None of the agents of this attractive strategy has provided satisfactory results so far. The dosing and combinations have to be worked out to extract maximum effects out of these shocking agents. As most of the shocking agents are related to anti-cancer drugs, they are likely to have a significant adverse effect profile. The activators of the NF-κB pathway are notorious for triggering a plethora of cytokines and can cause a fatal cytokine storm if administered at higher concentrations. Another important drawback is that, even if an efficient shocking agent is identified, killing of the actively replicating virions depends on anti-retroviral drugs which are expected to lose their efficacy in the future due to the evolution and dissemination of resistant viral population. Nevertheless, this strategy has immense potential in eradicating viral reservoirs if the various setbacks are addressed over time [130].

Apart from the trial of different compounds, techniques of gene therapy have also been tried out to activate viral reservoirs with limited success. Herpes virus and lentiviral vectors loaded with genes coding for key viral proteins involved in replication were found to induce replication and release of the provirus from the latent CD4 T-cells [131]. Problems with *in vivo* administration, lack of specificity in targeting the cellular reservoir, low frequency of recombination are the various setbacks which have withheld the progress of this technology in reservoir elimination [132].

5.3. Selective cytolysis without viral reactivation

Another interesting finding pertaining to reservoir eradication is the property of the gold complex drug 'auranofin' to selectively destroy the retroviral cellular reservoir. Although developed and used as an anti-rheumatic agent, the unique 'anti-memory T-cell effect' of auranofin has kindled interest in its possible role against HIV. Auranofin exerts its cytocidal action by inducing intracellular oxidative stress. The memory T-cells with low antioxidant defenses are highly vulnerable to the oxidative stress induced by auranofin and perish along with the integrated provirus. Combination of auranofin and buthionine sulfoximine, an inhibitor of glutathione synthesis is found to act synergistically by causing further imbalance in the redox pathways [133].

Auranofin has shown promising results in studies utilizing the simian AIDS model. Simian immunodeficiency virus (SIV) infected macaques, treated with a combination regimen of auranofin, buthionine and HAART have not only shown a prolonged post treatment drug free control of viremia but also developed enhanced cell mediated immunity with SIV specific cytotoxic CD8 T-cells following treatment suspension [134, 135]. However, well designed human clinical trials are required to know more about this anti-HIV reservoir compound before its flamboyance could be translated to practicality.

5.4. Repression of latency

With the mechanism exactly opposite to the shock and kill strategy, this strategy aims at achieving viremic control by keeping the viral reservoirs continually in the inactive state. As mentioned under the shock and kill strategy, concurrent activation of the gatekeeper kinase and NF-κB favours reactivation of the provirus. The compound Jun N-terminal protein kinase inhibitor-5 which is a potent inhibitor of the gatekeeper kinase strongly prevents viral reactivation even upon strong stimulation of the NF-κB pathway under *in vitro* conditions. Inhibitors of the NF-κB pathway such as aloisine A and roscovitine also inhibit HIV reactivation to a lesser extent [128]. Various other molecules such as C-terminal truncated STAT5, Staf 50, prothymosin α, thioredoxin reductase, glucosamine and OKT-18 zinc finger protein have been identified to prolong the proviral repression. As the HIV protein 'Tat' activates proviral transcription after getting itself activated by acetylation, molecules that could specifically inhibit host cell acetylases which, eventually subdues the activity of the Tat peptide, can serve as attractive candidates for continuing viral repression [136]. Also, molecules that enhance the activity of the histone deacetylase if identified, could serve as suitable agents for this strategy [137].

5.5. Genome editing

Genome editing techniques confer the possibility of excising out specific genetic sequences from the whole genome. This novel concept is currently being used for research involving in eukaryotic genome manipulation to produce gene knockout animals. The ability of this technology to specifically excise the integrated provirus from the genome of the latent reservoir cells is being evaluated.

Three different genome editing systems are currently available such as the zinc finger nuclease (ZFN) system, the transcription activator like-effector nucleases (TALEN) system and the clustered regularly interspaced short palindromic repeat (CRISPR) with CRISPR-associated protein-9 (Cas9) known as the CRISPR/Cas9 system (Table-5). Of the three systems, the ZFN and the CRISPR/Cas9 system are being tried in the genome editing of the latent reservoir cells. *In vitro* studies employing the CRISPR/Cas9 system have demonstrated the ability of the technique to remove the HIV internal genes and suppress proviral reactivation in T cells [138]. Alternatively, studies employing the ZFN system have demonstrated the ability of the technique to excise the full length HIV proviral DNA from the infected human T cell genome [139].

This advanced technology also has its own drawbacks. The efficacy of genome editing strategies observed with different *in vitro* studies is about 30% though research work is still ongoing, addressing the challenges and improving on the efficacy. Suitable transport systems are yet to be developed for *in vivo* delivery of the editing machinery to the viral reservoir cells. All genetic editing systems have a certain proportion of 'off-target activity' where they excise out genes unrelated to the targeted site. As this can result in undesired gene modification events, the genome editing systems must be made more specific before its utilization for anti-HIV treatment [140].

6. Strategies enhancing target cell resilience to HIV infection

6.1. Replacement therapy

The discovery of HIV cure by replacement therapy happened by chance from the observations made on Timothy Brown, widely referred as the 'Berlin patient'. The patient was seropositive for HIV and had undergone an allogenic bone marrow transplant on developing acute myelogenous leukemia. Incidentally, the transplanted donor stem cells carried a homozygous

CCR5Δ32 deletion and produced T-cells with a truncated chemokine receptor CCR5 conferring resistance to infection with CCR5 utilizing virus. The patient had discontinued HAART after the transplant yet has had no detectable viremia for over five years [141]. The experiences with the Berlin patient, introduced the concept of 'sterilizing cure' which essentially comprises of eradicating all replication competent viruses from the body including the ones inside the latent reservoirs.

Replacement with resilient target cells alone does not suffice to achieve a sterilizing cure. As seen with the Berlin patient, the replacement therapy must be preceded by eradication of latent reservoirs. This has been effectively achieved in the Berlin patient by the myelo-ablative procedures prior to bone marrow transplant and continued by the graft versus host disease which occurred following the transplant [142].

Attempts to replicate the cure of the Berlin patient have not been successful so far. A similar treatment provided for two adults in Boston resulted in a brief period of aviremic state, subsequently followed by rebound viremia in both the patients. A few reasons have been postulated for the failure of sterilizing cure in the Boston patients. The first reason being, the initial myelo-ablative procedure was milder than that which was given to the Berlin patient and hence would have not effectively destroyed the viral reservoirs. Also, the donor cells transplanted to the Boston patients carried a heterozygous CCRΔ32 deletion which might allow HIV infection, when compared to the more resilient homozygous mutant cells transplanted to the Berlin patient [143].

Although well substantiated, the concept of sterilizing cure still has many lacunae. The exact correlates of protection involved in pre-transplant reservoir ablation, establishment of a graft versus host disease and homozygous versus heterozygous CCR5Δ32 deletion are yet to be identified. It has been observed that CCR5Δ32 deletion is associated with increased susceptibility to infections with West Nile virus. There may be other serious adverse effects which are to be identified before using defective CCR5 as replacement therapy for HIV infection. Another thought provoking issue is the ability of defective CCR5 in protecting infections caused by CXCR4 tropic viruses [144].

Apart from the above mentioned hurdles, the major setback which could limit the reality of this strategy is the availability of matched donors with the required mutation. Autologous bone marrow transplant has been considered to overcome these stringent requirements of allogenic transplants. Transplants of uninfected haematopoietic stem cells harvested earlier from the same person and made resilient to HIV infection by *in vitro* genetic modification (discussed below) do not confer as much protection as their allogenic counterparts. The poor performance of autologous transplants is attributed to the lack of the 'allo-effect' in clearing the infected reservoirs by establishing a graft versus host disease [145]. Hence it has to be borne in mind that replacement with resilient target cells is not a stand-alone strategy and must be compulsorily preceded by reservoir eradication procedures, in order to achieve an effective sterilizing cure.

http://dx.doi.org/10.5772/60961

6.2. DNA manipulation

Techniques of DNA manipulation have immense potential and offer a wide scope in tackling HIV. Apart from their use in peptide delivery and in the shock and kill and the genome editing strategies for reservoir elimination, the different techniques of genetic manipulation can be exploited to confer resilience to the natural target cells against HIV infection. DNA manipulatory techniques can confer CD4 T-cells with resilience to HIV infection by either modification of the natural cellular components which are utilized by HIV or by the administration of engineered genetic material which get expressed to produce HIV inhibitory peptides. The techniques utilized for this purpose include gene therapy and genome editing.

Although the term 'gene therapy' is interchangeably used to denote all the DNA and RNA based techniques, this much earlier developed technique actually involves the delivery of specific genetic elements to the target cells by a suitable vector. This is followed by homologous recombination of the transferred genetic element with the recipient cell genome and its eventual participation in transcription and translation to express the desired phenotype. However attractive it may be, the success of this technique depends on the effective recombination of the foreign gene with the target cell genome. Low frequency of recombination is the principal drawback faced with this technology [146].

The more recent gene editing techniques as mentioned earlier, comprises excising specific portions of genetic material from the target cell genome. The principle of this technology makes it a good strategy for reservoir elimination as it can cut off the unwanted proviral genes without any subsequent untoward effect. Although when used for host cell genetic manipulation, the success of these techniques relies on the identification of suitable sub-cellular targets, which on manipulation cause significant impairment of HIV replication without affecting the normal cellular function. These novel techniques are found to have a higher success rate than other dated techniques of gene therapy [140].

Though the functional mechanism differ in the techniques, they still have several processes in common. Firstly, both techniques require an effective carrier-delivery system called vectors which can deposit the genetic elements / editing machinery specifically to the cells that are to be modified. Various viral vectors utilizing adenovirus, baculovirus, canary pox virus or lentivrus have been developed for this purpose. *In vivo* use of viral vectors face the problem of antibody mediated clearance. To overcome this challenge, non viral vectors based on nanoparticles like dendrimers are being developed. Cell electroporation is yet another technique that has been developed for the *in vitro* delivery of nucleic acids into target cells [147]. The second common feature is that, both the techniques can be developed for either *in vitro* or *in vivo* use. The *in vitro* methods involve in harvesting of the cells of interest, genetic modification in laboratory conditions followed by transfusion of the modified cells to the recipient, while the *in vivo* methods rely on vector mediated delivery by active targeting of the cells of interest. Another feature of the genetic manipulation procedures is that they could be performed on either mature cells or stem cells. Modification of mature CD4 T-cells confers protection only during their life span and warrant the need for repetitive transfusions over time. On the other hand, genetically modified stem cells such as the CD34+ haematopoietic stem cells can be effective with a single transplantation as exemplified with replacement therapy [148].

Both techniques attempt to make the target cells resilient to HIV infection by either modifying the cell surface components required for HIV entry or by altering the intracellular contents which are utilized by the virus during replication, or a combination of both. Strategies involved in limiting viral entry by surface component modification possess certain remarkable advantages. It has been detected that among all HIV related cell death events, over 95% are caused by apoptosis initiated by the cells immediately after viral entry [149]. Hence, the target cells can be saved from committing 'suicide' if they are made impervious to viral entry.

With the serendipitous discovery of its curative effects in the Berlin patient, CCR5 which acts as the co-receptor for HIV entry is the most sought-after target for genetic modification. A homozygous deletion of a specific 32 base pair sequence from the CCR5 gene confers complete protection, while a heterozygous deletion of the same nucleic acids confers partial protection from HIV entry, without causing any glaring change in the CD4 T-cell function. All the three systems of gene editing namely the ZFN, the TALEN and the CRISPR/Cas9 system are being evaluated for this purpose and are found to have nearly 50% efficacy in disrupting CCR5 in mature CD4 T-cells and around 25% efficacy in adult haematopoietic stem cells. In this regard, it is intriguing to use induced pluripotent stem (iPS) cells to introduce delta32-like mutation and test their viral resistance. *In vitro* studies of CXCR4 disruption has also shown promising results but this might not serve the purpose *in vivo*, as the deletion is expected to cause functional derangement.[140]. Yet another instance of gene therapy under human trials is the SB-728-T, a zinc finger DNA-binding transcription factor. It binds to the DNA of target cells and disrupts the gene responsible for CCR5 co-receptor production [150]. Apart from the ones mentioned here, there are numerous other techniques of DNA manipulation, RNA based and peptide based techniques being tried to harness the potential of CCR5 alteration in curtailing HIV infection (Table 5).

The target cells can also be made resistant to HIV infection by increasing the expression of intracellular factors that restrict the viral replication process. TRIM5α, APOBEC3G and tetherin are the well known restriction factors of HIV infection. TRIM5α is a cytoplasmic protein which inhibits HIV by binding with the incoming capsid and preventing further the process of replication. The APOBEC3 family of mRNA editing proteins, especially the APOBEC3G inhibits HIV replication by introducing lethal mutations during reverse transcription. Tetherin is another host cellular protein involved in HIV restriction by preventing the release of viral progeny from the infected cell.[151] As the vif and vpu proteins of the virus neutralize the effect of APOBEC3G and tetherin respectively, they can be made resistant to their respective viral proteins by introducing point mutations. Single amino acid substitution, D128K in APOBEC3G and T45I in tetherin makes them overcome the viral factors vif and vpu respectively. Gene therapy techniques to increase the expression of TRIM5α and mutated APOBEC3G and tetherin in CD4 T-cells are known to enhance their resilience to HIV infection. Mov 10 and CPSF6 are the newer restriction factors that are being considered for development in this strategy [106, 152]. Recently, the interferon inducible family of proteins called the myxovirus resistance proteins (Mxs) have been identified as potent restriction factors which

http://dx.doi.org/10.5772/60961

act by inhibiting HIV uncoating [153]. Also, TSG-101 the intracellular protein derivative of tumor susceptibility gene has been identified to inhibit the HIV protein p6 thereby blocking viral budding and release [154]. These proteins could possibly serve as candidates for anti-retroviral gene therapy.

Administration and expression of extraneous genetic material can also confer resistance to the target cells against HIV. Much of recent interest is towards the surface modification using the synthetic peptide 'C46'. When expressed on the CD4 T-cell surface, this peptide binds with gp41 of the approaching virions and prevents envelope fusion. Stable expression of C46 can be achieved on CD4 T-cells following delivery of the corresponding gene using retroviral vectors. As the cells made resilient by CCR5 alteration alone remain vulnerable to CXCR4 tropic viruses and the reverse also holds good, C46 can be effectively used to inhibit infection with both of the viral strains [152]. Extraneously administered genetic material coding for dominant negative inhibitory proteins of HIV replication such as the M-10 and those coding for intrabodies and intrakines can also cause favourable intracellular modifications in the T-cells making them resistant to HIV infection [148].

Newer studies advocate the combination of both surface and intracellular modifications of the target cells to obtain improved resilience against HIV [147]. Apart from their role in enhancing resilience to HIV infection, techniques of genetic manipulation are also useful in conferring resistance to viral integration and thereby restricting the reservoir formation [155]. Although the techniques of genetic manipulation has numerous setbacks; poor frequency of recombination faced with gene therapy, unwanted off-target effects and double strand break induced apoptosis occurring with gene editing are the principal challenges that have to be overcome. Nevertheless, few of these techniques have entered into clinical trials and give hope for a promising future [152]. Apart from their use in therapeutic strategies, techniques of gene therapy are being evaluated in DNA vaccines for prophylactic use and also in some of the strategies of 'immune therapy' [156].

6.3. RNA based mechanisms

Studies employing RNA based therapeutics such as antisense oligonucleotides, RNAi, ribozymes and aptamers have shown to be effective in down-regulation of CCR5 and subsequent inhibition of HIV replication in humanized mice [106, 157]. Of all the above mentioned technqiues, silencing of CCR5 using RNAi is the most widely studied. RNAi techniques have also been studied for the downregulation of other cellular factors of HIV replication such as CXCR4, CD4, NF-κB, LEDGF/p75 and DDX-3 [158].

RNAi techniques for host cell modulation are devoid of the problem of viral escape mutants that is faced, when the same technique is employed for inhibiting viral targets. However, the adverse effects faced with these techniqiues are due to loss of other essential functions of the target cell as a consequence of cellular factor silencing. Increased susceptibility to West Nile virus infections has been observed with the loss of CCR5 function. CXCR4 downregulation can disrupt the homeostasis of the lymphopoietic pathway as these receptors are essential for the homing of stem cells into bone marrow and their subsequent differentiation into T-cells [159].

Hence, the success of this strategy depends on the identification of suitable cellular co-factors of HIV infection which can be down regulated without altering the normal cellular physiology. In the search for such targets, genome wide profiling studies have revealed numerous previously unknown cellular factors that participate in HIV infection. Subsequent knock down studies have validated the effectiveness of silencing these factors for limiting HIV replication [160-162]. Further studies are needed to reveal the adverse effects following the knock down of these novel cellular factors.

The technique related pitfalls are the same as the ones mentioned earlier, which include the problems faced with delivery of inhibitory RNAs into specific target cells, off-target effects of the inhibitory RNAs and cytotoxicity to the administered cell. As of date, only one RNAi technique has entered clinical trial. The technique was designed to inhibit both viral (tat protein and TAR RNA) and cellular factors (CCR5). However, the trial was terminated in phase-0 and the results were not disclosed [163]. Table-5 broadly summarizes all the nucleic acid based therapeutics that are currently being tried against HIV.

Type	**Cells targeted**	**Phase acted on**	**Mechanism**		**Technique employed**
DNA based techniques	Infected reservoirs (In vivo)	Elimination of latent reservoirs	Direct excision of integrated proviral DNA		Genome editing systems - CRISPR/Cas9, ZFN and TALEN
			Activation of viral replication (Shock and kill)		Gene therapy - Vectors based delivery of genes coding for viral proteins of replication
	Uninfected susceptible cells (In vivo / In vitro)	Diversion of natural course of infection to make the target cells resilient	Modification of normal cellular components	Cell surface modifications	Genome editing systems - CRISPR/Cas9, ZFN and TALEN to knock out cellular co-factors that support HIV replication
				Intracellular modifications	
			Expression of novel protective proteins	Cell surface expression	Gene therapy - Vector based delivery of cDNA of novel peptides followed by their recombination and expression
				Intracellular expression	
RNA based techniques	Actively infected cells (In vivo)	Inhibition of active viral replication	Inhibition of viral mRNA		Agents of RNA interference (siRNA and shRNA) and to a lesser extent other RNA based techniques (Antisense oligonucleotides, ribozymes and aptamers) delivered in viral / non-viral vectors to the desired target cells by active targeting
			Inhibition of host cellular factors involved in viral replication		
	Uninfected susceptible cells (*In vivo / In vitro*)	Diversion of natural course of infection to make the target cells resilient	Modification of normal cellular components	Cell surface modifications	
				Intracellular modifications	

Table 5. Nucleic acid based therapeutics for HIV infection

7. The 'receptor decoy' strategy

The receptor decoy strategy is a novel concept which helps to salvage the natural target cells of HIV by diverting the virus to infect decoy particles, thereby altering the natural course of HIV infection. This involves the usage of decoy cells termed 'cancellers', which possess HIV entry receptors on their surface and do not contain the machinery required for retro-viral replication. The cancellers (Figure-2) intend to function as decoys and get infected by the free HIV virions thereby preventing the infection of the natural target cells. Apart from protection of the natural target cells, the cancellers also serve to limit viremia as the trapped virions cannot replicate inside the cancellers due to the absence of replication machinery. Optionally, the trapped virions could be destroyed by packing anti-viral agents within the cancellers [164].

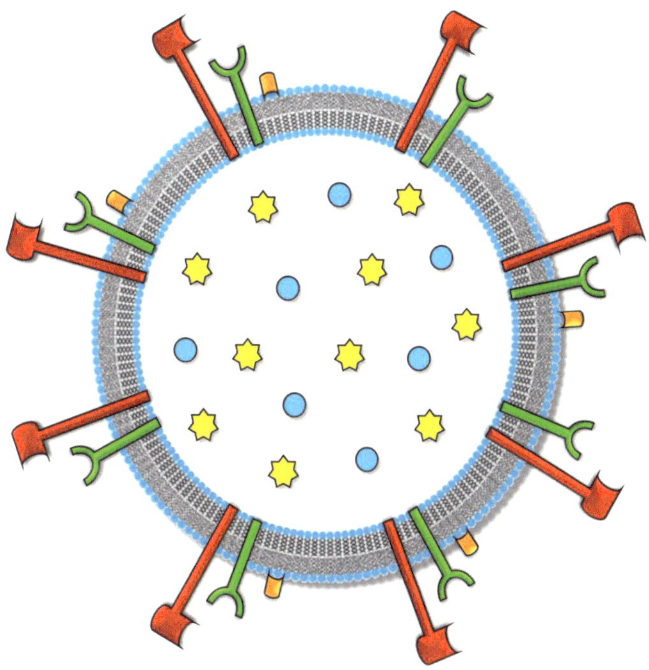

Figure 2. Schematic representation of a canceller particle. RBC particle reconstituted with receptors on the membrane surface and loaded with various molecules. CD4 (red) and CCR5 (green) receptors are involved in the active targeting of HIV virions. Accessory surface molecules (orange) may be added to enhance the fusion process and/or to prevent elimination of the canceller by reticulo-endothelial system. Molecules capable of viral destruction (blue spheres and yellow stars) such as protein and RNA damaging agents are packed within the canceller.

The superiority of the receptor decoy strategy over the conventional anti-retroviral drugs is that it mimics natural conditions and is thereby devoid of the 'adverse factor' effect in selecting out resistance. This attractive strategy is in the concept phase and more discussions and comments could be made only after its implementation. Similar strategies employing modified erythrocytes or nanoparticles as viral traps are being studied for their use against HIV [164].

8. Immune based therapies

Since the discovery of HIV repeated attempts to achieve effective protection using conventional methods of immunoprophylaxis have resulted in outright failure. The failure of the preventive strategies has lead to the concept of 'immunotherapy' or 'immune based therapy'. This strategy involves in the manipulation of the immune system in a therapeutic motive to eliminate the already acquired infection, rather than preventing new infection. The immune based therapies involve in enhancing the potency of the immune system to counteract HIV by reducing inflammation, preventing immune activation by HIV-1 or promoting effective immune responses against HIV. The different modalities used to achieve this effect can be broadly classified into non-HIV antigen specific therapies and those which use the HIV antigens (Table-6)[6, 165].

None of the immune based therapies have provided satisfactory results so far. Among the available methods of immunotherapy, HIV specific CTL induction using the dendritic cells is of recent interest and appears to be a promising strategy. Recent studies reveal that a therapeutic vaccine using autologous monocyte-derived dendritic cells pulsed with heat-inactivated whole HIV, stimulated anti-HIV immune response and shifted the virus/host balance in favor of the host when administered to patients on HAART with CD4+ T-cell count >450 cells/mm. At week 12 after ART interruption, 55% of people in the vaccinated group represented decrease of their viral load by at least 10-fold or 90%, compared with just 9% in the control group receiving non-pulsed DCs. These proportions dropped to 35% and 0%, respectively at week 24. This significant decrease in plasma viral load observed in vaccinated recipients was associated with a consistent increase in HIV-1-specific T cell responses. These data indicate that HIV-1-specific immune responses are elicited by the therapeutic DC vaccination. This could significantly reduce plasma viremia after ART interruption in HIV patients chronically infected but controlled with sufficiently high CD4 numbers. Thus, this study warrants further investigation with new candidates and/or new optimized strategies of vaccination toward the final goal to achieve a functional cure of HIV infection. Although heat-inactivated whole HIV was used as the antigen in this strategy, direct expression of the mRNA derived from patient's cells can also be considered using DCs in the immune therapy which expects highly precise antiviral efficacy targeting not only HIV but also non-viral antigens [166].

9. Complementary and alternative therapies

It is a common feature that people living with HIV or AIDS across the world resort to products and practices that are not presently considered to be part of conventional anti-retroviral medicine. When these are used together with conventional anti-retroviral medications, they are referred to as complementary therapies and if used as a stand-alone modality instead of conventional medications, they are referred to as alternative therapies [167]. A plethora of complementary and alternative strategies are available from all over the world which predominantly involves the use of natural products and/or mind and body practices. Herbal

http://dx.doi.org/10.5772/60961

Types	Components	Examples	Mechanism
Non-antigen specific therapies	Cytokines	Interleukin-2 (Proleukin)	Augmentation of CD4 T-cell proliferation and cytolytic function of CD8 T-cells
		Interleukin-7	Improvement of T-cell homeostasis
		Interleukin-12	Enhancement of Th1 response and increasing the cytotoxic activity of T-cells and NK cells against virally infected cells
		Interleukin-15	Expansion of effector and memory subsets of CD* T-cells
		Interleukin-21	Proliferation and enhancement of the cytolytic potential of effector CD8 T-cells
	Drugs	Chloroquine	Reduction of IFN-α in order to reduce the immune activation to prevent depletion of CD4 T-cells and progression to AIDS
		Hydroxy chloroquine	
		Aspirin	Reduction of T-cell activation due to its broad anti-inflammatory property
		Celecoxib	Inhibition of cyclo-oxygenase type-2 enzyme to reduce T-cell activation
	Antibodies	Anti-CD4 (Ibalizumab)	Competitive inhibition of viral entry receptors
		Anti-CCR5	Competitive inhibition of viral entry receptors
		Anti-PD-1	Blockage of the negative co-stimulatory molecules PD-1 and CLTA4 on the surface of T-cells to prevent CD8 T-cell dysfunction and enhancement of CD4 T-cell proliferation
		Anti-CLTA4	
	Prebiotics and probiotics		Modulation of the gut microbiome and amelioration of HIV induced mucosal damage
Antigen specific therapies	Vaccines	Inactivated whole virus	gp120 depleted, inactivated HIV strain with incomplete Freund's adjuvant
		Antigenic sub-units of HIV	Recombinant immunodominant proteins of HIV with suitable adjuvants
		Viral vectors expressing HIV antigens	Various HIV specific antigens expressed on different viral vectors
		DNA	Plasmids containing one or more genetic determinants coding for HIV proteins
		Dendritic cell	Delivery of viral antigens to dendritic cells to ensure activation of both CD4 and CD8 T-cells

Table 6. Immune based therapies being developed against HIV

remedies derived from the ancient medical science forms of different countries are the most widely sought after modality of complementary or alternative therapies. The various mind and body techniques include spirituality, meditation, yoga and other body manipulatory procedures, acupuncture and energy therapies [168].

Observations across the globe reveal that 30 - 90% of the HIV infected patients seek for complementary or alternative therapies of which, majority are females and educated individuals [169, 170]. The usefulness of these therapies is controversial. Spiritual methods such as prayer, faith healing and meditation are found to improve the psychological state by helping to overcome anxiety, depression and stress thereby providing a feeling of well being [171]. The compound IGM-1, obtained from herbs used in traditional medicine was observed to alleviate the symptoms of HIV infection but did not have any effect in reduction of viremia or improving the immune status. Many of the other Chinese herbal medicines tested were found to be unsatisfactory in altering the viral and immune parameters [172]. To much despair, several studies have highlighted the deleterious effects of complementary and alternative medicines. Recent reports indicate that patients on concurrent complementary therapy have reduced adherence rate to conventional anti-retroviral therapeutic regimens [173]. Homeopathy, a traditional health system has been proven ineffective for the treatment of HIV infection and has been disregarded by the WHO [174]. Herbal preparations containing St. John's Wort and those containing garlic extracts reduce the therapeutic levels of conventional anti-retrovirals. Apart from reducing the efficacy, many other herbal preparations have also been observed to increase the HAART related side effects [169].

Despite these assumptions, complementary and alternative therapies cannot be totally overlooked. This is due to the fact that natural compounds with antiretroviral property such as indirubin monoxime and tanshinone II A have been isolated from herbal medications [80, 81]. Meta analyses on the efficacy of herbal preparations have yielded only inconclusive results but not ineffective [172, 175]. Hence rigorous clinical trials including large study population are required to refute or accept the potential benefits of these therapeutic modalities. National Centre for Complementary and Alternative medicine, a division of the National Institute of Health, USA is an organization dedicated for research in alternative and complementary medicines and thus provides funding to various studies in this field [167].

10. Conclusions

The HAART has played its crucial role in curtailing the HIV pandemic so far. However, its inability to eliminate the infection and the rise of resistant mutants is a fundamental challenge. This has initiated the frantic search for novel compounds and strategies to counteract HIV. Desperate measures have resulted in the discovery of a plethora of anti-retroviral compounds and strategies, but none could be unanimously agreed upon as completely reliable. The much hyped functional cure concept has taken a big blow with the occurrence of rebound viremia in the Mississippi baby. Moreso, studies to replicate the sterilizing cure of the Berlin patient have provided disappointing results. Despite the development of various novel antiviral

http://dx.doi.org/10.5772/60961

compounds, HIV is well set before-hand to readily evolve and overcome all anti-viral actions. Novel techniques such as gene therapy, gene editing, RNA interference, anti-retroviral peptides may have sound concepts and appear attractive but in reality they face numerous roadblocks. By virtue of the ability to undergo rapid genetic evolution and the tendency to establish latent reservoirs, HIV has thwarted all the overcoming attempts. Currently, efforts are being stepped-up by scientist globally to overcome the challenges discussed herein, though the strategy(ies) may face limitations today but they still have the potential to achieve the required success of sustained functional cure.

Acknowledgements

This work was supported by NUS SoM Start-up Grant (R-182-000- 160-733, R-182-000-160 -133) to N.Y.

Author details

Jeremiah Stanley[1*] and Naoki Yamamoto[2]

*Address all correspondence to: naoki_yamamoto@nuhs.edu.sg

1 Department of Microbiology, Velammal Medical College Hospital and Research Institute, Anuppanadi, Madurai, Tamil Nadu, India

2 Translational ID Laboratory, Department of Mcirobiology, National University of Singapore, #-02 Centre for Translational Medicine, Singapore

References

[1] Williams SA, Greene WC: Regulation of HIV-1 latency by T-cell activation. *Cytokine* 2007, 39(1):63-74.

[2] Kulkosky J, Pomerantz RJ: Approaching eradication of highly active antiretroviral therapy-persistent human immunodeficiency virus type 1 reservoirs with immune activation therapy. *Clin Infect Dis* 2002, 35(12):1520-1526.

[3] Harada S, Koyanagi Y, Yamamoto N: Infection of HTLV-III/LAV in HTLV-I-carrying cells MT-2 and MT-4 and application in a plaque assay. *Science* 1985, 229(4713): 563-566.

[4] Matsuyama T, Kobayashi N, Yamamoto N: Cytokines and HIV infection: is AIDS a tumor necrosis factor disease? *Aids* 1991, 5(12):1405-1417.

[5] Tanvir FA, Spivak AM: HIV beyond HAART: Current Strategies for HIV Eradication. *J AIDS Clinic Res* 2012, S6-001:1-6.

[6] Vanham G, Van Gulck E: Can immunotherapy be useful as a "functional cure" for infection with Human Immunodeficiency Virus-1? *Retrovirology* 2012, 9:72.

[7] Researchers describe first 'functional HIV cure' in an infant. *J Miss State Med Assoc* 2013, 54(4):111-112.

[8] Persaud D, Gay H, Ziemniak C, Chen YH, Piatak M, Jr., Chun TW, Strain M, Richman D, Luzuriaga K: Absence of detectable HIV-1 viremia after treatment cessation in an infant. *N Engl J Med* 2013, 369(19):1828-1835.

[9] Saez-Cirion A, Bacchus C, Hocqueloux L, Avettand-Fenoel V, Girault I, Lecuroux C, Potard V, Versmisse P, Melard A, Prazuck T *et al*: Post-treatment HIV-1 controllers with a long-term virological remission after the interruption of early initiated antiretroviral therapy ANRS VISCONTI Study. *PLoS Pathog* 2013, 9(3):e1003211.

[10] vanLunzen J, zurWiesch JS, Schumacher U, Hauber I, Hauber J: Functional cure after long term HAART initiated during early HIV infection: a comprehensive case study. In: *7th IAS conference on HIV pathogenesis, treatment and prevention: 2013; Kuala Lumpur, Malaysia.*

[11] Dolgin E: New, intensive trials planned on heels of Mississippi HIV 'cure'. *Nat Med* 2013, 19(4):380-381.

[12] Siliciano JD, Siliciano RF: AIDS/HIV. Rekindled HIV infection. *Science* 2014, 345(6200):1005-1006.

[13] Parboosing R, Maguire GE, Govender P, Kruger HG: Nanotechnology and the treatment of HIV infection. *Viruses* 2012, 4(4):488-520.

[14] Murray JM, Kelleher AD, Cooper DA: Timing of the components of the HIV life cycle in productively infected CD4+ T cells in a population of HIV-infected individuals. *J Virol* 2011, 85(20):10798-10805.

[15] Siccardi M, Martin P, McDonald TO, Liptrott NJ, Giardiello M, Rannard S, Owen A: Nanomedicines for HIV therapy. *Ther Deliv* 2013, 4(2):153-156.

[16] Lenjisa JL, Woldu MA, Satessa GD: New hope for eradication of HIV from the body: the role of polymeric nanomedicines in HIV/AIDS pharmacotherapy. *J Nanobiotechnology* 2014, 12:9.

[17] Sharma P, Garg S: Pure drug and polymer based nanotechnologies for the improved solubility, stability, bioavailability and targeting of anti-HIV drugs. *Adv Drug Deliv Rev* 2010, 62(4-5):491-502.

[18] FDA-Approved HIV Medicines [http://aidsinfo.nih.gov/education-materials/fact-sheets/21/58/fda-approved-hiv-medicines](accessed 24th October 2014).

[19] AIDSinfo Drug Database. In.: National Institute of Health; 2014. http://aidsinfo.nih.gov/drugs.

[20] Flexner C, Saag M: The antiretroviral drug pipeline: prospects and implications for future treatment research. *Curr Opin HIV AIDS* 2013, 8(6):572-578.

[21] Saag MS: New and investigational antiretroviral drugs for HIV infection: mechanisms of action and early research findings. *Top Antivir Med* 2012, 20(5):162-167.

[22] Cohen CJ, Meyers JL, Davis KL: Association between daily antiretroviral pill burden and treatment adherence, hospitalisation risk, and other healthcare utilisation and costs in a US medicaid population with HIV. *BMJ Open* 2013, 3(8).

[23] Bodiwala HS, Sabde S, Gupta P, Mukherjee R, Kumar R, Garg P, Bhutani KK, Mitra D, Singh IP: Design and synthesis of caffeoyl-anilides as portmanteau inhibitors of HIV-1 integrase and CCR5. *Bioorg Med Chem* 2011, 19(3):1256-1263.

[24] Zeldin RK, Petruschke RA: Pharmacological and therapeutic properties of ritonavir-boosted protease inhibitor therapy in HIV-infected patients. *J Antimicrob Chemother* 2004, 53(1):4-9.

[25] Mathias AA, German P, Murray BP, Wei L, Jain A, West S, Warren D, Hui J, Kearney BP: Pharmacokinetics and pharmacodynamics of GS-9350: a novel pharmacokinetic enhancer without anti-HIV activity. *Clin Pharmacol Ther* 2010, 87(3):322-329.

[26] Lori F, Foli A, Groff A, Lova L, Whitman L, Bakare N, Pollard RB, Lisziewicz J: Optimal suppression of HIV replication by low-dose hydroxyurea through the combination of antiviral and cytostatic ('virostatic') mechanisms. *Aids* 2005, 19(11):1173-1181.

[27] Lori F, Foli A, Kelly LM, Lisziewicz J: Virostatics: a new class of anti-HIV drugs. *Curr Med Chem* 2007, 14(2):233-241.

[28] Hossain MM, Margolis DM: Inhibition of HIV replication by A77 1726, the active metabolite of leflunomide, in combination with pyrimidine nucleoside reverse transcriptase inhibitors. *J Acquir Immune Defic Syndr* 2001, 28(2):199-201.

[29] Read SW, DeGrezia M, Ciccone EJ, DerSimonian R, Higgins J, Adelsberger JW, Starling JM, Rehm C, Sereti I: The effect of leflunomide on cycling and activation of T-cells in HIV-1-infected participants. *PLoS One* 2010, 5(8):e11937.

[30] Zhou N, Nowicka-Sans B, McAuliffe B, Ray N, Eggers B, Fang H, Fan L, Healy M, Langley DR, Hwang C *et al*: Genotypic correlates of susceptibility to HIV-1 attachment inhibitor BMS-626529, the active agent of the prodrug BMS-663068. *J Antimicrob Chemother* 2014, 69(3):573-581.

[31] Hanna GJ, Lalezari J, Hellinger JA, Wohl DA, Nettles R, Persson A, Krystal M, Lin P, Colonno R, Grasela DM: Antiviral activity, pharmacokinetics, and safety of BMS-488043, a novel oral small-molecule HIV-1 attachment inhibitor, in HIV-1-infected subjects. *Antimicrob Agents Chemother* 2011, 55(2):722-728.

[32] Liu T, Huang B, Zhan P, De Clercq E, Liu X: Discovery of small molecular inhibitors targeting HIV-1 gp120-CD4 interaction drived from BMS-378806. *Eur J Med Chem* 2014, 86:481-490.

[33] Duong YT, Meadows DC, Srivastava IK, Gervay-Hague J, North TW: Direct inactivation of human immunodeficiency virus type 1 by a novel small-molecule entry inhibitor, DCM205. *Antimicrob Agents Chemother* 2007, 51(5):1780-1786.

[34] Takeda-Hirokawa N, Neoh LP, Akimoto H, Kaneko H, Hishikawa T, Sekigawa I, Hashimoto H, Hirose S, Murakami T, Yamamoto N *et al*: Role of curdlan sulfate in the binding of HIV-1 gp120 to CD4 molecules and the production of gp120-mediated TNF-alpha. *Microbiol Immunol* 1997, 41(9):741-745.

[35] Mosi RM, Anastassova V, Cox J, Darkes MC, Idzan SR, Labrecque J, Lau G, Nelson KL, Patel K, Santucci Z *et al*: The molecular pharmacology of AMD11070: an orally bioavailable CXCR4 HIV entry inhibitor. *Biochem Pharmacol* 2012, 83(4):472-479.

[36] Murakami T, Nakajima T, Koyanagi Y, Tachibana K, Fujii N, Tamamura H, Yoshida N, Waki M, Matsumoto A, Yoshie O *et al*: A small molecule CXCR4 inhibitor that blocks T cell line-tropic HIV-1 infection. *J Exp Med* 1997, 186(8):1389-1393.

[37] Ichiyama K, Yokoyama-Kumakura S, Tanaka Y, Tanaka R, Hirose K, Bannai K, Edamatsu T, Yanaka M, Niitani Y, Miyano-Kurosaki N *et al*: A duodenally absorbable CXC chemokine receptor 4 antagonist, KRH-1636, exhibits a potent and selective anti-HIV-1 activity. *Proc Natl Acad Sci U S A* 2003, 100(7):4185-4190.

[38] Lamorte L, Titolo S, Lemke CT, Goudreau N, Mercier JF, Wardrop E, Shah VB, von Schwedler UK, Langelier C, Banik SS *et al*: Discovery of novel small-molecule HIV-1 replication inhibitors that stabilize capsid complexes. *Antimicrob Agents Chemother* 2013, 57(10):4622-4631.

[39] Li J, Chen J, Zhang L, Wang F, Gui C, Qin Y, Xu Q, Liu H, Nan F, Shen J *et al*: One novel quinoxaline derivative as a potent human cyclophilin A inhibitor shows highly inhibitory activity against mouse spleen cell proliferation. *Bioorg Med Chem* 2006, 14(16):5527-5534.

[40] Blair WS, Pickford C, Irving SL, Brown DG, Anderson M, Bazin R, Cao J, Ciaramella G, Isaacson J, Jackson L *et al*: HIV capsid is a tractable target for small molecule therapeutic intervention. *PLoS Pathog* 2010, 6(12):e1001220.

[41] Shi J, Zhou J, Shah VB, Aiken C, Whitby K: Small-molecule inhibition of human immunodeficiency virus type 1 infection by virus capsid destabilization. *J Virol* 2011, 85(1):542-549.

[42] Kortagere S, Madani N, Mankowski MK, Schon A, Zentner I, Swaminathan G, Princiotto A, Anthony K, Oza A, Sierra LJ *et al*: Inhibiting early-stage events in HIV-1 replication by small-molecule targeting of the HIV-1 capsid. *J Virol* 2012, 86(16): 8472-8481.

[43] Gordon RK, Ginalski K, Rudnicki WR, Rychlewski L, Pankaskie MC, Bujnicki JM, Chiang PK: Anti-HIV-1 activity of 3-deaza-adenosine analogs. Inhibition of S-adenosylhomocysteine hydrolase and nucleotide congeners. *Eur J Biochem* 2003, 270(17): 3507-3517.

[44] Dapp MJ, Bonnac L, Patterson SE, Mansky LM: Discovery of novel ribonucleoside analogs with activity against human immunodeficiency virus type 1. *J Virol* 2014, 88(1):354-363.

[45] Evans D: KP-1461: a novel anti-HIV drug in limbo? *Beta* 2010, 22(2):9-11.

[46] Mathiesen S, Dam E, Roge B, Joergensen LB, Laursen AL, Gerstoft J, Clavel F: Long-term foscarnet therapy remodels thymidine analogue mutations and alters resistance to zidovudine and lamivudine in HIV-1. *Antivir Ther* 2007, 12(3):335-343.

[47] Mousseau G, Valente S: Strategies to Block HIV Transcription: Focus on Small Molecule Tat Inhibitors. *Biology (Basel)* 2012, 1(3):668-697.

[48] Schuller A, Suhartono M, Fechner U, Tanrikulu Y, Breitung S, Scheffer U, Gobel MW, Schneider G: The concept of template-based de novo design from drug-derived molecular fragments and its application to TAR RNA. *J Comput Aided Mol Des* 2008, 22(2):59-68.

[49] Zeng L, Li J, Muller M, Yan S, Mujtaba S, Pan C, Wang Z, Zhou MM: Selective small molecules blocking HIV-1 Tat and coactivator PCAF association. *J Am Chem Soc* 2005, 127(8):2376-2377.

[50] Ali A, Ghosh A, Nathans RS, Sharova N, O'Brien S, Cao H, Stevenson M, Rana TM: Identification of flavopiridol analogues that selectively inhibit positive transcription elongation factor (P-TEFb) and block HIV-1 replication. *Chembiochem* 2009, 10(12): 2072-2080.

[51] Biglione S, Byers SA, Price JP, Nguyen VT, Bensaude O, Price DH, Maury W: Inhibition of HIV-1 replication by P-TEFb inhibitors DRB, seliciclib and flavopiridol correlates with release of free P-TEFb from the large, inactive form of the complex. *Retrovirology* 2007, 4:47.

[52] Agbottah E, de La Fuente C, Nekhai S, Barnett A, Gianella-Borradori A, Pumfery A, Kashanchi F: Antiviral activity of CYC202 in HIV-1-infected cells. *J Biol Chem* 2005, 280(4):3029-3042.

[53] Debebe Z, Ammosova T, Breuer D, Lovejoy DB, Kalinowski DS, Kumar K, Jerebtsova M, Ray P, Kashanchi F, Gordeuk VR *et al*: Iron chelators of the di-2-pyridylketone thiosemicarbazone and 2-benzoylpyridine thiosemicarbazone series inhibit HIV-1 transcription: identification of novel cellular targets--iron, cyclin-dependent kinase (CDK) 2, and CDK9. *Mol Pharmacol* 2011, 79(1):185-196.

[54] Mantelingu K, Reddy BA, Swaminathan V, Kishore AH, Siddappa NB, Kumar GV, Nagashankar G, Natesh N, Roy S, Sadhale PP *et al*: Specific inhibition of p300-HAT

alters global gene expression and represses HIV replication. *Chem Biol* 2007, 14(6): 645-657.

[55] Hole AJ, Baumli S, Shao H, Shi S, Huang S, Pepper C, Fischer PM, Wang S, Endicott JA, Noble ME: Comparative structural and functional studies of 4-(thiazol-5-yl)-2-(phenylamino)pyrimidine-5-carbonitrile CDK9 inhibitors suggest the basis for isotype selectivity. *J Med Chem* 2013, 56(3):660-670.

[56] Chugh P, Bradel-Tretheway B, Monteiro-Filho CM, Planelles V, Maggirwar SB, Dewhurst S, Kim B: Akt inhibitors as an HIV-1 infected macrophage-specific anti-viral therapy. *Retrovirology* 2008, 5:11.

[57] Tremblay-Letourneau M, Despins S, Bougie I, Bisaillon M: Virtual high-throughput screening identifies mycophenolic acid as a novel RNA capping inhibitor. *PLoS One* 2011, 6(9):e24806.

[58] Daelemans D, Afonina E, Nilsson J, Werner G, Kjems J, De Clercq E, Pavlakis GN, Vandamme AM: A synthetic HIV-1 Rev inhibitor interfering with the CRM1-mediated nuclear export. *Proc Natl Acad Sci U S A* 2002, 99(22):14440-14445.

[59] Soto-Rifo R, Rubilar PS, Ohlmann T: The DEAD-box helicase DDX3 substitutes for the cap-binding protein eIF4E to promote compartmentalized translation initiation of the HIV-1 genomic RNA. *Nucleic Acids Res* 2013, 41(12):6286-6299.

[60] Maga G, Falchi F, Radi M, Botta L, Casaluce G, Bernardini M, Irannejad H, Manetti F, Garbelli A, Samuele A *et al*: Toward the discovery of novel anti-HIV drugs. Second-generation inhibitors of the cellular ATPase DDX3 with improved anti-HIV activity: synthesis, structure-activity relationship analysis, cytotoxicity studies, and target validation. *ChemMedChem* 2011, 6(8):1371-1389.

[61] Lemke CT, Titolo S, von Schwedler U, Goudreau N, Mercier JF, Wardrop E, Faucher AM, Coulombe R, Banik SS, Fader L *et al*: Distinct effects of two HIV-1 capsid assembly inhibitor families that bind the same site within the N-terminal domain of the viral CA protein. *J Virol* 2012, 86(12):6643-6655.

[62] Khoury G, Ewart G, Luscombe C, Miller M, Wilkinson J: Antiviral efficacy of the novel compound BIT225 against HIV-1 release from human macrophages. *Antimicrob Agents Chemother* 2010, 54(2):835-845.

[63] Martin DE, Salzwedel K, Allaway GP: Bevirimat: a novel maturation inhibitor for the treatment of HIV-1 infection. *Antivir Chem Chemother* 2008, 19(3):107-113.

[64] Charvat TT, Lee DJ, Robinson WE, Chamberlin AR: Design, synthesis, and biological evaluation of chicoric acid analogs as inhibitors of HIV-1 integrase. *Bioorg Med Chem* 2006, 14(13):4552-4567.

[65] Ali A, Wang J, Nathans RS, Cao H, Sharova N, Stevenson M, Rana TM: Synthesis and structure-activity relationship studies of HIV-1 virion infectivity factor (Vif) inhibitors that block viral replication. *ChemMedChem* 2012, 7(7):1217-1229.

[66] Nathans R, Cao H, Sharova N, Ali A, Sharkey M, Stranska R, Stevenson M, Rana TM: Small-molecule inhibition of HIV-1 Vif. *Nat Biotechnol* 2008, 26(10):1187-1192.

[67] Zuo T, Liu D, Lv W, Wang X, Wang J, Lv M, Huang W, Wu J, Zhang H, Jin H *et al*: Small-molecule inhibition of human immunodeficiency virus type 1 replication by targeting the interaction between Vif and ElonginC. *J Virol* 2012, 86(10):5497-5507.

[68] Ejima T, Hirota M, Mizukami T, Otsuka M, Fujita M: An anti-HIV-1 compound that increases steady-state expression of apoplipoprotein B mRNA-editing enzyme-catalytic polypeptide-like 3G. *Int J Mol Med* 2011, 28(4):613-616.

[69] Li J, Tan Z, Tang S, Hewlett I, Pang R, He M, He S, Tian B, Chen K, Yang M: Discovery of dual inhibitors targeting both HIV-1 capsid and human cyclophilin A to inhibit the assembly and uncoating of the viral capsid. *Bioorg Med Chem* 2009, 17(8): 3177-3188.

[70] Tian B, He M, Tang S, Hewlett I, Tan Z, Li J, Jin Y, Yang M: Synthesis and antiviral activities of novel acylhydrazone derivatives targeting HIV-1 capsid protein. *Bioorg Med Chem Lett* 2009, 19(8):2162-2167.

[71] Ceragenix Enters into Agreement to License CSA-54 and other Ceragenin Compounds To Biopharmaceutical Company for HIV and STD App. In: *FierceBiotech.* 2014.

[72] Hanauske-Abel HM, Saxena D, Palumbo PE, Hanauske AR, Luchessi AD, Cambiaghi TD, Hoque M, Spino M, D'Alliessi Gandolfi D, Heller DS *et al*: Drug-induced reactivation of apoptosis abrogates HIV-1 infection. *PLoS One* 2013, 8(9):e74414.

[73] Dang Z, Ho P, Zhu L, Qian K, Lee KH, Huang L, Chen CH: New betulinic acid derivatives for bevirimat-resistant human immunodeficiency virus type-1. *J Med Chem* 2013, 56(5):2029-2037.

[74] Khan MTH, Ather A: Lead Molecules from Natural Products, Discovery and New Trends, First edn. New York: Elsevier; 2006.

[75] De Clercq E: Current lead natural products for the chemotherapy of human immunodeficiency virus (HIV) infection. *Med Res Rev* 2000, 20(5):323-349.

[76] Ma SK, Wu KZ, Li AX: Virtual screening for natural product inhibitors of HIV-1 integrase. *Interdiscip Sci* 2011, 3(1):17-21.

[77] Zhang HS, Wu TC, Sang WW, Ruan Z: EGCG inhibits Tat-induced LTR transactivation: role of Nrf2, AKT, AMPK signaling pathway. *Life Sci* 2012, 90(19-20):747-754.

[78] Hauber I, Hohenberg H, Holstermann B, Hunstein W, Hauber J: The main green tea polyphenol epigallocatechin-3-gallate counteracts semen-mediated enhancement of HIV infection. *Proc Natl Acad Sci U S A* 2009, 106(22):9033-9038.

[79] Ovenden SP, Yu J, Wan SS, Sberna G, Tait RM, Rhodes D, Cox S, Coates J, Walsh NG, Meurer-Grimes BM: Globoidnan A: a lignan from Eucalyptus globoidea inhibits HIV integrase. *Phytochemistry* 2004, 65(24):3255-3259.

[80] Heredia A, Natesan S, Le NM, Medina-Moreno S, Zapata JC, Reitz M, Bryant J, Redfield RR: Indirubin 3'-monoxime, from a Chinese traditional herbal formula, suppresses viremia in humanized mice infected with multidrug-resistant HIV. *AIDS Res Hum Retroviruses* 2014, 30(5):403-406.

[81] Zhang HS, Chen XY, Wu TC, Zhang FJ: Tanshinone II A inhibits tat-induced HIV-1 transactivation through redox-regulated AMPK/Nampt pathway. *J Cell Physiol* 2014, 229(9):1193-1201.

[82] Helfer M, Koppensteiner H, Schneider M, Rebensburg S, Forcisi S, Muller C, Schmitt-Kopplin P, Schindler M, Brack-Werner R: The root extract of the medicinal plant Pelargonium sidoides is a potent HIV-1 attachment inhibitor. *PLoS One* 2014, 9(1):e87487.

[83] Lee EO, Kim SE, Park HK, Kang JL, Chong YH: Extracellular HIV-1 Tat upregulates TNF-alpha dependent MCP-1/CCL2 production via activation of ERK1/2 pathway in rat hippocampal slice cultures: inhibition by resveratrol, a polyphenolic phytostilbene. *Exp Neurol* 2011, 229(2):399-408.

[84] Ainslie GR, Wolf KK, Li Y, Connolly EA, Scarlett YV, Hull JH, Paine MF: Assessment of a Candidate Marker Constituent Predictive of a Dietary Substance-Drug Interaction: Case Study with Grapefruit Juice and CYP3A4 Drug Substrates. *J Pharmacol Exp Ther* 2014, 351(3):576-584.

[85] Micewicz ED, Cole AL, Jung CL, Luong H, Phillips ML, Pratikhya P, Sharma S, Waring AJ, Cole AM, Ruchala P: Grifonin-1: a small HIV-1 entry inhibitor derived from the algal lectin, Griffithsin. *PLoS One* 2010, 5(12):e14360.

[86] Xue J, Hoorelbeke B, Kagiampakis I, Demeler B, Balzarini J, Liwang PJ: The griffithsin dimer is required for high-potency inhibition of HIV-1: evidence for manipulation of the structure of gp120 as part of the griffithsin dimer mechanism. *Antimicrob Agents Chemother* 2013, 57(8):3976-3989.

[87] Mehbub MF, Lei J, Franco C, Zhang W: Marine sponge derived natural products between 2001 and 2010: trends and opportunities for discovery of bioactives. *Mar Drugs* 2014, 12(8):4539-4577.

[88] Bharate SB, Manda S, Mupparapu N, Battini N, Vishwakarma RA: Chemistry and biology of fascaplysin, a potent marine-derived CDK-4 inhibitor. *Mini Rev Med Chem* 2012, 12(7):650-664.

[89] Ellithey MS, Lall N, Hussein AA, Meyer D: Cytotoxic and HIV-1 enzyme inhibitory activities of Red Sea marine organisms. *BMC Complement Altern Med* 2014, 14:77.

[90] Ellithey MS, Lall N, Hussein AA, Meyer D: Cytotoxic, cytostatic and HIV-1 PR inhibitory activities of the soft coral Litophyton arboreum. *Mar Drugs* 2013, 11(12): 4917-4936.

[91] Barrientos LG, Gronenborn AM: The highly specific carbohydrate-binding protein cyanovirin-N: structure, anti-HIV/Ebola activity and possibilities for therapy. *Mini Rev Med Chem* 2005, 5(1):21-31.

[92] Bokesch HR, O'Keefe BR, McKee TC, Pannell LK, Patterson GM, Gardella RS, Sowder RC, 2nd, Turpin J, Watson K, Buckheit RW, Jr. *et al*: A potent novel anti-HIV protein from the cultured cyanobacterium Scytonema varium. *Biochemistry* 2003, 42(9): 2578-2584.

[93] Fleta-Soriano E, Martinez JP, Hinkelmann B, Gerth K, Washausen P, Diez J, Frank R, Sasse F, Meyerhans A: The myxobacterial metabolite ratjadone A inhibits HIV infection by blocking the Rev/CRM1-mediated nuclear export pathway. *Microb Cell Fact* 2014, 13:17.

[94] Wolff B, Sanglier JJ, Wang Y: Leptomycin B is an inhibitor of nuclear export: inhibition of nucleo-cytoplasmic translocation of the human immunodeficiency virus type 1 (HIV-1) Rev protein and Rev-dependent mRNA. *Chem Biol* 1997, 4(2):139-147.

[95] Henrich TJ, Hu Z, Li JZ, Sciaranghella G, Busch MP, Keating SM, Gallien S, Lin NH, Giguel FF, Lavoie L *et al*: Long-term reduction in peripheral blood HIV type 1 reservoirs following reduced-intensity conditioning allogeneic stem cell transplantation. *J Infect Dis* 2013, 207(11):1694-1702.

[96] Chen Y, Cao L, Zhong M, Zhang Y, Han C, Li Q, Yang J, Zhou D, Shi W, He B *et al*: Anti-HIV-1 activity of a new scorpion venom peptide derivative Kn2-7. *PLoS One* 2012, 7(4):e34947.

[97] Nakashima H, Yamamoto N, Masuda M, Fujii N: Defensins inhibit HIV replication in vitro. *Aids* 1993, 7(8):1129.

[98] Gordon YJ, Romanowski EG, McDermott AM: A review of antimicrobial peptides and their therapeutic potential as anti-infective drugs. *Curr Eye Res* 2005, 30(7): 505-515.

[99] Qureshi A, Thakur N, Kumar M: HIPdb: a database of experimentally validated HIV inhibiting peptides. *PLoS One* 2013, 8(1):e54908.

[100] Castel G, Chteoui M, Heyd B, Tordo N: Phage display of combinatorial peptide libraries: application to antiviral research. *Molecules* 2011, 16(5):3499-3518.

[101] Gentilucci L, De Marco R, Cerisoli L: Chemical modifications designed to improve peptide stability: incorporation of non-natural amino acids, pseudo-peptide bonds, and cyclization. *Curr Pharm Des* 2010, 16(28):3185-3203.

[102] Peters BM, Shirtliff ME, Jabra-Rizk MA: Antimicrobial peptides: primeval molecules or future drugs? *PLoS Pathog* 2010, 6(10):e1001067.

[103] Fjell CD, Hiss JA, Hancock RE, Schneider G: Designing antimicrobial peptides: form follows function. *Nat Rev Drug Discov* 2012, 11(1):37-51.

[104] Burnett JC, Rossi JJ: RNA-based therapeutics: current progress and future prospects. *Chem Biol* 2012, 19(1):60-71.

[105] Nakashima H, Shoji Y, Kim SG, Shimada J, Mizushima Y, Ito M, Yamamoto N, Takaku H: Anti-human immunodeficiency virus type 1 activity of phosphorothioate analogs of oligodeoxynucleotides: penetration and localization of oligodeoxynucleotides in HIV-1-infected MOLT-4 cells. *Nucleic Acids Res* 1994, 22(23):5004-5010.

[106] Bennett MS, Akkina R: Gene therapy strategies for HIV/AIDS: preclinical modeling in humanized mice. *Viruses* 2013, 5(12):3119-3141.

[107] Kim D, Rossi J: RNAi mechanisms and applications. *Biotechniques* 2008, 44(5):613-616.

[108] Torrecilla J, Rodriguez-Gascon A, Solinis MA, del Pozo-Rodriguez A: Lipid nanoparticles as carriers for RNAi against viral infections: current status and future perspectives. *Biomed Res Int* 2014, 2014:161794.

[109] Boden D, Pusch O, Lee F, Tucker L, Ramratnam B: Human immunodeficiency virus type 1 escape from RNA interference. *J Virol* 2003, 77(21):11531-11535.

[110] Senserrich J, Pauls E, Armand-Ugon M, Clotet-Codina I, Moncunill G, Clotet B, Este JA: HIV-1 resistance to the anti-HIV activity of a shRNA targeting a dual-coding region. *Virology* 2008, 372(2):421-429.

[111] Centlivre M, Legrand N, Klamer S, Liu YP, Jasmijn von Eije K, Bohne M, Rijnstra ES, Weijer K, Blom B, Voermans C *et al*: Preclinical in vivo evaluation of the safety of a multi-shRNA-based gene therapy against HIV-1. *Mol Ther Nucleic Acids* 2013, 2:e120.

[112] Herrera-Carrillo E, Liu YP, Berkhout B: The impact of unprotected T cells in RNAi-based gene therapy for HIV-AIDS. *Mol Ther* 2014, 22(3):596-606.

[113] Schopman NC, ter Brake O, Berkhout B: Anticipating and blocking HIV-1 escape by second generation antiviral shRNAs. *Retrovirology* 2010, 7:52-64.

[114] Scarborough RJ, Levesque MV, Boudrias-Dalle E, Chute IC, Daniels SM, Ouellette RJ, Perreault JP, Gatignol A: A Conserved Target Site in HIV-1 Gag RNA is Accessible to Inhibition by Both an HDV Ribozyme and a Short Hairpin RNA. *Mol Ther Nucleic Acids* 2014, 3:e178.

[115] Castanotto D, Rossi JJ: The promises and pitfalls of RNA-interference-based therapeutics. *Nature* 2009, 457(7228):426-433.

[116] Yates A, Stark J, Klein N, Antia R, Callard R: Understanding the slow depletion of memory CD4+ T cells in HIV infection. *PLoS Med* 2007, 4(5):e177.

[117] Siliciano RF, Greene WC: HIV latency. *Cold Spring Harb Perspect Med* 2011, 1(1):a007096.

[118] Mallipeddi R, Rohan LC: Progress in antiretroviral drug delivery using nanotechnology. *Int J Nanomedicine* 2010, 5:533-547.

[119] Phillips NC, Tsoukas C: Liposomal encapsulation of azidothymidine results in decreased hematopoietic toxicity and enhanced activity against murine acquired immunodeficiency syndrome. *Blood* 1992, 79(5):1137-1143.

[120] Kinman L, Brodie SJ, Tsai CC, Bui T, Larsen K, Schmidt A, Anderson D, Morton WR, Hu SL, Ho RJ: Lipid-drug association enhanced HIV-1 protease inhibitor indinavir localization in lymphoid tissues and viral load reduction: a proof of concept study in HIV-2287-infected macaques. *J Acquir Immune Defic Syndr* 2003, 34(4):387-397.

[121] Kinman L, Bui T, Larsen K, Tsai CC, Anderson D, Morton WR, Hu SL, Ho RJ: Optimization of lipid-indinavir complexes for localization in lymphoid tissues of HIV-infected macaques. *J Acquir Immune Defic Syndr* 2006, 42(2):155-161.

[122] Gomes MJ, Neves J, Sarmento B: Nanoparticle-based drug delivery to improve the efficacy of antiretroviral therapy in the central nervous system. *Int J Nanomedicine* 2014, 9:1757-1769.

[123] Kreuter J, Shamenkov D, Petrov V, Ramge P, Cychutek K, Koch-Brandt C, Alyautdin R: Apolipoprotein-mediated transport of nanoparticle-bound drugs across the blood-brain barrier. *J Drug Target* 2002, 10(4):317-325.

[124] Archin NM, Bateson R, Tripathy MK, Crooks AM, Yang KH, Dahl NP, Kearney MF, Anderson EM, Coffin JM, Strain MC *et al*: HIV-1 expression within resting CD4+ T cells after multiple doses of vorinostat. *J Infect Dis* 2014, 210(5):728-735.

[125] Sgarbanti M, Battistini A: Therapeutics for HIV-1 reactivation from latency. *Curr Opin Virol* 2013, 3(4):394-401.

[126] Matsuyama T, Hamamoto Y, Okamoto T, Shimotohno K, Kobayashi N, Yamamoto N: Tumour necrosis factor and HIV: a note of caution. *Lancet* 1988, 2(8624):1364.

[127] Okamoto T, Matsuyama T, Mori S, Hamamoto Y, Kobayashi N, Yamamoto N, Josephs SF, Wong-Staal F, Shimotohno K: Augmentation of human immunodeficiency virus type 1 gene expression by tumor necrosis factor alpha. *AIDS Res Hum Retroviruses* 1989, 5(2):131-138.

[128] Wolschendorf F, Bosque A, Shishido T, Duverger A, Jones J, Planelles V, Kutsch O: Kinase control prevents HIV-1 reactivation in spite of high levels of induced NF-kappaB activity. *J Virol* 2012, 86(8):4548-4558.

[129] Katlama C, Deeks SG, Autran B, Martinez-Picado J, van Lunzen J, Rouzioux C, Miller M, Vella S, Schmitz JE, Ahlers J *et al*: Barriers to a cure for HIV: new ways to target and eradicate HIV-1 reservoirs. *Lancet* 2013, 381(9883):2109-2117.

[130] Shan L, Siliciano RF: From reactivation of latent HIV-1 to elimination of the latent reservoir: the presence of multiple barriers to viral eradication. *Bioessays* 2013, 35(6): 544-552.

[131] Turner LS, Tsygankov AY, Henderson EE: StpC-based gene therapy targeting latent reservoirs of HIV-1. *Antiviral Res* 2006, 72(3):233-241.

[132] Macias D, Oya R, Saniger L, Martin F, Luque F: A lentiviral vector that activates latent human immunodeficiency virus-1 proviruses by the overexpression of tat and that kills the infected cells. *Hum Gene Ther* 2009, 20(11):1259-1268.

[133] Chirullo B, Sgarbanti R, Limongi D, Shytaj IL, Alvarez D, Das B, Boe A, DaFonseca S, Chomont N, Liotta L *et al*: A candidate anti-HIV reservoir compound, auranofin, exerts a selective 'anti-memory' effect by exploiting the baseline oxidative status of lymphocytes. *Cell Death Dis* 2013, 4:e944.

[134] Shytaj IL, Chirullo B, Wagner W, Ferrari MG, Sgarbanti R, Corte AD, LaBranche C, Lopalco L, Palamara AT, Montefiori D *et al*: Investigational treatment suspension and enhanced cell-mediated immunity at rebound followed by drug-free remission of simian AIDS. *Retrovirology* 2013, 10:71-85.

[135] Lewis MG, DaFonseca S, Chomont N, Palamara AT, Tardugno M, Mai A, Collins M, Wagner WL, Yalley-Ogunro J, Greenhouse J *et al*: Gold drug auranofin restricts the viral reservoir in the monkey AIDS model and induces containment of viral load following ART suspension. *Aids* 2011, 25(11):1347-1356.

[136] Gatignol A, Jeang KT: Tat as a transcriptional activator and a potential therapeutic target for HIV-1. *Adv Pharmacol* 2000, 48:209-227.

[137] Abbas W, Herbein G: Molecular Understanding of HIV-1 Latency. *Adv Virol* 2012, 2012:574967.

[138] Ebina H, Misawa N, Kanemura Y, Koyanagi Y: Harnessing the CRISPR/Cas9 system to disrupt latent HIV-1 provirus. *Sci Rep* 2013, 3:2510-16.

[139] Qu X, Wang P, Ding D, Wang X, Zhang G, Zhou X, Liu L, Zhu X, Zeng H, Zhu H: Zinc finger nuclease: a new approach for excising HIV-1 proviral DNA from infected human T cells. *Mol Biol Rep* 2014, 41(9):5819-5827.

[140] Manjunath N, Yi G, Dang Y, Shankar P: Newer gene editing technologies toward HIV gene therapy. *Viruses* 2013, 5(11):2748-2766.

[141] Hutter G, Nowak D, Mossner M, Ganepola S, Mussig A, Allers K, Schneider T, Hofmann J, Kucherer C, Blau O *et al*: Long-term control of HIV by CCR5 Delta32/Delta32 stem-cell transplantation. *N Engl J Med* 2009, 360(7):692-698.

[142] Allers K, Hutter G, Hofmann J, Loddenkemper C, Rieger K, Thiel E, Schneider T: Evidence for the cure of HIV infection by CCR5Delta32/Delta32 stem cell transplantation. *Blood* 2011, 117(10):2791-2799.

http://dx.doi.org/10.5772/60961

[143] Hopes of HIV cure in 'Boston patients' dashed [http://www.nature.com/news/hopes-of-hiv-cure-in-boston-patients-dashed-1.14324](accessed on 24th October 2014)

[144] Yukl SA, Boritz E, Busch M, Bentsen C, Chun TW, Douek D, Eisele E, Haase A, Ho YC, Hutter G *et al*: Challenges in detecting HIV persistence during potentially curative interventions: a study of the Berlin patient. *PLoS Pathog* 2013, 9(5):e1003347.

[145] Younan P, Kowalski J, Kiem HP: Genetic modification of hematopoietic stem cells as a therapy for HIV/AIDS. *Viruses* 2013, 5(12):2946-2962.

[146] Yu M, Poeschla E, Wong-Staal F: Progress towards gene therapy for HIV infection. *Gene Ther* 1994, 1(1):13-26.

[147] Peterson CW, Younan P, Jerome KR, Kiem HP: Combinatorial anti-HIV gene therapy: using a multipronged approach to reach beyond HAART. *Gene Ther* 2013, 20(7): 695-702.

[148] Hoxie JA, June CH: Novel cell and gene therapies for HIV. *Cold Spring Harb Perspect Med* 2012, 2(10).pii: a007179.

[149] Doitsh G, Cavrois M, Lassen KG, Zepeda O, Yang Z, Santiago ML, Hebbeler AM, Greene WC: Abortive HIV infection mediates CD4 T cell depletion and inflammation in human lymphoid tissue. *Cell* 2010, 143(5):789-801.

[150] SangamoBiosciences: Dose Escalation Study of Cyclophosphamide in HIV-Infected Subjects on HAART Receiving SB-728-T. In: *ClinicalTrialsgov NCT01543152*. National Institue of Health; 2014.

[151] Miyakawa K, Sawasaki T, Matsunaga S, Tokarev A, Quinn G, Kimura H, Nomaguchi M, Adachi A, Yamamoto N, Guatelli J *et al*: Interferon-induced SCYL2 limits release of HIV-1 by triggering PP2A-mediated dephosphorylation of the viral protein Vpu. *Sci Signal* 2012, 5(245):ra73.

[152] Kitchen SG, Shimizu S, An DS: Stem cell-based anti-HIV gene therapy. *Virology* 2011, 411(2):260-272.

[153] Fricke T, White TE, Schulte B, de Souza Aranha Vieira DA, Dharan A, Campbell EM, Brandariz-Nunez A, Diaz-Griffero F: MxB binds to the HIV-1 core and prevents the uncoating process of HIV-1. *Retrovirology* 2014, 11:68-81.

[154] Demirov DG, Ono A, Orenstein JM, Freed EO: Overexpression of the N-terminal domain of TSG101 inhibits HIV-1 budding by blocking late domain function. *Proc Natl Acad Sci U S A* 2002, 99(2):955-960.

[155] Fadel HJ, Morrison JH, Saenz DT, Fuchs JR, Kvaratskhelia M, Ekker SC, Poeschla EM: TALEN knockout of the PSIP1 gene in human cells: analyses of HIV-1 replication and allosteric integrase inhibitor mechanism. *J Virol* 2014, 88(17):9704-9717.

[156] Kitchen SG, Levin BR, Bristol G, Rezek V, Kim S, Aguilera-Sandoval C, Balamurugan A, Yang OO, Zack JA: In vivo suppression of HIV by antigen specific T cells derived from engineered hematopoietic stem cells. *PLoS Pathog* 2012, 8(4):e1002649.

[157] Watanabe S, Terashima K, Ohta S, Horibata S, Yajima M, Shiozawa Y, Dewan MZ, Yu Z, Ito M, Morio T *et al*: Hematopoietic stem cell-engrafted NOD/SCID/IL2Rgamma null mice develop human lymphoid systems and induce long-lasting HIV-1 infection with specific humoral immune responses. *Blood* 2007, 109(1):212-218.

[158] Eekels JJ, Berkhout B: Toward a durable treatment of HIV-1 infection using RNA interference. *Prog Mol Biol Transl Sci* 2011, 102:141-163.

[159] von Eije KJ, Berkhout B: RNA-interference-based gene therapy approaches to HIV type-1 treatment: tackling the hurdles from bench to bedside. *Antivir Chem Chemother* 2009, 19(6):221-233.

[160] Genovesio A, Kwon YJ, Windisch MP, Kim NY, Choi SY, Kim HC, Jung S, Mammano F, Perrin V, Boese AS *et al*: Automated genome-wide visual profiling of cellular proteins involved in HIV infection. *J Biomol Screen* 2011, 16(9):945-958.

[161] Zhou H, Xu M, Huang Q, Gates AT, Zhang XD, Castle JC, Stec E, Ferrer M, Strulovici B, Hazuda DJ *et al*: Genome-scale RNAi screen for host factors required for HIV replication. *Cell Host Microbe* 2008, 4(5):495-504.

[162] Eekels JJ, Geerts D, Jeeninga RE, Berkhout B: Long-term inhibition of HIV-1 replication with RNA interference against cellular co-factors. *Antiviral Res* 2011, 89(1):43-53.

[163] Gene Transfer for HIV Using Autologous T Cells - NCT01153646. In: *ClinicalTrials-gov.* U.S. National Institutes of Health; 2011.

[164] Jeremiah SS, Yamamoto N, Ohba K: Cancellers - Exploring the Possibility of Receptor Decoy Traps as a Superior Anti-Retroviral Strategy. *Curr Drug Target*, In Press.

[165] Smith PL, Tanner H, Dalgleish A: Developments in HIV-1 immunotherapy and therapeutic vaccination. *F1000Prime Rep* 2014, 6:43-54.

[166] Garcia F, Climent N, Guardo AC, Gil C, Leon A, Autran B, Lifson JD, Martinez-Picado J, Dalmau J, Clotet B *et al*: A dendritic cell-based vaccine elicits T cell responses associated with control of HIV-1 replication. *Sci Transl Med* 2013, 5(166):166ra162.

[167] Munoz-Barroso I, Salzwedel K, Hunter E, Blumenthal R: Role of the membrane-proximal domain in the initial stages of human immunodeficiency virus type 1 envelope glycoprotein-mediated membrane fusion. *J Virol* 1999, 73(7):6089-6092.

[168] Markosyan RM, Cohen FS, Melikyan GB: Time-resolved imaging of HIV-1 Env-mediated lipid and content mixing between a single virion and cell membrane. *Mol Biol Cell* 2005, 16(12):5502-5513.

[169] Lorenc A, Robinson N: A review of the use of complementary and alternative medicine and HIV: issues for patient care. *AIDS Patient Care STDS* 2013, 27(9):503-510.

[170] Agnoletto V, Chiaffarino F, Nasta P, Rossi R, Parazzini F: Use of complementary and alternative medicine in HIV-infected subjects. *Complement Ther Med* 2006, 14(3): 193-199.

[171] Peltzer K, Preez NF, Ramlagan S, Fomundam H: Use of traditional complementary and alternative medicine for HIV patients in KwaZulu-Natal, South Africa. *BMC Public Health* 2008, 8:255-68.

[172] Liu JP, Manheimer E, Yang M: Herbal medicines for treating HIV infection and AIDS. *Cochrane Database Syst Rev* 2005(3):CD003937.

[173] Ekwunife OI, Oreh C, Ubaka CM: Concurrent use of complementary and alternative medicine with antiretroviral therapy reduces adherence to HIV medications. Int J Pharm Pract 2012, 20(5):340-343.

[174] Mashta O: WHO warns against using homoeopathy to treat serious diseases. Bmj 2009, 339:b3447.

[175] Hu J, Zhang J, Zhao W, Zhang Y, Zhang L, Shang H: Cochrane systematic reviews of Chinese herbal medicines: an overview. PLoS One 2011, 6(12):e28696.